Decision making in health and medicine
Integrating evidence and values

Decision making in health care involves navigating through a complex and tangled web of diagnostic and therapeutic uncertainties, patient preferences and values, and costs. Medical therapies have side-effects, surgery may lead to undesirable complications, and diagnostic technologies may produce false or inconclusive results. In many clinical and health policy decisions it is necessary to counterbalance benefits and risks, and to trade off competing objectives such as maximizing life expectancy vs. optimizing quality of life vs. minimizing the resources required.

This user-friendly text will help everyone involved in health care and medical decision making to plot a clear course through these complex and conflicting variables. It clearly explains and illustrates tools for integrating quantitative evidence-based data and subjective outcome values in making clinical and health policy decisions. The book will be of immense practical value for all those charged with the responsibility of decision making in medicine, including practitioners and trainees, and for students studying clinical decision analysis, evidence-based medicine, and clinical epidemiology.

The book includes numerous helpful features:
- clear definitions of key terms and phrases
- step-by-step approach which guides the reader quickly and clearly to the heart of the issue
- practical and problem solving: uses a very varied selection of clinical cases and examples drawn from all areas of medicine and health policy to highlight real-life applications
- superbly illustrated throughout
- exercises at the end of each chapter help to reinforce key messages
- includes a CD-ROM with supplementary reference material

Decision making in health and medicine
Integrating evidence and values

M.G. Myriam Hunink
Paul P. Glasziou

Joanna E. Siegel, Jane C. Weeks
Joseph S. Pliskin, Arthur S. Elstein,
Milton C. Weinstein

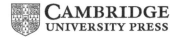

CAMBRIDGE
UNIVERSITY PRESS

CAMBRIDGE
UNIVERSITY PRESS

University Printing House, Cambridge CB2 8BS, United Kingdom

Published in the United States of America by Cambridge University Press, New York

Cambridge University Press is part of the University of Cambridge.

It furthers the University's mission by disseminating knowledge in the pursuit of education, learning and research at the highest international levels of excellence.

www.cambridge.org
Information on this title: www.cambridge.org/9780521770293

First published 2001
13th printing 2014

Printed in the United Kingdom by the CPI Group Ltd, Croydon CR0 4YY

A catalogue record for this publication is available from the British Library

Library of Congress Cataloguing in Publication data

Decision making in health and medicine: integrating evidence and values /
M.G. Myriam Hunink . . . [et al.]
    p. cm.
Includes bibliographical references and index.
ISBN 0 521 77029 7 (pbk.)
1. Medicine – Decision making.   2. Medical care – Decision making.   3. Evidence-based
medicine.   4. Values.   I. Hunink, M.G. Myriam, 1958–
[DNLM: 1. Decision Making.   2. Delivery of Health Care.   3. Evidence-Based Medicine.
W 84.1 D2938 2001]
R723.5.D39 2001
610–dc21   2001025537

ISBN 978-0-521-77029-3 Paperback

Contents

About the authors

M.G. Myriam Hunink received her MD degree from the University of Leiden, trained as a radiologist in Amsterdam, and received her PhD degree in clinical decision analysis from the Erasmus University, Rotterdam. Currently, she holds appointments as radiologist and Professor of Clinical Epidemiology at the Erasmus University Medical Center Rotterdam, the Netherlands, and as Adjunct Professor of Health Policy and Management at the Harvard School of Public Health, Boston. She is currently President of the Society for Medical Decision Making.

Paul P. Glasziou is Professor of Evidence-based Medicine at the University of Queensland, Australia, and a general practitioner at the Inala Community Health Centre. He teaches evidence-based practice to medical students and other health care workers. He holds honorary positions as adjunct Associate Professor at the Harvard School of Public Health, and adjunct Associate Professor at the NHMRC Clinical Trials Centre, Sydney University. Dr Glasziou is the co-editor of the BMJ's *Journal of Evidence-Based Medicine.*

Joanna E. Siegel is Director of the Research Initiative in Clinical Economics at the Agency for Healthcare Research and Quality (AHRQ), US Department of Health and Human Services. She received her masters in health policy and doctorate in health decision sciences at Harvard School of Public Health; her undergraduate training is in nursing.

Jane C. Weeks is an Associate Professor of Medicine at the Dana–Farber Cancer Institute and Harvard Medical School and the Director of the Center for Outcomes and Policy Research at the Dana–Farber Cancer Institute. She is a medical oncologist and health services researcher whose work focuses on evaluating the outcomes and cost-effectiveness of cancer prevention and treatment strategies.

Joseph S. Pliskin is the Sidney Liswood Professor of Health Care Management at Ben-Gurion University of the Negev, Beer-Sheva, Israel. He is chairman of the Department of Health Systems Management and is a member of the Department of Industrial Engineering and Management. He is also an Adjunct Professor at the Department of Health Policy and Management at the Harvard School of Public Health, Boston, US. He is currently the President of the European Society for Medical Decision Making.

Arthur S. Elstein is a professor in the Department of Medical Education, University of Illinois College of Medicine at Chicago. He was editor-in-chief of the journal *Medical Decision Making* from 1995 to 1999. He is a co-author of *Medical Problem Solving: An Analysis of Clinical Reasoning* (1978), *Clinical Decision Analysis* (1980), and co-editor of *Professional Judgment: A Reader in Clinical Decision Making* (1988), and is past President of the Society for Medical Decision Making.

Milton C. Weinstein is the Henry J. Kaiser Professor of Health Policy and Management and Biostatistics at the Harvard School of Public Health, Professor of Medicine at the Harvard Medical School, and Director of the Program on Economic Evaluation of Medical Technology in the Harvard Center for Risk Analysis. He is Vice President of Innovus Research, Inc. He is also past President of the Society for Medical Decision Making.

Foreword

...high Arbiter *Chance* governs all.

John Milton, *Paradise Lost*, book II, lines 909–10

When the predecessor to this book was being prepared in the late 1970s (Weinstein et al., 1980), medical decision making seemed to have become more complicated than ever before. The number of diagnostic and therapeutic options dwarfed those of an earlier generation, and the costs of care were growing relentlessly. Increasing numbers of patients expected to play an active role in decisions that affected their lives, and many physicians were acclimating themselves to a less authoritarian doctor–patient relationship. The tools of decision analysis permitted the clinician and patient to break down the complexity of a medical situation into its constituent parts, to identify and assess the pertinent uncertainties and values, and to reassemble the pieces into a logical guide to action.

Today, a generation later, the dilemma of medical decision making seems even more problematic. This is not merely the result of scientific and technologic advances – ingenious new devices, pharmaceuticals, surgical possibilities, and other interventions. The environment of decision making has itself become confounded by government agencies and service delivery systems playing a more direct (and directive) role in decision making. Today, not only are the costs of care a prime concern, so, too, is the quality of care. Patients no longer need rely mainly on their physicians to gain access to medical information – the internet has given millions a direct line to abundant information, though of variable accuracy and pertinence. In light of progress in mapping the human genome, clinicians may soon face profound ethical questions that only a generation ago were the stuff of science fiction.

These dynamic changes in medicine, in science, and in the health-care environment make this new book more valuable than ever. This volume conveys both fundamental and sophisticated methods that can render complex health-care situations more comprehensible. It would be a mis-take, however, to think that the methods described in this volume apply only to the exceptional case, to the rare clinical encounter. The task of integrating scientific knowledge, clinical evidence, and value judgments into coherent decisions remains the daily task of medical care.

Much of what counts for differences in outcome related to medicine comes not from failure to access experimental and expensive technology. It comes rather from the failure to deploy relatively inexpensive and proven technology to all those who need it: vaccine against pneumonia for those at risk, beta-blockers in the period following myocardial infarction, appropriate screening for cancer, and much more. The challenge for quality improvement is not the extraordinary case and exceptional decision so much as the challenge to implement systematically the preventive, diagnostic, and therapeutic measures for all who would benefit at reasonable cost. The lessons in this book can reinforce the case for sounder everyday decisions in medicine and health care.

Regardless of how far science and health care advance, the element of chance will remain a fixture in medical encounters. A refined understanding of causation and prognosis will alter how much we know about the likelihood of certain consequences, but uncertainty will persist. Much of medical learning can be interpreted as an effort to reduce the range of uncertainty in medical care. The ideas and methods provided in this volume teach how to make informed decisions in the face of the uncertainty which inevitably remains.

The methods in this book to aid decision makers are simply tools. They are tools for the willing clinician. They are tools for the worried patient. They are tools for the concerned policy maker and payer. They will not make a hazardous situation safe, nor will they make a lazy or incompetent clinician into a superior caregiver. If the methods do not eliminate controversy, they can clarify the reasons for differences of opinion. In dealing with the realities and uncertainties of life and illness, they will enable the thoughtful clinician, the honest patient, and the open-minded policy maker to reach more reasoned conclusions.

Provost, Harvard University   **Harvey V. Fineberg**

REFERENCE

Weinstein, M.C., Fineberg, H.V., Elstein, A.S. et al. (1980). *Clinical Decision Analysis.* Philadelphia: W.B. Saunders.

Preface

How often do you find yourself struggling with a decision, be it a medical decision, a policy decision, or a personal one? In clinical medicine and health-care policy, making decisions has become a very complicated process: we have to make trade-offs between risks, benefits, costs, and preferences. We have to take into account the rapidly increasing evidence – some good, some poor – presented in scientific publications, on the worldwide web, and by the media. We have to integrate the best available evidence with the values relevant to patient and society; and we have to reconcile our intuitive notions with rational analysis.

In this book we explain and illustrate tools for integrating quantitative evidence-based data and subjective outcome values in making clinical and health-policy decisions. The book is intended for all those involved in clinical medicine or health-care policy who would like to apply the concepts from decision analysis to improve their decision-making process. The audience we have in mind includes (post-)graduate students and health-care professionals interested in medical decision making, clinical decision analysis, clinical epidemiology, evidence-based medicine, technology assessment in health care, and health-care policy.

The authors' backgrounds ensure that this is a multidisciplinary text. Together we represent general practice, radiology, oncology, mathematics, decision sciences, psychology of decision making, and health-care policy and management. The examples in the book are taken from both clinical practice and from health policy.

There is a previous version of this book (Weinstein et al., 1980), but the name of the book has changed, the content is 80% different, the publisher has changed, and the list of authors has changed. The color of the cover is, however, the same! And the main message is the same: decisions in clinical medicine and health care in general can benefit from a proactive approach to decision making in which evidence and values are integrated into one framework.

The book comes with a CD-rom. The book itself can, however, be read without immediate access to the CD-rom, that is, in a comfortable chair or on a couch! The CD-rom supplies additional materials: solutions to the exercises, decision-analytical software, examples of the decision models in the book programmed using the software, supplementary materials for the chapters including some useful spreadsheets, and the references with abstracts.

We hope you enjoy reading. Good (but calculated) luck with your decision making!

April 2001   **M.G. Myriam Hunink**
                                                                      Paul P. Glasziou

REFERENCE

Weinstein, M.C., Fineberg, H.V., Elstein, A.S. et al. (1980). *Clinical Decision Analysis.* Philadelphia: WB Saunders.

Acknowledgments

A book never gets prepared by the authors only. Numerous people helped to make this book come into being. We would like to thank especially those who reviewed the manuscript, edited, revised, and helped prepare the exercises, solutions, and reference material: Karen Visser, Majanka Heijenbrok, Galied Muradin, Rogier Nijhuis, Ylian Liem, Ankie Verstijnen, Miraude Adriaensen, and Karen Kuntz. Helpful comments on the draft manuscript were given by April Levin, Alan Schwartz, Julie Goldberg, Edwin Oei, Jeroen Nikken, Marc Kock, Liang Wang, YiXiang Wang, and Rick van Rijn. The technical editing performed by Anne Bosselaar was appreciated.

But writing a book consists not only of putting text on paper and making illustrations. The thoughts, ideas, and intellectual input from many, too numerous to list, have played a role in getting this book together. We would especially like to acknowledge the contributions of the authors of the previous version of the book who were not directly involved this time: Harvey V. Fineberg, Howard S. Frazier, Duncan Neuhauser, Raymond R. Neutra, and Barbara J. McNeil. Furthermore, we are grateful for the intellectual input from members of the Society for Medical Decision Making, and the students and postgraduates at Harvard School of Public Health, University of Queensland, and the Erasmus University Medical Center Rotterdam.

Finally, we'd like to thank our families, and especially Nancy, Steven, and Peter Glasziou and Marijn and Laura Franx, for being supportive and giving us the opportunity to spend time working on the book during many evenings and weekends.

Abbreviations

ACP	American College of Physicians
ASR	age–sex–race
CABG	coronary artery bypass grafting
CDC	Centers for Disease Control and Prevention
CEA	carotid endarterectomy
CEA	cost-effectiveness analysis
CE25	certainty equivalent 25
CE50	certainty equivalent 50
CE ratio	cost-effectiveness ratio
CI	confidence interval
CPI	Consumer Price Index
CRC	colorectal cancer
CT	computed tomography
DALY	disability-adjusted life year
DRG	diagnostic-related group
DVT	deep venous thrombosis
EBCT	electron beam computed tomography
EKG	electrocardiogram
EQ-5D	EuroQol with five dimensions
EU	expected utility
EVCI	expected value of clinical information
EVPI	expected value of perfect information
FNR	false-negative ratio
FOBT	fecal occult blood test
FPR	false-positive ratio
HBV	hepatitis B virus
HDL	high-density lipoprotein
HIV	human immunodeficiency virus
HMO	health maintenance organization
HUI	Health Utilities Index
IV	intravenous
LE	life expectancy

LR	likelihood ratio
MeSH	Medical Subject Headings
MI	myocardial infarction ('heart attack')
MISCAN	Microsimulation of Screening for Cancer
MRA	magnetic resonance angiography
NHB	net health benefit
OME	otitis media with effusions ('glue ear')
OR	odds ratio
ORS	oral rehydration solution
PAD	peripheral arterial disease
PAT	paroxysmal atrial tachycardia
PE	pulmonary embolism
PIOPED	Prospective Investigation of Pulmonary Embolism Diagnosis
PTA	percutaneous transluminal angiography
PV	present value
QALE	quality-adjusted life expectancy
QALY	quality-adjusted life year
QWB	Quality of Well-Being
RCT	randomized controlled trial
ROC	receiver operating characteristic
RR	relative risk
RRR	relative risk reduction
RRTO	risk–risk trade-off
RS	rating scale
SF-36	36-Item Short Form
SG	standard gamble
SIP	Sickness Impact Profile
TNR	true-negative ratio
TPR	true-positive ratio
VAS	visual analog scale
V/Q scan	ventilation–perfusion scan
WTP	willingness to pay

Elements of decision making in health care

And take the case of a man who is ill. I call two physicians: they differ in opinion. I am not to lie down and die between them: I must do something.

Samuel Johnson

1.1 Introduction

How are decisions made in practice, and can we improve the process? Decisions in health care can be particularly awkward, involving a complex web of diagnostic and therapeutic uncertainties, patient preferences and values, and costs. It is not surprising that there is often considerable disagreement about the best course of action. One of the authors of this book tells the following story (Hunink, 2001):

Being a vascular radiologist, I regularly attend the vascular rounds at the University Hospital. It's an interesting conference: the Professor of Vascular Surgery really loves academic discussions and each case gets a lot of attention. The conference goes on for hours. The clinical fellows complain, of course, and it sure keeps me from my regular work. But it's one of the few conferences that I attend where there is a real discussion of the risks, benefits, and costs of the management options. Even patient preferences are sometimes (albeit rarely) considered.

And yet, I find there is something disturbing about the conference. The discussions always seem to go along the same lines. Doctor R. advocates treatment X because he recently read a paper that reported wonderful results; Doctor S. counters that treatment X has a substantial risk associated with it, as was shown in another paper published last year in the world's highest-ranking journal in the field; and Doctor T. says that given the current limited health-care budget maybe we should consider a less expensive alternative or no treatment at all. They talk around in circles for 10–15 min, each doctor reiterating his or her opinion. The Professor, realizing that his fellows are getting irritated, finally stops the discussion. Practical chores are waiting; there are patients to be cared for. And so the Professor concludes: 'All right. We will offer the patient treatment X.' About 30% of those involved in the decision-making process nod their heads in agreement; another 30% start bringing up objections which get stifled quickly by the fellows who *really* do not want an encore, and the remaining 40% are either too tired or too flabbergasted to respond, or are more concerned about another objective, namely their job security.

The authors of this book are all familiar with conferences like this. We suspect our readers also recognize the scenario and that they too have wondered, 'Isn't there a better way to make clinical decisions? Isn't there a better way for health professionals, policy makers, patients, and the general public to communicate with each other and talk things out when the going gets tough?'

This book is about our answer to these questions. The methods it presents are addressed to the needs of all decision makers in the health-care arena – patients; physicians, nurses, and other providers of clinical services; public health and hospital administrators; health-care payers in both the private and public sectors – and to the clinical and public health researchers whose job it is to offer all of these constituencies wise and reasoned counsel.

Health-care decisions have become complex. As recently as a century ago, a physician had only a narrow range of possible diagnoses, a handful of simple tests, and a few, mostly ineffective, treatments to choose from. For example, the first edition of the justly famous *Merck Manual* (1899) ran to 192 pages. Since then our understanding of disease processes and our ability to control them have vastly increased, but so too has the complexity of health-care decisions. The 1999 centennial edition of the *Merck Manual* runs to 2833 pages, although it is unquestionably only a digest of what is now known (Beers and Berkow, 1999).

While new treatments have improved the outcome for many conditions, and even eliminated some diseases such as smallpox, many treatments are 'half-way' technologies that improve a condition but do not cure. For example, in cancer, there are many new, useful but sometimes taxing treatments that improve the prognosis without curing. Along with this increase in management options, we now contemplate treatment in a broader range of diseases, from mild hypertension to major disfigurement. This combination of a broad range of illnesses and imperfect treatment options increases our potential to help, but it also increases costs and makes decision making more complex and difficult. In this chapter, we outline a systematic approach to describing and analyzing decision problems. This approach, decision analysis, is intended to improve the quality of decisions and of communication between physicians, patients, and other health professionals. Decision analysis is designed to deal with choice under uncertainty and so it is naturally suited to the clinical setting. We believe that decision analysis is a valuable tool for physicians and others concerned with clinical decision making, both for decisions affecting individual patients and for health policy decisions affecting populations of patients. The ability of physicians collectively to command a vast array of powerful and expensive diagnostic and therapeutic interventions carries with it a social responsibility to use these resources wisely. Decision analysis is a systematic, explicit, quantitative way of making decisions in health care that can, we believe, lead to both enhanced communication about clinical controversies and better decisions. At a minimum, the methods we expound can illuminate what we disagree about and where better data or clearer goals are needed. At best, they may assure us that the decisions we make are the logical consequences of the evidence and values that were the inputs to the decision. That is no small achievement.

1.2 Decision making and uncertainty

Unlike most daily decisions, many health-care decisions have substantial consequences, and involve important uncertainties and trade-offs. The uncertainties may be about the diagnosis, the accuracy of available diagnostic tests, the natural history of the disease, the effects of treatment in an individual patient or the effects of an intervention in a group or population as a whole. With such complex decisions, it can be difficult to comprehend all options 'in our heads,' let alone to compare them. We need to have some visual or written aids. Hence a major purpose of decision analysis is to assist in comprehension of the problem and to give us insight into what variables or features of the problem should have a major impact on our decision. It does this by allowing and encouraging the decision maker to divide the logical structure of a decision problem into its components so that they can be analyzed individually and then recombine them systematically so as to suggest a decision. Here are two representative clinical situations that can be addressed with this approach:

Example 1	As a member of the State Committee for common childhood diseases, you have been asked to help formulate a policy on the management of chronic otitis media with effusions (also known as 'glue ear'). Glue ear is the most common cause of hearing problems in childhood and can lead to delayed language development. It has been recognized for over a century, but in the 1900s the only available treatments were ineffective. For example, the British surgeon Astley Cooper recognized that an incision of the eardrum temporarily relieved the deafness, but the incision closed rapidly despite attempts to keep it open by inserting, among other things, a lead wire, fish bones, and a gold ring. We now have many treatment choices, including grommets (ventilation tubes; there are at least two major types), antibiotics, corticosteroids, and

hearing aids (Rosenfeld and Bluestone, 1999). However, since glue ear usually resolves spontaneously, you might also choose to do nothing, at least initially. Given these various treatment options, should your committee recommend monitoring for hearing loss, treatment with grommet insertion, or the use of hearing aids? For example, tympanometry, which measures the eardrum's ability to move, can be used as a monitoring tool, though an audiogram is needed to confirm the degree of any hearing loss. How do you proceed with formulating a recommendation? How can you systematically approach such a decision?

Example 2

A 70-year-old man with coronary artery disease is being evaluated for coronary artery bypass grafting (CABG). An ultrasound demonstrates an asymptomatic stenosis (a narrowing) of one of the carotid arteries leading to the brain. The decision faced by the team of physicians is whether to:

(a) perform bypass surgery without further diagnostic workup or treatment of the carotid artery stenosis;

(b) perform a special X-ray, a carotid angiography, and then a carotid endarterectomy (i.e., surgery to clear the obstruction in the carotid artery) prior to coronary artery bypass surgery;

(c) perform angiography and then perform carotid endarterectomy during the same procedure as the bypass surgery.

Medical decisions must be made, and they are often made under conditions of uncertainty. Uncertainty about the current state of the patient may arise from erroneous observation or inaccurate recording of clinical findings or misinterpretation of the data by the clinician. For example, was the carotid artery stenosis really asymptomatic? Did the patient ever have a transient ischemic attack (temporary symptoms due to loss of blood flow to a region of the brain) that went unnoticed or that he interpreted as something else?

Uncertainty may also arise due to ambiguity of the data or variations in interpretation of the information. For example, if you repeated the ultrasound examination, would you get the same result? Uncertainty exists too about the correspondence between clinical information and the presence or absence of disease. The ultrasound is not perfect: how accurately does it indicate the presence or absence of a carotid artery stenosis? Some patients with a stenosis may be falsely classified as not having the disease, and some patients without a stenosis may be falsely classified as having the disease. Does our patient really have a carotid artery stenosis?

Finally, the effects of treatment are uncertain. In Example 1, there is essentially no diagnostic uncertainty, but there is uncertainty about the outcomes of treatment and about whether a trial of watchful waiting might allow the glue ear to clear up without medical or surgical intervention and without harm to the child. An important uncertainty, therefore, is the natural history of the disease. In Example 2, there would be uncertainty about the outcome of treatment, even if the diagnosis is certain and the treatment is well established. The rate of treatment failure may be known, but in whom it will fail is unpredictable at the time the treatment is initiated. For our 70-year-old patient we cannot predict whether performing a carotid endarterectomy will really protect him from a stroke during the CABG (Ali et al., 1998).

To deal with the uncertainties associated with the decision problem you need to find the best available evidence to support or refute your assumptions, and you need a framework for combining all of these uncertainties into a coherent choice. In a decision analysis process we first make the problem and its objectives explicit; then we list the alternative actions and how these alter subsequent events with their probabilities, values, and trade-offs; and finally we synthesize the balance of benefits and harms of each alternative. We shall refer to this as the PROACTIVE approach (problem – reframe – objectives – alternatives – consequences and chances – trade-offs – integrate – value – explore and evaluate) to health-care decision making. This has three major steps, each with three substeps. (The steps are a modification of the PrOACTive approach suggested by Hammond et al. (1999) in their book *Smart Choices*.) Though we present this as a linear process, you should be aware that often iteration through some steps will be required, and that sometimes the solution will be apparent before all steps are complete.

1.3 Step 1 – PROactive: the problem and objectives

You should begin by making sure you are addressing the right problem. This first requires that you make explicit what the possible consequences are that you are seeking to avoid or achieve. This may not be straightforward, as there are often different ways of viewing the problem and there may be competing objectives. Exploring these dimensions before analyzing the alternative actions is important to steer the analysis in the right direction. After the initial attempt at defining the *problem*, you should *reframe* the problem from other perspectives, and finally, identify the fundamental *objectives* for any course of action.

1.3.1 P: Define the problem

What are your principal concerns? A good way to clarify management problems is to begin by asking, 'What would happen if you took no immediate action?' This simple question seeks to uncover the outcomes that you might wish to avoid or achieve. Carefully answering this question should lead to a description of the possible sequences of events in the natural history of the condition. You may need to follow up by asking 'and what then?' several times. For example, a common cause of a very rapid heart beat is paroxysmal atrial tachycardia or PAT (episodes of rapid heart beat initiated by the conducting system in the upper heart chambers). A patient with PAT will typically experience a sudden onset of rapid heart beat (around 200 beats/min), which ceases suddenly after minutes to hours. It is usually accompanied by some anxiety, since patients worry that there is something very wrong with their heart, but it usually causes no other physical discomfort. If a patient presents after such an episode, you may analyze the problem by asking: 'What would happen if you took no immediate action?' Patients with PAT are often concerned that it signals a problem with their heart. However, long-term follow-up studies of patients with PAT show that their risk of dying from heart disease is no different from that of the rest of the population (Aronow et al., 1995). So the natural history tells us that the real issue is not the risk of a heart attack or death, but the risk of recurrent episodes of PAT and the anxiety they induce.

Of course, many medical problems have much more serious consequences. Other problems we will consider as illustrative examples in later chapters include severe chest pain, abdominal aortic aneurysms (dilatation of the main abdominal artery), management of needlestick injuries, testing for the BrCa1 gene for breast cancer, and atrial fibrillation (an irregular heart beat that greatly increases the risk of stroke). Each of these problems has a complex sequence of uncertain but potentially serious consequences. Visual aids that help describe the problem include decision trees, state-transition diagrams, influence diagrams, and survival plots. These descriptions are necessarily schematic: just as a map is useful to describe a territory, these visual aids help chart the possible course of events. They are helpful in describing and communicating the consequences and hence help navigate the decision-making process. The most straightforward tool to begin with is a *consequence table*, i.e., a tabulation of the principal concerns. Table 1.1 shows this for the management options for glue ear.

DEFINITION

A *consequence table* tabulates the consequences of a choice and considers all relevant perspectives and important dimensions.

Table 1.1 Consequence table for the wait-and-see option for the problem of otitis media with effusion (glue ear)

Consequences	Wait-and-see option
Hearing	Slow improvement over months to years
Behavior	Poor hearing may lead to disruptive behavior
Language development	Delayed articulation and comprehension (with possible long-term consequences)
Acute middle-ear infections	Recurrent episodes
Long-term complications	Possible conductive problems

Source: Rosenfeld and Bluestone (1999).

1.3.2 R: Reframe from multiple perspectives

Does the problem look different from different perspectives? You should understand how the problem you are dealing with appears to others. In the clinical setting this requires that you broaden, at least temporarily, your focus from a disease framework to one that includes the concerns for the patient. In the context of public health this requires broadening your perspective to include the aggregate limits on resources, as well as the individual perspectives of the patient, the provider, the payer, and the public policy maker.

How does the problem of glue ear appear from different perspectives? You might consider different disciplinary perspectives. For example, biologically, glue ear is a problem of microbes, immune responses, and anatomical dysfunctions. From a psychological perspective, it is one of difficulties in language development. From a sociological perspective, it might be seen to be a problem of classroom behavior and family interactions. The child, the parents, the clinician, the teacher, and the health system will all view the problem differently and have overlapping objectives but with different emphases.

1.3.3 O: Focus on the objective

The main objective of health care is to avert or diminish the consequences of a disease. Sometimes this means prevention or cure; sometimes it may be slowing the disease's progress or preventing the disease's complications; sometimes it may be only the alleviation of symptoms or dysfunction. In our first example, only time will 'cure' the age-related anatomical problem with the Eustachian tube that leads to glue ear, but meanwhile you may alleviate the major problem – deafness – by removing fluid from the middle ear, or you may simply use a hearing aid.

If you framed and reframed the problem appropriately, the pivotal concerns and objectives should have become apparent. However, before proceeding to develop and evaluate options, you should check that you have a clear idea of the objectives. What elements are of most concern to the patient or population? What are the short-term and long-term objectives and concerns, and how do these vary between patients? Sometimes these objectives are straightforward. For example, the objective of immunization decisions is to reduce morbidity and mortality from infectious diseases. However, often there are multiple competing objectives. For example, in managing patients with advanced cancer there may be competing objectives of comfort, function, and length of life, and these may be different for patient and caregivers. If there are trade-offs between the objectives, it is obviously important to understand what the objectives are.

When listing the objectives, you should clearly distinguish between *means objectives* and *fundamental objectives.* A means objective is an intermediate goal but which is only a stepping stone to what we truly value. In our second example, the coronary artery bypass surgery is not a goal in itself, but a means of achieving the fundamental objectives of improved quality of life (less angina, i.e., chest pain) and avoidance of early mortality.

The nature of objectives may be clarified by repeatedly asking 'why.' In our first example, you might consider that insertion of a ventilation tube will achieve the objective of resolving the glue ear, which may appear to be an objective. Why do you want the glue ear to resolve? Because that will lead to normal hearing. And why do you want normal hearing? Hearing is both an end in itself, and important for proper language development. Why do you want proper language development? That is something we intrinsically value, and hence it is a fundamental objective. Thus resolving the glue ear is a means objective, whereas normal hearing is both a fundamental objective (it has its own intrinsic value) and a means objective (it is needed for normal language development).

Understanding the fundamental objectives can help us generate options that achieve such objectives through different means. For example, focusing on hearing instead of the fluid in the middle ear suggests a hearing aid as one alternative to consider. Similarly, with the coronary artery bypass graft, you may need to step back and reconsider other options to manage the angina, such as angioplasty (balloon dilatation of stenosis of the coronary arteries) or better medical management. Committing too early to

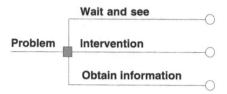

Figure 1.1   Generic decision tree for the initial decision node.

a means objective rather than the fundamental objectives can unnecessarily narrow our view of the possible options.

1.4 Step 2 – proACTive: the alternatives, consequences, and trade-offs

1.4.1 A: Consider all relevant alternatives

To be able to choose the best alternative in a particular circumstance, you need to know the range of reasonable alternatives. This list may be very long, so it is helpful to have a generic list. All alternatives may be placed in one of three categories: (i) a wait-and-see, watchful waiting, or a 'do-nothing' policy; (ii) initiate an intervention, e.g., treatment now; or (iii) obtain more information before deciding, such as ordering a diagnostic test or doing a population survey. These alternatives are illustrated in the decision tree of Figure 1.1.

The initial line is labeled with the population or problem you are considering (such as glue ear or coronary artery disease). The square represents a *decision node* at which just one of the several alternative actions, represented by the subsequent lines, must be chosen. At the decision node, the decision maker is in control. From each alternative action, there will usually be a subsequent chance node (the circles), with branches representing the possible outcomes of each option. The probabilities of events and outcomes will depend on the alternative chosen. The consequences of the other alternatives will be examined in the next step. We will have more to say about decision trees in Chapters 2 and 3.

You may have already developed the chance tree for the wait-and-see policy when describing the problem in Step 1. The consequences of the other alternatives will be examined in the next step. Before doing that, let us look in more detail at each of the three generic alternatives.

DEFINITION

A *decision tree* is a visual representation of all the possible options and the consequences that may follow each option.

1.4.1.1 Wait-and-see, watchful waiting, or do-nothing policy

A wait-and-see, watchful waiting, or do-nothing policy may take several forms. You may decide to do nothing about the condition. For example, this might be a reasonable choice for benign skin lesions or other variants of 'normal.' However, usually you will have a contingent policy that requires action depending on the disease course over time. The contingencies may be classified as either *monitoring*, where a regular check is made, or *triggering*, where you wait for a change in the type or severity of symptoms.

With monitoring, a check is made at fixed times to see whether the condition has improved, remained the same, or become worse. Action is then based on this progression. You may decide not to treat patients with mild hypertension until their blood pressure increases or they develop other risk factors; the criterion for action is the condition becoming worse. For the glue ear case, you may decide that action is required if no improvement is seen at 2 months; the criterion is either no change in the condition or a worsening. If a condition is unchanged, why should its persistence indicate a need for action? Imagine that there are two types of the condition: those that spontaneously resolve and those that never resolve. Waiting will allow us to differentiate these. Effectively this is a test of time. In reality, the groups will not be so distinct, and the test-of-time will be imperfect. So there will be a trade-off: delay may reduce the benefits for the persistent case but avoid the harm of unnecessary treatment for those who would resolve spontaneously. We will look at this trade-off more formally in Chapter 6.

With triggering, the patient is advised to return if particular events occur. If a patient has PAT, you may take action if the episodes become very frequent or if they are associated with chest pain or breathlessness (indicating that the heart is not coping with the rapid heart rate). In family practice this method is known as safety netting – a patient is instructed in the criteria required to catch a potentially ominous change. Clearly, wait-and-see is a strategy rather than a single action. Thus a *strategy* is a sequence of choices at decision nodes, contingent on the observed events at previous chance nodes. In some cases it may be useful to consider several different wait-and-see strategies.

1.4.1.2 Intervention

The next step is to list the active intervention alternatives, refraining from any evaluation of their merit at this point so that the full range of options can be considered. In the glue ear example, intervention would be treatment which may be aimed at cure, at arresting the progress of the disease, at preventing complications, or at alleviating the symptoms. As described earlier, glue ear may be managed by attempting to resolve the effusion (cure), or by use of a hearing aid, which would alleviate the principal symptom and its consequences.

Where do you get the list of alternatives? Current knowledge, discussions with colleagues and experts, textbooks, and literature searches all contribute. An important component is a search of controlled trials, since these are often the source of the best-quality evidence on the benefits and risks of interventions. The Cochrane Controlled Trials Registry contains references and abstracts of many of the hundreds of thousands of controlled trials in health care. A search of the Registry for 'otitis media with effusion' (performed in 1999) provided 195 references with trials that include: (i) antibiotics, such as ceftibuten, cefixime, amoxicillin, and co-trimoxazole; (ii) oral corticosteroids, such as betamethasone, prednisolone, and prednisone; (iii) intranasal corticosteroids such as beclometasone; (iv) nonsteroidal antiinflammatory drugs, such as naproxen and tranilast; (v) ventilation tubes (grommets) with two major different types; (vi) adenoidectomy; (vii) mucolytics such as carboxymethylcysteine and bromhexine; (viii) autoinflation (mechanical maneuvers which force air up the Eustachian tube); (ix) decongestants and antihistamines; and (x) hearing aids. Some of these options, such as antihistamines, are clearly ineffective. Others, such as mucolytics, autoinflation, and nonsteroidal antiinflammatory drugs, are of doubtful or uncertain value. The remaining treatments show a range of effectiveness and harms, which need to be compared in the next step.

1.4.1.3 Obtain information

If you are uncertain about the prognosis or diagnosis, further information, such as from a diagnostic test, may help in selecting the best intervention. In the area of public health, obtaining information may imply, for example, determining the prevalence of disease, doing a population survey, or measuring the level of a toxin. Useful information for making a clinical diagnosis may include symptoms, signs, laboratory tests, or imaging tests. Most tests will, however, produce some false-positive and false-negative results. In Chapters 5, 6, and 7, we will look in detail at interpreting such imperfect tests.

When the diagnosis is clear, testing may still help to clarify the prognosis or the responsiveness to treatment. With glue ear, the test-of-time helps by identifying those who are likely to have a sustained problem. Some tests specifically help to identify those most likely to respond. In women with

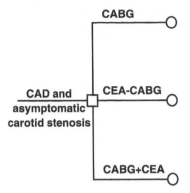

Figure 1.2   Decision tree fragment for Example 2: asymptomatic carotid artery stenosis in a male planned for coronary artery bypass grafting (CABG) for coronary artery disease (CAD). The options are: perform CABG only; perform carotid endarterectomy (CEA) and then CABG (CEA-CABG); or perform CABG and CEA in a combined procedure (CABG + CEA).

breast cancer, for example, the estrogen receptor status (i.e., whether or not the tumor cells have hormone receptors) of the cancer identifies cancers more likely to respond to hormonal treatments such as tamoxifen (Bland, 1999).

Figure 1.2 shows the start of a decision tree for our second example. In this example, the do-nothing option is to refrain from treating the carotid artery stenosis and proceed directly to CABG. There are at least two alternative treatment options: to either do a combined procedure, or to do the carotid endarterectomy first and then proceed to CABG.

1.4.2 C: Model the consequences and estimate the chances

You need to think through the sequence of consequences of each decision option and the chances of each event. Both short-term and long-term consequences should be considered. For each consequence you need to find the best available evidence to support your arguments. Having listed the alternatives, you next need to consider the consequences of each. This was partly accomplished when you outlined the natural history in Step 1, since natural history outlines the consequences of the do-nothing option. In Chapter 2 we will detail the types of probabilities you will encounter in decision making. These include the risks and benefits of interventions (Chapters 3, 8) and the accuracy and interpretation of diagnostic test information (Chapters 5, 6, and 7). Depending on the type of decision, the

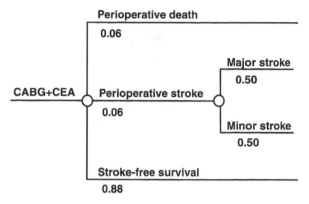

Figure 1.3   Chance tree for combined coronary artery bypass grafting (CABG) and carotid endarterectomy (CEA) (Example 2).

relevant outcomes may be identified based on the patient's values and preferences (Chapter 4) and/or the resource costs (Chapter 9).

Each alternative will lead to a different distribution of outcomes which need to be quantified. The relevant outcomes depend on the particular problem at hand. It may be the number of days of illness avoided or deaths prevented by a vaccine for influenza; or the chances of permanent hearing loss if glue ear is untreated; or the chances of 5- or 10-year stroke-free survival for the 70-year-old man with coronary artery disease and asymptomatic carotid artery stenosis. Some of the consequences may be better described in diagrams than words. For example, the possible consequences following the combined CABG and carotid endarterectomy operation for our patient in Example 2 might be described as in Figure 1.3, which shows one representation of the *chance tree*.

The round circles (chance nodes) are used to indicate time points at which there are two or more possible outcomes. Several sequences of chance nodes may be needed to describe a problem. For Example 2, choosing to do the combined CABG and carotid endarterectomy might result in one of three possible outcomes. Which of the three occurs is beyond our control. However, the likelihood of each can be indicated by the probabilities shown below the branches emanating from the chance node. We will return to the simple mathematics of probability in Chapter 2; for now, note that the probabilities are all between 0 and 1 (or between 0% and 100%, if expressed as percentages), and the sum of the probabilities of all of the branches from a single chance node adds up to 1 (that is, 100%). This reflects the fact that one, and only one, of the possibilities at each chance node may occur. From each chance arm, there may either be a

DEFINITION

A *chance tree* is a visual representation of a series of random discrete linked events. It visualizes the chance that each event can occur.

DEFINITION

A *clinical balance sheet* tabulates the consequences of different options and considers all relevant perspectives and important dimensions.

further division into possible outcomes, such as the major or minor stroke shown in Figure 1.3, or further decisions to be made. The decision tree thus assists in structuring the sequence of choices and outcomes over time.

Sometimes consequences are simple. For example, in patients who have had ventricular fibrillation (a fatal arrhythmia unless resuscitation is given), the main concern is sudden death from a recurrence. Decisions about appropriate drugs or implantable defibrillators will focus around this obviously important outcome. Many disease conditions, however, involve multiple consequences. For these, comparison of the benefits and harms across different options is assisted by a clinical balance sheet.

Table 1.2 provides an example of a balance sheet for some of the alternatives for managing glue ear. Usually, the first alternative will be a wait-and-see strategy and the balance sheet will then incorporate the consequence table from Step 1 (Table 1.1). The subsequent columns will show the consequences of each alternative. Note that the probabilities of uncertain outcomes are also included, e.g., the spontaneous resolution rate and the complication rates.

The balance sheet can be assembled by either describing the outcomes with each alternative, or by describing the relative effects of each alternative (relative to the wait-and-see strategy). Both methods are reasonable, and often one will be more convenient than the other. However, only one method should be used within a single table to insure consistent interpretation of the information presented.

The table will also describe the potential harms and resource costs of treatment alternatives. These harms and costs will include: (i) the direct burden or discomfort from the intervention; (ii) the complications and adverse effects of the intervention; and (iii) the cost to the health-care system, patients, and their families, including management of any complications. The direct burden may vary considerably. This burden might also include changes in the patient's self-perception. For example, the burden of a diagnosis of hypertension includes not just the taking of a daily medication but also the change in self-perception which has been shown to result in increased sick days taken and poorer career progress. The complications can range from minor dose-related side-effects to major surgical complications or drug reactions. Finally, the burden to the health-care system is the cost of the intervention, including personnel, materials, overheads, and costs to patients and families (see Chapter 9).

Table 1.2. Clinical balance sheet for some options for managing glue ear

	Alternatives		
	Monitor (wait-and-see)	Grommet insertion (short-term tube)	Hearing aid
Potential treatment benefits			
Improve hearing and behavior	Slow improvement of months to years (resolution at 1, 3, and 6 months is 60%, 74%, and 88%)	Rapid improvement with grommet until it falls out in 8 months (range 6–12 months)	Immediately improved
Language development	Delayed (possibly permanent)	'Normal'	'Normal'
Acute middle-ear infections	1–2 episodes per year	Reduced by 0.5 episodes per year	1–2 episodes per year
Long-term complications of glue ear	Uncertain: possible conductive problems	Uncertain effects	Uncertain: possible conductive problems
Potential treatment harms and costs			
Long-term complications of treatment	None	Tympanosclerosis (scarred drum): 40% Retraction: 18% Grommet lost into middle ear^a: 0.4% Perforation^a: 0.4%	None
Restrictions	None	(Some) swimming restrictions while grommet in place	Need to wear hearing aid
Short-term complications	None	Ear discharge: Brief: 40% Chronic: 5%	None
Cost	Low	$2400	$600–1500

^{a}These complications will require further surgery to retrieve the grommet or patch the perforation.

1.4.3 T: Identify and estimate the value trade-offs

Valuation of consequences becomes important when there is more than one type of consequence. If you are only concerned with a single adverse consequence, such as mortality, then the issue is simply a question of which alternative offers the lowest (expected) probability of that consequence or the highest probability of survival. If there are several disparate consequences, however, the choice of alternative might depend on how we value them. With the alternatives for managing glue ear, the inconvenience and perhaps embarrassment of wearing a hearing aid must be weighed against the small probability of complications from grommet insertion. Such trade-offs require clarification of the values involved. In some problems values can be clarified by trying out one of the alternatives. For example, a child with glue ear might borrow a hearing aid to test practicality and satisfaction with the results. Information about the experience of others may also be helpful in deciding whether an alternative is worth trying. In a study of 48 English children with glue ear, 71% reported complete satisfaction with a hearing aid and experienced improved speech and hearing.

Many decisions do not allow such a trial period. A common dilemma is a treatment that offers relief of symptoms but at a small risk of serious adverse consequences. Example 2 is a vivid illustration of this issue. There is a measurable risk of perioperative mortality to be balanced against the better quality of life and longevity to be gained with successful surgery. Other examples include: total hip replacement for severe arthritis, a procedure which relieves pain and can restore mobility but has a small risk of operative mortality or major complications; nonsteroidal antiinflammatory drugs, which provide relief for several conditions but with a very small risk of stomach bleeding; and a blood transfusion which may relieve symptoms of anemia but at small risks of a transfusion reaction or bloodborne infection. Because of the processes for drug and device approval in place in most of the industrialized world, the benefits are likely to outweigh the adverse consequences for most commonly used treatments. However, the balance will depend on the individual's prognosis and severity as well as on the magnitude of the potential harms and the strength of each individual's outcome preferences. For example, women with the BrCa1 gene are at greatly increased risk of breast cancer, and this risk may be decreased by undergoing bilateral mastectomy. Clearly this is an individual decision and women may have very different values and attitudes about the risks and outcomes of each choice. Methods for quantifying preferences and values are discussed in Chapter 4. Resource constraints limit the ability of health care to meet all the needs of patients and society and the method of cost-effectiveness analysis (also known as cost–utility analysis) is the topic of Chapter 9.

1.5 Step 3 – proactIVE: integration and exploration

Once the probabilities and values of each outcome have been identified, it is time to figure out which option is best. To do this we may need to calculate the expected value, that is, the average value gained from choosing a particular alternative. The option with the highest expected value will generally be chosen, provided we have captured the major decision elements in the analysis. However, you should also explore how sensitive the decision is to the exact probabilities and values chosen. Let us look at these three subcomponents.

1.5.1 I: Integrate the evidence and values

After explicitly formulating the problem, the options, and the associated risks, benefits, and values, it sometimes becomes obvious which option is optimal. Further analysis is unnecessary. But this is not always the case. If there are multiple dimensions, a useful next step is to focus on the important differences between options. To do this with the clinical balance sheet you might first rank the issues in order of importance. The rearranged table on glue ear – with only the two active treatment options – is shown in Table 1.3, with the rankings done separately within the benefits and harms. Next, those rows for which the consequences are fairly even may be struck out. These consequences can be ignored, as they are not altered by the available choices. For the treatment of glue ear, the simplified table suggests that grommet insertion has more complications and slightly greater expense than a hearing aid but reduces the number of acute middle-ear infections.

The balance sheet can help tease out the different dimensions of a problem. However, for some dimensions the sequence of events is complex and will be better represented by a chance tree. To summarize the consequences will require a formal calculation of the expected value of each option. In addition, in problems that involve both valuations and probabilities, the decision can be aided by calculating the expected value.

The process of calculating expected values is described further in Chapter 3. Furthermore, we may want to take quality of life into account, and calculate the expected quality-adjusted life years, which will be described in Chapter 4. Sometimes we will want to consider two different dimensions of the outcomes simultaneously and separately calculate the expected value for each. For example, in Chapter 9 we will incorporate costs, separately

DEFINITION

The *expected value* of an option is the sum of the values of all the consequences of that option, each value weighed by the probability that the consequence will occur.

Table 1.3. Balance sheet with rows in order of importance

	Alternatives	
	Grommet insertion (short-term tube)	Hearing aid
Potential treatment benefits		
Language development	~~Normal~~	~~Normal~~
Improve hearing and behavior	Rapid improvement with grommet until it falls out in 8 months (range 6–12 months)	Immediately improved
Long-term complications of glue ear	~~Uncertain effects~~	~~Uncertain: possible conductive problems~~
Acute middle-ear infections	Reduced by 0.5 episodes per year	1–2 episodes per year
Potential treatment harms and costs		
Long-term complications of treatment	Tympanosclerosis (scarred drum): 40% Retraction: 18% Grommet lost into middle ear[a]: 0.4% Perforation[a]: 0.4%	None
Restrictions	~~(Some) swimming restrictions while grommet in place~~	~~Need to wear hearing aid~~
Short-term complications	Ear discharge: Brief: 40% Chronic: 5%	None
Cost	$2400	$600–1500

[a]These complications will require further surgery to retrieve the grommet or patch the perforation.

calculating expected benefits and expected economic costs, allowing us to calculate the cost per unit of benefit gained.

1.5.2 V: Optimize the expected value

You have now evaluated each alternative, but which should you choose? Decision analysis employs an explicit principle for making choices: maximize expected utility. The complex and sometimes conflicting information about outcomes, harms, and benefits represented in our list are combined and integrated by a multiplication-and-addition procedure: the probability of each outcome is multiplied by its value, and for each alternative, these products are added. You obtain an expected value for each alternative, and these expectations are the basis for recommending one.

In theory, you should prefer the alternative with the best net expected benefit, that is, the one that appears to give the best overall utility taking into account both the chances and value of each consequence. If the outcome values have been expressed as desirable values, we would want to maximize the expected value. If the outcome values have been expressed as undesirable values, we would want to minimize the expected value. Other decision goals are defensible, especially if you think that some especially important objectives or features of the problem have not been included in the analysis. For example, in some situations, some decision makers prefer to minimize the chance of the worst outcome (a minimax strategy). This 'fear-of-flying' strategy focuses on avoiding a single catastrophic outcome without regard to its probability. It would rule out total hip replacement for hip arthritis because of the small risk of operative mortality, and would eschew medication for anything but life-threatening illnesses because of the small risk of an adverse reaction that was worse than the illness being treated. Precedent, authority, habit, religious considerations, or local consensus may also play a part in making a decision. We think that the approach we have described, which leads to the maximum net expected benefit, should generally be preferred because it balances considerations of the harms and benefits of all outcomes, weighed by the probability that they will occur.

1.5.3 E: Explore the assumptions and evaluate uncertainty

The approach we have described uses numbers to talk about both the probabilities and values of treatment outcomes. Clearly some of these numbers will be well established in the clinical literature, while others may be very 'soft.' You may not be sure they are really right. You may be uncertain about whether some probabilities retrieved from the literature apply to our patient, or, if you have to estimate some key probabilities, you may be uncertain about the accuracy of our estimates or concerned about various cognitive biases that have been shown to affect probability estimates (Bogardus et al., 1999; Chapman and Elstein, 2000). If you have consulted patients to elicit their values and preferences, you may be uncertain about the stability of the numbers obtained from these inquiries, especially if the patients have been asked to evaluate health states they have not yet experienced (Fischhoff et al., 1980; Christensen-Szalanski, 1984). What if some or all of these numbers were different? Would our decision change? How much change in any of these numbers will change the recommended decision? Or is the recommendation insensitive to any plausible change in either the probabilities or the utilities?

To understand the effects of these uncertainties on our decision, you should perform a 'what-if' analysis, also known as a *sensitivity analysis*. By varying the uncertain variables over the range of values considered plausible, you can calculate what the effect of that uncertainty is on the decision. If the decision is not sensitive to a plausible change in a parameter value, then the precise value of that parameter is irrelevant. If the decision does change, this warrants further study to find out more precisely what the value is. In Example 2, a sensitivity analysis for age and perioperative risk in a published decision analysis (Cronenwett et al., 1997) could enable a decision maker to apply the results to her particular case, or to gain confidence that her decision was best. A quantitative, formal sensitivity analysis permits us to gain insight into what particular variables really drive a decision. If the key variables causing changes are probabilities, we say the decision is 'probability-driven.' More research may be needed to get better or more updated evidence. If the decision hinges on values and preferences, it is said to be 'utility-driven.' These uncertainties cannot be resolved by better evidence, because they are not about the facts. But they can be ameliorated by values clarification: whose values are at issue? How clear are the decision makers about what they really want? Do they understand the trade-offs that may be involved? Many recently developed decision aids for patients aim to assist in clarifying the patient's values and understanding of the treatment options.

1.6 Using the results

What is the end product of this decision process? You might consider that 'the decision' is the major outcome. However, the insight gained will be useful for other similar decisions. So you should explicitly consider how to capture this insight for future use.

So, how can you apply the results of an analysis to other patients or target populations? Future patients may differ in many ways, so it is not usually the decision that is reapplied but rather the analysis process. Elements of the problem that, if different, are likely to change the decision are the critical factors in applying the decision analysis more broadly. Probabilities, such as the likelihood of having a disease, the likelihoods of observing various test results given the presence or absence of a disease, and the responses to treatments, are among the most important factors. Also important, and often more important, are the values attached to the various dimensions of outcome, such as survival, functional status, and symptoms. Consideration of these factors is assisted by sensitivity and threshold analysis, which we shall cover in several chapters, particularly 3 and 6. Here we shall look briefly at how the results of an analysis might be summarized as a guideline for future decisions.

1.6.1 Guidelines for specific clinical decisions

A clinically useful decision guide (or aid) should meet two requirements. First, it should give the clinician information about how outcomes of a recommended practice are likely to vary with different patient characteristics. Second, the outcomes should be presented in a way that permits incorporating patients' preferences. For example, a summary showing how quality-adjusted life years (see Chapter 4) vary with predictors is helpful for decision making at the level of public health, but it is insufficient at the bedside, as it does not allow each patient's unique values to be incorporated. In constructing a decision guide that will fulfill these two requirements and take account of individual prognosis and values, a decision analyst needs to be mindful of the practicalities and constraints of using a guide in clinical practice: the more it provides for individually tailoring to an individual patient, the more time it will take to use it, and so it may be less used as its complexity increases. On the other hand, insufficient flexibility also threatens its acceptability in clinical practice.

Decision guides have several formats. These vary in the degree to which they satisfy our two requirements. The most common guide is the section on management in clinical textbooks. These will generally describe some of the alternatives and heuristics for making a choice, along the lines of: 'unless the patient is allergic to penicillin, the first-line treatment should be...'. However, these texts are usually not written with the requirements outlined and rarely meet them. There are two other major formats for decision guides: clinical algorithms and clinical balance sheets.

1.6.2 Clinical algorithms

A clinical algorithm consists of a structured sequence of questions and recommended actions based on the answers to those questions. They are

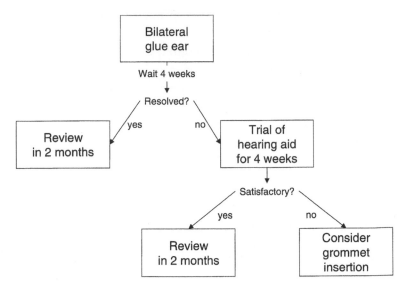

Figure 1.4   A possible clinical algorithm for the management of glue ear (Example 1).

also called clinical protocols, clinical pathways, or flow charts. The questions will divide patients into subgroups based on features such as disease severity, allergies, other diseases, etc., which will then lead to a sequence of actions such as investigation or treatment. These algorithms are usually represented as a tree of questions and actions, as illustrated in Figure 1.4.

If we were to develop a decision tree, then prune away the suboptimal alternatives at each decision node and leave out the probability and value estimates, the result would be a clinical algorithm. Thus, decision analysis can be used to develop a clinical algorithm, but not all clinical algorithms are developed using decision analysis. Indeed, most are not.

Algorithms may be developed in different ways, using the opinions and recommendations of individual experts, or of a hospital guideline committee, or of a national consensus group. The development process may be informal or formal, using methods such as the PROACTIVE approach. Clinical algorithms are particularly useful to assist rapid and consistent decision making when patient preferences are not crucial. For example, clinical algorithms are common and helpful for the management of cardiac arrests, treatment of anaphylaxis, or preparation for bowel surgery.

A drawback of simply pruning away the nonoptimal alternatives is that we cannot readily adapt the steps to different circumstances and patient values. Thus clinical algorithms do not usually satisfy either of our requirements, and therefore have a price in flexibility. An algorithm is usually devised for a well-defined set of circumstances, and it is difficult to broaden it to cover others, even if they are plausibly related to the base condition. For example, if a magnetic resonance imaging scan is recommended, what do you do when the local machine is unavailable for 24 h and the nearest alternative is 300 km away? Without an estimate of the consequences of following or disregarding a recommendation, we have no guide to action. Thus, not specifying the outcomes used to construct the algorithm limits its applicability. This limitation is most relevant for a decision in which patient values are crucial, such as the choice of contraception, or whether to use hormone replacement therapy, or treatments for prostate and breast cancer. These decisions have no single 'right' choice but depend on the patient's view of the consequences. Algorithms can neglect patients' preferences, however, and still be useful, even in these instances. For example, an algorithm for hormonal replacement therapy for postmenopausal women was based on maximizing life expectancy as the outcome criterion, which provides at least one perspective on the decision problem, and avoids the complexities of measuring patients' values (Col et al., 1997). We return to these issues in Chapter 4.

1.6.3 Clinical balance sheets

An alternative format for a decision guide is the clinical balance sheet. Whether this is in the form of a table (such as Table 1.2) or a graph, the aim is to present quantitative estimates of the consequences of the different reasonable alternatives. It may or may not make a specific recommendation, but it does present the data needed for an informed choice. Hence, we should be able to see the consequences of deviation from the recommended alternative.

1.6.4 Patient-oriented decision aids

For value-sensitive decisions, informing patients adequately may take considerable time that is not available in practice. To break free of this constraint, several investigators have developed patient decision aids that use paper, video, or interactive computer-guided information that describe the problem, the alternatives, and the consequences (O'Connor et al., 1999). The informed patient and clinician can then meet to make a final decision. Many of these patient-oriented decision aids are based on the principles expounded in the following chapters, but they generally avoid making a formal recommendation based on expected-utility maximization. Instead, they concentrate on explaining the harms and benefits of each alternative treatment, and leave the decision up to the patients and their clinicians.

1.7 Why are these tools helpful?

What do the tools we have discussed add to decision making in health care? Surely patients, physicians, and public policy makers think in terms of risks and benefits when making medical decisions? The tools enable us to lay out our assumptions, the evidence, and our goals explicitly and systematically, and they help us overcome some well-documented cognitive limitations. A major problem in making decisions without some kind of aid, even one as simple as a consequence table, is that our capacity to deal with complex problems is limited (Newell and Simon, 1972; Redelmeier et al., 1993). We tend to think we can manage more information at once than is really possible (Miller, 1956; Dawson and Arkes, 1987). So we are inclined to hone in on one particular piece of the problem, and it is difficult to consider the other parts in a balanced way at the same time. We focus first on one aspect, then move on to another, and so on. By the time we have reviewed the entire set of choices, we may have forgotten what was said (or thought) at the beginning. Even if we remember all of the steps in our deliberations, it is difficult to fit all of the pieces together into a coherent package. We run the risk of going round in circles and getting stuck in our thinking and our discussions. We may focus on optimizing one tiny piece and forget to think about whether optimizing that piece serves our global goal, or we may respond to minor variations in the formulation of the problem, features that should not affect our decision (Tversky and Kahneman, 1974, 1981). Or we may be influenced by the sheer number of available alternatives (Redelmeier and Shafir, 1995). Visual aids and other logical thinking tools help us take a broad perspective. They help us to think through the problem from all angles, to identify conflicting objectives and trade-offs, and to think and communicate in a systematic logical way. It is like 'going to the balcony' and getting a general overview of what's happening.

1.7.1 But are they practical?

How practical are these tools and this sequence of steps and substeps? Not all substeps will be required for every decision. Sometimes the first few substeps will be sufficient. For example, with the problem of PAT, knowing the natural history will usually be sufficient and defining the problem will be enough. The evidence of a good clinical follow-up study (Aronow et al., 1995) demonstrated that mortality for patients with PAT was the same as for those with normal heart rhythms. Hence, if a patient has no other signs of cardiac problems and is not unduly disturbed by these episodes, our decision process might end here; we have enough information to know that 'it ain't broke,' so we do not need to know the alternatives for 'fixing it.' For the glue ear example, on the other hand, more steps are needed because of the complex trade-off between the consequences. Many other decisions can be resolved by finding the evidence about the effects of different alternatives and clearly describing the consequences.

To complete all three major steps, each with its three substeps, usually takes far more time than is available for the typical health-care decision. Hence, we suggest that for 'once-only' decisions, it is advisable to check the evidence and draw a rough consequence table, even if there is not enough time to draw a complete decision tree. If the decision is one that you or your colleagues will face repeatedly, then spending the time to do all the steps and develop a decision guide for future cases may improve decisions, help with patient education and communication, and reduce future decision-making time. Finally, with the growth of clinical guidelines, it is worth understanding the steps and asking whether the guidelines you employ have used a similar process and presentation, or whether they can be supplemented or replaced using the techniques described in this book.

The basic concepts and tools of decision analysis, however, are useful in many situations and are valuable in day-to-day practice even when a decision analysis cannot be fully worked out. We hope that these fundamental concepts become part of your entire approach to clinical reasoning and decision making. We have tried to show how these tools grow out of a formal theory of decision making, even if they do not invoke it explicitly or employ all of the steps involved in a complete decision analysis.

1.8 Summary

We have outlined a systematic rational approach to decision making in health care. The process itself helps health-care decision makers to gain an overview of the issues and think beyond the perspective most of us are most inclined to take. Table 1.4 presents these steps, summarized with a convenient mnemonic – PROACTIVE.

Table 1.4. The PROACTIVE (problem – reframe – objectives – alternatives – consequences and chances – trade-offs – integrate – value – explore and evaluate) approach to decision making

Problem: Define the problem
What exactly is the problem? Is there a problem? What will happen if I take no immediate action? What are the possible consequences? How likely are these? When may they occur? How serious is each consequence?

Reframe: Reframe from multiple perspectives
Whose perspective do I represent? Who else is involved in the decision-making process? Who is affected by the decision? What do they think and feel? What is important from the perspectives of the patient, physician, department, hospital, payer, and the public policy maker?

Objective: Focus on the objective
What is the goal of an intervention? Why is this important? Examine all important dimensions, or attributes, of the problem, including medical effectiveness, economics, psychosocial, political, ethical, and philosophical aspects. Is this a means objective or a fundamental objective? What do I really hope to attain?

Alternatives: Consider all relevant alternatives
Do I know all the reasonable alternatives? Consider wait-and-see, intervention, and obtaining information. Can I expand the number of options? List all possible options – brainstorm first, decide later

Consequences and chances: Model the consequences and estimate the chances
Which diseases could the patient possibly have? What events may occur over time? What are the chances?

Trade-offs: Identify and estimate the value trade-offs
How do the benefits and harms compare for each possible outcome? What are the values and value trade-offs? How do patients value the consequences? What are the monetary costs?

Integrate: Integrate the evidence and values
Can I qualitatively integrate the evidence and values or do I need a quantitative estimate of expected value? If there are uncertainties, what is the overall expected value of each alternative?

Value: Optimize expected value
How do I optimize the decision? Are the outcomes desirable or undesirable? Do I need to choose the option with the maximum or minimum expected value? Can I combine the desirable and undesirable outcomes into one multiattribute outcome? Are there any intangible factors that we have omitted?

Explore and evaluate: Explore the assumptions and evaluate uncertainty
What if I have a different patient consult me? Can I generalize the results to other patients? What if the population for which I am choosing a public health program is somewhat different? What if the estimates in my model are not quite accurate? Would plausible changes in any variable change the recommended action? What if my modeling assumptions are inaccurate?

Decision analysis may appear to be a serial process, i.e., the steps are followed consecutively. This is because we can only describe it sequentially. In reality the process is far more a recursive circular process with feedback loops. For example, we structure the problem and consider all the possible options. Subsequently, as we search the literature for evidence, we may find other diagnostic or treatment options that we had not yet considered, or we realize that the way we structured the problem does not accurately reflect the best available evidence. We then have to go back and adjust our initial formulation of the problem and expand the list of options. Analogously, after completing the analysis we may find ourselves confronted with varying cases and conditions that force us to adjust our assumptions and estimates. A conflict between the plan we had in mind before the analysis and that recommended by the model may cause us to consider whether important variables have been omitted from our analysis or if our thinking has been inconsistent. Thus, the analytic process helps us continually to reflect on the important trade-offs and issues involved in the decision problem.

Time is needed for a full-fledged decision analysis involving all of these steps. Consequently, a complete decision model is generally developed only for commonly recurring problems that necessitate and justify detailed analysis. A detailed analysis is necessary if there are competing diagnostic or treatment strategies, where consensus has not been established, and where there is considerable uncertainty. In these circumstances, decision analyses can help formulate a clinical guideline or health policy statement for health-care practice or at least clarify the issues at the heart of the controversy.

1.9 Overview of the book

In Chapter 2, we expand on the treatment of uncertainty by developing fundamental rules of probability and the concept of expected value. We show how to calculate the expected value of simple monetary lotteries, as a preparation for calculating expected value in more complex clinical situations, involving life expectancy, quality of life, and health states between perfect health and death.

Chapter 3 discusses the proactive approach to a clinical problem and explains the use of decision trees to determine the best treatment under diagnostic uncertainty. Maximization of expected utility is employed as the criterion for decision making under uncertainty.

Chapter 4 outlines utility assessment. It discusses different methods that are employed to quantify outcome values, for both individual clinical decision making and for health policy or population-based decisions.

Chapter 5 develops Bayes' theorem, the basic tool of decision analysis for revising opinion with imperfect information. The theorem is widely used in clinical diagnosis, to revise diagnostic opinion with physical findings, tests, or laboratory studies that we know are not 100% accurate. We begin with an analysis of tests with dichotomous results (positive and negative).

Chapter 6 revisits decision trees, this time adding Bayes' theorem. We shall explore a family of decision problems with three options – do not treat, treat without further testing, and test-and-treat – and show how to determine in which region you are operating.

Chapter 7 deepens the analysis of tests, moving from dichotomous test results to tests with multiple results and deals with combining results from multiple tests. Some of the material covered in this chapter is fairly advanced and can be skipped without loss of the general flow of the text of the book. The advanced material is marked with an asterisk.

In Chapter 8, we will discuss techniques for rapidly identifying the best available relevant data and how to manage the limitations of such data.

Chapter 9 discusses the problems of societal decision making with limited financial resources. It introduces cost-effectiveness analysis and cost–utility analysis and shows how to apply decision analytic principles to select among health-care programs using a cost-effectiveness criterion.

Chapter 10 introduces an additional complexity, showing how to model clinical situations in which a patient or population moves from one state to another over time. Examples are the development of lung cancer after many years of smoking, or the development of breast cancer after years of hormonal replacement therapy. Decision trees do not handle these situations conveniently, but state-transition models do, and we shall discuss these models in some detail.

Chapter 11 discusses methods to explore and evaluate variability and uncertainty. Several approaches to estimation, including Monte Carlo simulation, are developed and explained. This chapter covers advanced material and would not be recommended for an introductory course.

Chapter 12 reviews the PROACTIVE steps, putting each step in a broader context, examining strengths and limitations of this approach, and suggesting possible future developments.

Exercises

Exercise 1.1

Consider a decision problem that you have been faced with recently. It may be a clinical problem, a health policy problem, or a personal problem. Go through the steps of the PROACTIVE approach and try to apply each step to your own case problem. For the time being do this qualitatively. As you read this book try to apply the quantitative techniques it teaches to your own case.

Sometimes the specific technique taught will not be useful for your initially chosen case example. Think of other decision problems that you have been confronted with as you read. As you work through the book try to find problems in your own day-to-day work situation or personal life in which the technique described may be useful, whether simply through the concept it teaches or through a formal analysis.

Exercise 1.2

Imagine that you are an epidemiologist in the public health service in Ecuador. A cholera epidemic has broken out, spreading from a neighboring country. Rural villages close to the border and on the highlands appear to be at increased risk. You are asked to intervene to avoid further spread of the disease.

The population of Ecuador is approximately 10 million. At the time you are consulted, approximately 2% of the population is infected. The incubation time of cholera is 2 days on average, with a range from 6 h to 5 days. Sixty-five percent of cases are mild and resolve spontaneously. Thirty percent are moderate and respond well to oral rehydration solution (ORS). Without ORS, moderate cases progress to severe cases. Five percent of cases are severe from the onset. Patients with severe cholera die if untreated. Intravenous fluid saves patients with severe cholera but costs 40 times as much as ORS and is not available everywhere, certainly not in the rural areas.

Measures that you could consider include vaccination, making the water supply safe, antibiotic prophylaxis, ORS, and educating the public.

Use the proactive approach to decision making to get a handle on the problem.

P How would you define the problem?

R Reframe the problem from various perspectives.

O What is the objective of intervention?

A What are your alternatives?

C What could be the possible consequences of each alternative and what are the chances?

T What are the value trade-offs?

I Synthesize the information qualitatively by integrating the evidence and values.

V What decision criterion would you choose in deciding what to do?

E Explore how your decision may change if the probabilities or values were slightly different than you had initially estimated.

Exercise 1.3

Imagine that you are a clinical epidemiologist with a background in radiology. You are consulted by the Ministry of Health to give your expert advice on whether a randomized controlled trial for the screening of lung cancer among smokers and former smokers should be initiated given the extremely optimistic results of screening using spiral computed tomography (CT) reported in a paper in 1999:

Henschke, C.I., McCauley, D.I., Yankelevitz, D.F. et al. (1999). Early Lung Cancer Action Project: overall design and findings from baseline screening. *Lancet*, **354**, 99–105.

Background: The Early Lung Cancer Action Project (ELCAP) is designed to evaluate baseline and annual repeat screening by low-radiation-dose computed tomography (low-dose CT) in people at high risk of lung cancer. We report the baseline experience.

Methods: ELCAP has enrolled 1000 symptom-free volunteers, aged 60 years or older, with at least 10 pack-years of cigarette smoking and no previous cancer, who were medically fit to undergo thoracic surgery. After a structured interview and informed consent, chest radiographs and low-dose CT were done for each participant. The diagnostic investigation of screen-detected non-calcified pulmonary nodules was guided by ELCAP recommendations, which included short-term high-resolution CT follow-up for the smallest non-calcified nodules.

Findings: Non-calcified nodules were detected in 233 (23% [95% CI 21–26]) participants by low-dose CT at baseline, compared with 68 (7% [5–9]) by chest radiography. Malignant disease was detected in 27 (2.7% [1.8–3.8]) by CT and seven (0.7% [0.3–1.3]) by chest radiography, and stage I malignant disease in 23 (2.3% [1.5–3.3]) and four (0.4% [0.1–0.9]), respectively. Of the 27 CT-detected cancers, 26 were resectable. Biopsies were done on 28 of the 233 participants with non-calcified nodules; 27 had malignant non-calcified nodules and one had a benign nodule. Another three individuals underwent biopsy against the ELCAP recommendations; all had benign non-calcified nodules. No participant had thoracotomy for a benign nodule.

Interpretation: Low-dose CT can greatly improve the likelihood of detection of small non-calcified nodules, and thus of lung cancer at an earlier and potentially more curable stage. Although false-positive CT results are common, they can be managed with little use of invasive diagnostic procedures.

How would you go about formulating an advice for the Ministry of Health? Use the PROACTIVE approach to decision making. Don't hesitate to look up any information you may need. Note that many articles will probably have been published on this subject since the time the book went to print.

Exercise 1.4

A male friend of yours, 40 years of age, has bright red blood loss per rectum and undergoes a sigmoidoscopy. A polyp is found and removed. The procedure was very uncomfortable and your friend is anxious about having to undergo another endoscopic procedure in the future. But at the same time he is anxious about developing colorectal cancer. The pathology report says it is a tubular villous adenoma with atypical cells but no infiltrative spread. The adenoma has been totally removed. Your friend questions you about what the best management options are.

Use the PROACTIVE approach to decision making to give your advice. Look up any information you need.

REFERENCES

Ali, I.M., Cummings, B., Sullivan, J. & Francis, S. (1998). The risk of cerebrovascular accident in patients with asymptomatic critical carotid artery stenosis who undergo open-heart surgery. *Can. J. Surg.*, **41**, 374–81.

Aronow, W.S., Ahn, C., Mercando, A.D. & Epstein, S. (1995). Correlation of atrial fibrillation, paroxysmal supraventricular tachycardia, and sinus rhythm with incidences of new coronary events in 1359 patients, mean age 81 years, with heart disease. *Am. J. Cardiol.*, **75**, 182–4.

Beers, M.H. & Berkow, R. (eds) (1999). *The Merck Manual of Diagnosis and Therapy*, 17th edn. Whitehouse Station, NJ: Merck.

Bland, K.I. (1999). Future directions in endocrine treatment of advanced breast cancer. *Ann. Surg. Oncol.*, **6** (Suppl.), 14S–16S.

Bogardus, S.T., Homboe, E. & Jekel, J.F. (1999). Perils, pitfalls and possibilities in talking about medical risk. *J.A.M.A.*, **281**, 1037–41.

Chapman, G.B. & Elstein, A.S. (2000). Cognitive processes and biases in medical decision making. In: *Decision Making in Health Care*, ed. G.B. Chapman & F.A. Sonnenberg. New York: Cambridge University Press.

Christensen-Szalanski, J.J.J. (1984). Discount functions and the measurement of patients' values: women's decisions in childbirth. *Med. Decis. Making*, **4**, 47–58.

Col, N.F., Eckman, M.H., Karas, R.H. et al. (1997). Patient-specific decisions about hormone replacement therapy in postmenopausal women [see comments]. *J.A.M.A.*, **277**, 1140–7.

Cronenwett, J.L., Birkmeyer, J.D., Nackman, G.B. et al. (1997). Cost-effectiveness of carotid endarterectomy in asymptomatic patients. *J. Vasc. Surg.*, **25**, 298–311.

Dawson, N.V. & Arkes, H.R. (1987). Systematic errors in medical decision making: judgment limitations. *J. Gen. Intern. Med.*, **2**, 183–7.

Fischhoff, B., Slovic, P. & Lichtenstein, S. (1980). Knowing what you want: measuring labile values. In: *Cognitive Processes in Choice and Decision Behavior*, ed. T.S. Wallsten, pp. 117–41. Hillsdale, NJ: Erlbaum.

Hammond, J.S., Keeney, R.L. & Raiffa, H. (1999). *Smart Choices: A Practical Guide to Making Better Decisions*. Boston, MA: Harvard Business School Press.

Hunink, M.G.M. (2001). In search of tools to aid logical thinking and communicating about medical decision making. *Med. Decis. Making*, **21**, 267–77.

Merck's Manual of the Materia Medica (1899). *A Ready Reference Pocketbook for the Physician and Surgeon*. Merck.

Miller, G.A. (1956). The magical number seven, plus or minus two: some limits on our capacity for processing information. *Psychol. Rev.*, **63**, 81–97.

Newell, A. & Simon, H.A. (1972). *Human Problem Solving*. Englewood Cliffs, NJ: Prenticehall.

O'Connor, A.M., Rostom, A., Fiset, V. et al. (1999). Decision aids for patients facing health treatment or screening decisions: systematic review [see comments]. *Br. Med. J.*, **319**, 731–4.

Redelmeier, D.A. & Shafir, E. (1995). Medical decision making in situations that offer multiple alternatives. *J.A.M.A.*, **273**, 302–5.

Redelmeier, D.A., Rozin, P. & Kahneman, D. (1993). Understanding patients' decisions: cognitive and emotional perspectives. *J.A.M.A.*, **270**, 72–6.

Rosenfeld, R.M. & Bluestone, C.D. (1999). *Evidence-based Otitis Media*. Hamilton, Ontario: Decker.

Tversky, A. & Kahneman, D. (1974). Judgment under uncertainty: heuristics and biases. *Science*, **185**, 1124–34.

Tversky, A. & Kahneman, D. (1981). The framing of decisions and the psychology of choice. *Science*, **211**, 453–8.

Weinstein, M.C., Fineberg, H.V., Elstein, A.S. et al. (1980). *Clinical Decision Analysis*. Philadelphia: W.B. Saunders.

2

Managing uncertainty

Much of medical training consists of learning to cope with pervasive uncertainty and with the limits of medical knowledge. Making serious clinical decisions on the basis of conflicting, incomplete, and untimely data is routine.

J.D. McCue

2.1 Introduction

Despite our best efforts, much of clinical medicine and health care involves uncertainties. Better decisions will be made if we are open and honest about these uncertainties, and develop skills in estimating, communicating, and working with such uncertainties. What types of uncertainty exist? Consider the following example.

Example

Needlestick injury

It has been a hard week. It is time to go home when you are called to yet another heroin overdose: a young woman has been found unconscious outside your clinic. After giving intravenous (IV) naloxone (which reverses the effects of heroin), you are accidentally jabbed by the needle. After her recovery, despite your reassurances, the young woman flees for fear of the police. As the mêlée settles, the dread of human immunodeficiency virus (HIV) infection begins to develop. You talk to the senior doctor about what you should do. She is very sympathetic, and begins to tell you about the risks and management. The good news is that, even if the patient was HIV-positive, a needlestick injury *rarely* leads to HIV infection (about 3 per 1000). And if she was HIV-positive then antivirals such as zidovudine (AZT) are *likely* to be able to prevent most infections (perhaps 80%).

Unfortunately, the HIV status of the young woman who had overdosed is unknown. Since she was not a patient of your clinic, you are uncertain about whether she is infected, but think that it is *possible* since she is an IV drug user. The Centers for Disease Control and Prevention (CDC) guidelines suggest: 'If the exposure source is *unknown*, use of postexposure prophylaxis should be decided on a case-by-case basis. Consideration should include the severity of the exposure and the epidemiologic likelihood that the health care worker was exposed to HIV.' What do you do?

33

In the example above we are uncertain of the HIV status of the heroin user and both the possibility of HIV transmission and the effectiveness of prophylactic treatment are not certainties but must be expressed in terms of chances. Regardless of these uncertainties, we must make a choice. Even doing nothing is a choice; inaction should not be an evasion of decision making but a deliberate choice, which should be made only if it is better than the alternatives. Thus, in health care we are often reluctant 'gamblers,' who must place our stakes as wisely as possible in the face of multiple uncertainties. To enable us to choose wisely we must make these uncertainties explicit.

When communicating and reasoning about uncertainties, verbal expressions create problems. For example, what do the words 'rarely,' 'likely,' and 'possible' mean to you? Do they mean the same thing to a co-worker or patient? Unfortunately, several surveys demonstrate wide variation in the interpretation of such verbal expressions. This makes them a poor vehicle for communication about uncertainty, risk, and probability. For example, Figure 2.1 shows an assessment of these words by 100 mothers of infants and 50 doctors and medical students (Shaw and Dear, 1990).

To some extent we can predict people's differences in meaning for probabilistic terms. For example, patients with previous experience of an adverse event tend to ascribe its 'likely' occurrence a higher probability than those who have not experienced it (Woloshin et al., 1994). This is in line with a general tendency to give a higher probability to events that are more 'available' to us, that is, that we have seen more frequently or more recently or that are especially memorable. Similarly, patients' interpretations of 'rare' were higher if the event was more severe. However, such differences are not sufficiently predictable to enable repair of our faulty risk communication. We may know what we mean by a particular risk expression but we do not know what other people mean by the same expression. This can have undesirable consequences for important decisions involving uncertainty. Being explicit has practical advantages: doctors' agreement about decisions to treat hypothetical cases was improved when given numerical rather than verbal expressions of probability (Timmermans, 1994).

Patients generally express a desire for risk communication, and most prefer this to be quantitative. For example, of the mothers interviewed for the data in Figure 2.1, 53% wanted numerical statements of risk; 37% wanted a verbal expression; and 10% had no preference (Shaw and Dear, 1990). Despite this, doctors have been reluctant to communicate risk either quantitatively or qualitatively. Given the inevitability of uncertainties in

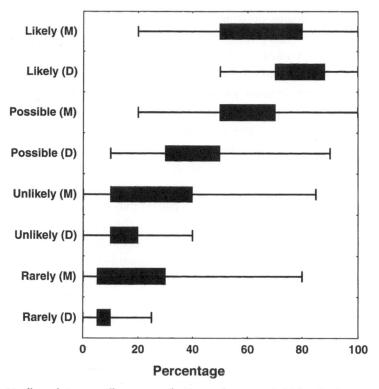

Figure 2.1   Median, interquartile range (box), and range (whiskers), for percentages assigned to expressions by 100 mothers (M) and 50 doctors and medical students (D). Reproduced from Shaw, N.J. & Dear, P.R. (1990). How do parents of babies interpret qualitative expressions of probability? *Arch. Dis. Child.*, **65**, 520–3, with permission of the BMJ Publishing Group.

many health-care decisions, we believe that both health-care workers and patients would be best served by learning how to express uncertainty numerically. If it is difficult to give a single figure, using a range still provides a clearer statement than a verbal expression. This approach requires that health-care workers develop skills in understanding, assessing, and manipulating information about probabilities.

Some physicians may question the use of probabilities for an individual patient and wonder whether any probability estimates, such as the probability that the patient has a particular disease or the likelihood that the patient will survive an illness, can possibly be valid and meaningful for a given individual. After all, one might argue that this patient either has the disease or does not and will either recover or not. There is no probability involved. Furthermore, the argument continues, since each patient is unique, probability estimates derived from experience with previous patients or from epidemiological studies cannot possibly apply to any individual case.

Unfortunately, decisions must be made in the present looking into the uncertain future, not looking back at the certain past. It is true that every patient is unique, either has the disease or does not, and will either recover or not. But in the situation we are discussing, both her underlying true state and future course of the illness (if any) are unknown and hence uncertain. What is important for a decision maker is the state of his or her beliefs and knowledge at the time of the decision and not what may then be – and perhaps may later emerge as – the truth. The assignment of probabilities to the case of an individual patient may be viewed as a measure of the decision maker's ignorance about all of the special characteristics of that unique individual. We must be cognizant of what we know and do not know about each patient, but a refusal to quantify our ignorance will not lessen it. We argue that a physician should use probabilities to help decide on a strategy for an individual patient.

This chapter will begin by looking at the most common probabilities in health care: diagnosis, prognosis, and the effects of treatment. We will then discuss how these probabilities can be combined and manipulated. In the next chapter we will look at how, when either diagnosis or outcome is uncertain, explicit probabilities can be combined with a quantitative assessment of the outcomes to make better decisions.

2.2 Types of probability

Uncertainty may be expressed quantitatively in several different ways: as probabilities, proportions, frequencies, odds, percentages, and rates (Table 2.1). Probabilities, by definition, range in value from 0.0 to 1.0. A probability of 0 means that the event is impossible; a probability of 1.0 means that it is certain. A probability of 0.5 means the event is equally as likely to occur as not to occur. Probabilities may also be expressed as percentages, where 0% corresponds to a probability of 0, and 100% corresponds to a probability of 1. A percentage expresses a probability as a frequency per 100, but other frequency expressions are common. For example, cancer incidence is often expressed as a frequency per 100 000. For consistency in this book, we will usually use probabilities rather than frequencies for working problems. However, since many people find frequencies easier to interpret, you should generally express final results as frequencies, particularly when communicating with patients.

We shall not concern ourselves here with two types of distinctions that

Table 2.1. Probability terms: definitions and relationships of various terms for probabilities

Term	Definition	Formula	Range
Probability	The chance of an event	P	0–1
Proportion	The relative frequency of a state	P	0–1
Prevalence	The proportion of a group with a specific disease	P	0–1
Percentage	Probability expressed as a frequency 'per 100'	$P \times 100$	0–100
Frequency	Probability expressed per sample (e.g., 1 per 1000)	P	0–denominator
Odds	The ratio of the probability of an event to its complement	$P/(1-P)$	0–infinity
Probability measures involving time			
Incidence (or hazard) rate	The occurrence of new disease cases or events per unit of person-time	P/t	0–infinity
Incidence proportion	The proportion of people who develop a new disease or have an event during a specified period of time	P	0–1
Risk	The probability that an individual develops a new disease or has an event during a specified period of time	P	0–1

become crucial at a more advanced level. One such distinction concerns 'frequencies' and 'probabilities.' One school of thought, known as 'frequentist,' holds that the only meaningful sense in which probability can be discussed is in terms of empirical frequencies in a sample of observations. Another school of thought, known as 'subjectivist' or 'Bayesian,' holds that probability is fundamentally a degree of belief, and that, while frequency data may inform estimates of probability, they are not themselves probabilities. Chapter 8 describes an approach to probabilities and the data that inform their estimation, incorporating a healthy respect for empirical data while retaining the view that, in the end, decision makers must act on the probabilities they believe.

A second, more technical distinction, which we do not belabor here, but to which we return in Chapter 10 in the context of state-transition models, concerns rates and probabilities. Technically, a rate is an instantaneous change in the cumulative probability of an outcome per unit of time, rather than an average change. The formal definition of a rate requires calculus, as it is the first derivative of a cumulative probability with respect to time. Until we get to Chapter 10, we will rather loosely use the term 'rate' to apply to the probability of an event in a specified time interval.

There are several types of uncertainty in the needlestick example at the beginning of this chapter: the diagnostic uncertainty of whether the heroin user has an HIV infection; the prognostic uncertainty of how often the development of HIV (seroconversion) would occur after a needlestick injury from an HIV-infected patient; and the uncertainty about the effectiveness of prophylactic treatment with antiviral drugs. It is important to have an understanding of the measures of and sources for these three common medical uncertainties, all of which can be quantified using probabilities.

2.3 Diagnostic uncertainty

Diagnosis is a very uncertain art. Studies comparing clinicians' diagnoses show disagreement is very common (Fleming, 1997). This is implicit in the differential diagnosis, which lists the possible causes of an individual illness. Skilled diagnosticians often generate a longer list, but also are better able to differentiate between the most and least likely causes. Good diagnosis depends on both knowing all the possibilities and accurately assessing their relative frequency. Diagnostic probabilities express our uncertainty about the list of differential diagnoses. For example, we might need to know the likelihood of different possible causes of sudden chest pain; or, in our needlestick example, we would like to know the chance that an IV drug user had a blood-borne infection such as HIV, hepatitis B, or hepatitis C.

2.3.1 The summation principle

There are some simple 'rules' that a differential diagnosis should follow. First, the differential diagnosis should include all possible single diseases and combinations of diseases and the sum of the probabilities of all possibilities must add up to 1 (the summation principle). Second, one and only one possibility must be true. This is a general requirement for the analysis of chance outcomes: they must be structured to be mutually exclusive (only one can occur) and collectively exhaustive (one must occur). For example, either a patient has HIV or not. The probabilities of these two possibilities add up to 1. In mathematical notation:

$$P(\text{HIV}) + P(\text{not HIV}) = 1 \tag{2.1}$$

where $P(\text{HIV})$ is shorthand which is read as 'the probability of HIV.' Thus, with our needlestick example, if the probability of HIV is 0.25 then the complement, $P(\text{not HIV})$, must be $1 - 0.25 = 0.75$.

It is common to assume that only one diagnosis is causing a problem. This is usually true, as the likelihood of two illnesses with similar presentations occurring simultaneously is low. However, for longer-term illness this will not be true and among the elderly, multiple diseases are common. If multiple diseases are possible we need to be explicit about this. For example, if we were considering the chances of HIV and hepatitis B, then we would need to consider each alone, both, or neither, so that:

$$P(\text{HIV only}) + P(\text{hepatitis B only}) + P(\text{HIV and hepatitis B})$$
$$+ P(\text{neither}) = 1 \tag{2.2}$$

More generally, the summation rule for n mutually exclusive possibilities may be written as:

$$P(\text{possibility 1}) + P(\text{possibility 2}) + \ldots + P(\text{possibility } n) = 1 \tag{2.3}$$

2.3.2 Conditional probabilities

Returning to our needlestick example, we need to assess the probability of HIV in the heroin user. We write this probability as $P(\text{HIV} \mid \text{IV drug use})$ which is read as 'the probability of HIV given IV drug use.' The symbol '$\mid$' is read as 'given' the particular group in whom we have estimated the probability.

DEFINITION

The probability that event E occurs, given that event F has occurred, is called the *conditional probability* of event E given event F. It is denoted by $P(E \mid F)$.

If this conditional information makes no difference to the probability, then we say the two factors are (statistically, or probabilistically) independent. For example, if gender made no difference to our estimate of the probability of HIV, that is, $P(\text{HIV} \mid \text{female}) = P(\text{HIV} \mid \text{male}) = P(\text{HIV})$, then HIV status and gender are said to be independent (this will be formally defined in the section on combining probabilities at the end of this chapter).

2.3.3 Sources of data

Where do diagnostic probabilities come from? We do not start with a blank slate: the patient's presenting problem, other symptoms and signs, his or her age, and gender all contribute to the likelihood of different possibilities. Estimates may come from (a combination of) personal experience, empirical data (the systematically collected experience of others), and our understanding of the different disease processes. The principal empirical information will be studies of consecutive patients with a particular presenting complaint. For example, if we wish to know the probabilities of different causes of headaches for patients in ambulatory care, then the ideal study (see Checklist A) will have collected a consecutive series of patients presenting with headache, then ascertained the cause through a standard protocol of tests and follow-up. However, our setting and individual patient will usually differ in several ways from this study, so, while it may provide a useful starting point, some mental adjustment will be needed to particularize the results. Estimates based on personal experience are often called subjective probabilities, while those based on data are sometimes called objective, data-based, or frequency-based probabilities. For our purposes in this book, it is important to note that the rules for combining these probabilities are exactly the same, regardless of the source.

Example (*cont.*) For our needlestick injury case, we need to know how likely an HIV infection is for an IV drug user. Clearly this will vary greatly in different locations. Ideally, we would like a recent serological survey of a representative sample of intravenous drug users in the local area. This is unlikely to be available. Our best data for US populations is probably from the CDC, which compiles data on HIV prevalence in many subgroups, including IV drug users. The 1997 statistics suggested an overall prevalence of about 15% among IV drug users. However, this varied widely over the 12 locations which had sufficient data: from 0% in Denver to 38% in Newark. Clearly, the local data are relevant, and we should be more concerned in Newark than in Denver.

2.4 Prognostic uncertainty

The television image of doctors suggests they are clairvoyant and can tell you that you have 3 months to live. Reality falls far short of this. For many conditions, the natural history is not well documented, and even when it is, the prediction is an average, which may not apply well to any single individual. For example, the average survival for a cancer may be 2 years, but the range of survival is wide and unpredictable, with some patients surviving only a few weeks and others many years. Prognostic uncertainty is uncertainty about future health states rather than current health states.

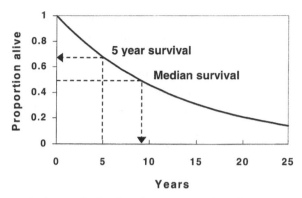

Figure 2.2   Survival curve indicating the 5-year and median survival.

For example, prognostic questions include the chance that someone who has survived a myocardial infarction (heart attack) will have another, or the long-term risk of liver failure in someone with hepatitis C. Thus prognosis involves probability over time. For example, cancer prognosis is often expressed as a 5-year survival rate. There is nothing special about 5 years; we might also want to know the 1-year and 20-year survival, though 5-year survival gives a single convenient 'snapshot.'

Because of the time element, prognosis is often expressed through incidence and hazard rates, which measure the probability per unit time, e.g., percent per year. Since the rate may change, the most complete description of prognosis will usually be a survival curve, which shows the effects of risk over time, not simply at a defined interval.

2.4.1 Survival curves

Though the calculations can be difficult, the concept of a survival curve is straightforward: it plots the probability of being alive over a period of time. Figure 2.2 shows an example of a survival curve. It begins at time 0, with all patients alive. As we follow the plot out over time, there is a progressive decrease in survival. As shown for the 5-year point in the figure, the proportion alive (5-year survival), and its complement, the proportion dead (5-year mortality), can be read off by drawing a line from the survival curve and then to the vertical axis.

The overall survival can be summarized in several ways. First, from the graph we can read off the median survival – the point at which exactly 50% of patients have died and 50% are still alive – by drawing a line from the 0.50 on the vertical axis across to the survival curve and then down to the time (horizontal) axis. In this example, the median survival is about 9 years. The expected value or mean (also called the life expectancy) is more difficult to calculate but corresponds to the area under the survival curve. We shall be returning frequently to the concept of life expectancy and its calculation, both in Chapter 4 on outcome values, and in Chapter 10, where we show how simple state-transition models can be used to generate estimates of life expectancy.

Survival curves can be constructed through published life tables, by applying so-called product-limit (Kaplan–Meier) estimators to empirical data, or by estimating the parameters of survival functions statistically from data. For a detailed description of survival analysis we refer the reader to textbooks and articles on the subject (Armitage and Berry, 1994; Collette, 1994).

2.4.2 Probability trees

In the most general sense, *prognosis* may be defined as the chance tree facing an individual, or population of individuals, given particular conditions. These conditions include *prognostic factors* (also called *risk factors*) and any health-care interventions that may be applied.

A survival curve is really a concise format for visually representing the chance tree of successive event rates (e.g., mortality rates) over time. For example, in Figure 2.2, the probability of dying during the first year can be calculated as the difference between the probability of being alive at year 0 (100%) and the probability of being alive at year 1 (approximately 91%), or about 0.09. This probability of dying in the first year could be represented as the first event in a sequence of chance nodes in a chance tree (Figure 2.3). The probabilities of dying in each successive year can be obtained similarly from the survival curve, taking care to divide each survival difference (between the nth year and the $(n-1)$th year) by the probability of being alive at year $n-1$. These annual probabilities of death would be represented as the remaining chance nodes in the chance tree that corresponds to the survival curve (Figure 2.3).

> **DEFINITION**
>
> An individual's *prognosis* is the chance tree describing future events, given a set of prognostic factors and interventions.

2.4.3 Prognostic factors

Everyone with the same disease does not have the same prognosis. Risk may be modified by many other factors, such as the stage of disease, and the patient's age and gender. Such prognostic factors enable us to refine our

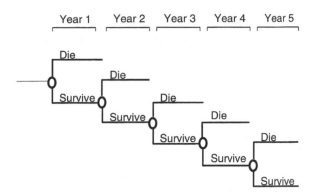

Figure 2.3   Chance tree indicating the probability of dying in the first 5 years.

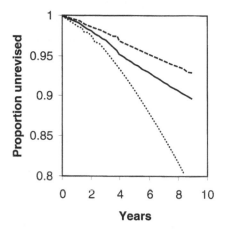

Figure 2.4   Proportion of total hip replacements that have not needed replacement at various points in time, for the subgroups cemented (dashed line) and uncemented (dotted line). The continuous line denotes both. Data based on Norwegian Arthroplasty Registry. Reproduced from Espehaug et al. (1999) with permission.

individual predictions. Again, when risk varies over time, the ideal description would be a survival curve for each particular subgroup. For example, for colorectal cancer the 5-year survival is 92% for patients whose colorectal cancer is detected at an early stage, 64% if there is spread to nearby organs or lymph nodes, and only 7% if there is spread (metastasis) to distant parts of the body such as the liver or lungs. Similarly, Figure 2.4 illustrates the time to replacement for cemented and uncemented hip prostheses. It also illustrates that survival curves are useful for presenting any data that involve the time to an event, not only mortality. For example, the duration of influenza, the time to cancer relapse, and the duration of pain in acute middle-ear infections have all been presented as 'survival' curves. In these cases 'survival' implies being event-free.

2.4.4 Sources of data

How can we obtain information on prognosis and prognostic factors? To understand the development of a disease over time, the ideal would be to have a large cohort of patients with all prognostic factors measured at the beginning of the disease, followed up to the end stage of the disease. This is usually referred to as an inception cohort. The important features to look for are given in Checklist B. Such studies may be found through literature searches of MEDLINE, but finding the better-quality studies can be difficult. PubMed's Clinical Queries, which is part of the internet version of MEDLINE, provides filters that assist in identifying the better prognostic studies. There are some useful compilations and summaries of prognostic studies, such as that provided by Best Evidence, which contains all previous editions of the American College of Physicians' (ACP) *Journal Club* and *Evidence-based Medicine*. Among the most widely used inception cohorts for decision analysis is the Framingham Heart Study, which measured numerous risk factors for cardiovascular disease every 2 years, and followed subjects for the occurrence of heart disease, stroke, and death at these intervals (Kannel, 2000).

Such a study will describe the prognosis of patients given their particular treatments. If they had no specific treatment, the prognosis is known as the natural history. However, if they had specific treatment that modified the disease process, then the study provides evidence on the prognosis conditional on those treatments. Natural history is important, as it gives us the probabilities we need to estimate along the 'no-intervention' branch of a decision tree. By comparing it with the prognosis in the absence of the disease, the natural history also enables us to calculate the individual's potential benefit from treatment.

In general, the potential benefit will be greater in those with more severe disease and/or those who are at higher risk. Unfortunately, most treatments are neither perfect cures nor harmless. Most treatments provide symptomatic relief or a chance of cure, but usually with the risk of some adverse effects. This means that the net benefit a patient derives from treatment is usually less (sometimes considerably so) than the potential benefit.

Integrating prognostic information as a function of patient characteristics is necessary when developing a guideline. For example, the guideline for managing cardiovascular risk shown in Figure 2.5

DEFINITION

The *potential benefit* is the difference between the expected outcome based on an individual's prognosis if a harmless curative treatment is available and the expected outcome based on his or her current prognosis without specific treatment.

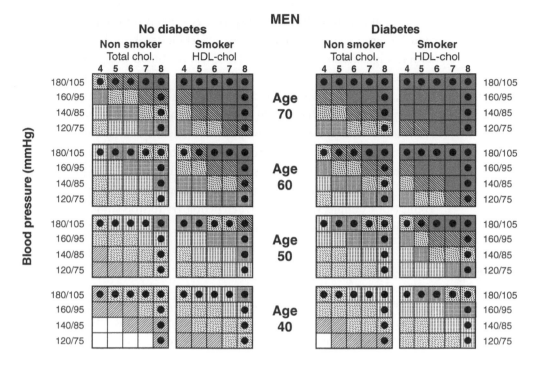

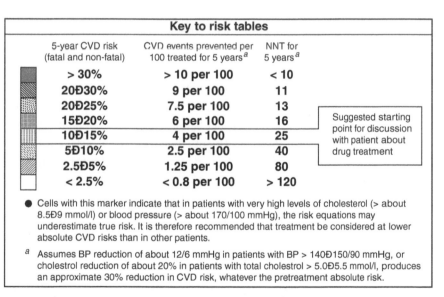

Figure 2.5   Guideline for managing cardiovascular risk. chol., cholesterol; HDL-chol., high-density lipoprotein cholesterol; CVD, cardiovascular disease; BP, blood pressure; NNT, number-needed-to-treat. Reproduced from Jackson (2000) with permission.

(Baker et al., 2000; Jackson, 2000) provides explicit information on individual prognosis using six risk factors: age, cholesterol (as the total cholesterol to high-density lipoprotein (HDL) ratio), blood pressure, smoking, diabetes, and gender (only the male chart is shown here). From these factors, the guide quantifies the 5-year risk of a cardiovascular event (first column of key), and the benefit of treatment alternatives in terms of the reduction in risk. The guide shows patients and clinicians by how much the risk of cardiovascular events is reduced through control of the risk factors that are manageable. We would suggest one additional step, to provide the 'harms' of the treatment alternatives, including the frequency of adverse events (for example, weight gain when people try to stop smoking) and the effort involved in compliance and monitoring.

2.5 Treatment uncertainty

Few treatments have the dramatic impact of insulin for juvenile-onset diabetes or penicillin for pneumococcal pneumonia. The efficacy of such 'miracle' cures is clear: without treatment, the disease is usually progressive, while treatment cures almost all patients and has few or no adverse effects. However, usually the disease fluctuates or a proportion remits spontaneously; in either case the treatment effect is incomplete. For example, the vast majority of people with high blood pressure (hypertension) will not have a stroke (prognostic uncertainty); and lowering blood pressure will not prevent all strokes (treatment uncertainty). The effects of such imperfect treatments need to be weighed against their harms, such as mild adverse effects and the occasional severe or even fatal reaction, such as anaphylaxis. For those treatments that are not 'miracle' cures, we need an accurate assessment of their incremental benefit for comparison with possible harms.

How can we best assess treatment effects? The ideal study would compare two large similar groups of patients, one treated and the other not, observing how treatment influences the course of illness. This is the aim of controlled clinical trials. For several reasons, however, the results may need to be adapted for application to individual patients. First, any individual's prognosis, and hence the potential benefit, may be quite different from the average patient in the trial. Second, the individual's concomitant illnesses and risk factors may be different, modifying the potential benefit. Third, the effectiveness and cost of the intervention may differ by setting; for example, experienced surgeons may get better results than less experienced ones, or follow-up and monitoring may be more difficult in a rural setting.

2.5.1 Sources of data

Randomized controlled trials provide the best type of information on which to base an analysis. If there are several such trials, a systematic review of these is ideal (see Chapter 8). For controlled trials, there are two principal design problems: establishing two comparable groups and unbiased observation of the outcomes.

How can we establish comparable groups? Allowing the clinician and patient to choose either treatment is likely to lead to systematic differences. For example, older patients or smokers might prefer one of the treatments, and hence both these prognostic factors (determinants in epidemiological terminology) and the treatment would influence the outcome. These imbalanced prognostic factors are said to *confound* the treatment comparison.

Statistical techniques can partly adjust for known prognostic factors but not for unknown prognostic factors. Randomization is the only secure method of obtaining balance between the treatment groups in both known and unknown prognostic factors. Since the first randomized trial of streptomycin for tuberculosis was published in 1948, over a quarter of a million randomized trials have been conducted.

How can we obtain unbiased observation of outcomes? As observers, we have a natural tendency to see what we want to see. The principal method of reducing observer bias is for the person assessing the outcome to be unaware of which treatment the patient was allocated to – known as *blinding*. Ideally, both patient and clinician will be unaware of the treatment allocation, known as a *double blind*. A common way to achieve this in pharmaceutical trials is using a placebo, which matches the active treatment for size, color, taste, and dosing schedule. If two pharmaceuticals are being compared, then either these need to match or each is provided with its own placebo (known as the double-dummy technique). Even when using a placebo is not feasible, one should ensure that the person assessing the outcome is unaware of the treatment allocation. For example, blinding in surgical and other nonpharmaceutical treatments is often very difficult, although not impossible, but blind outcome assessment is still achievable for some outcomes. The important features to consider when appraising a study of the effects of an intervention are summarized in Checklist C.

Not all treatments can be subjected to a double-blind randomized trial and, even when it is possible, it has not always been done. Although the aim is to use the best evidence available, decisions about individual treatment and policy need to be made even when 'perfect' evidence is lacking. To rank evidence from 'best' to 'worst,' several hierarchies of evidence for interventions have been developed (Table 2.2).

DEFINITION

A *confounder* is a prognostic factor that is associated both with the exposure to an intervention (or with another determinant of outcome) and with the outcome (or disease) but is not an intermediate in the causal chain.

Table 2.2. Levels of evidence used for preventive interventions

Level	Description
Level 1	Evidence obtained from at least one properly randomized controlled trial
Level 2-I	Evidence obtained from well-designed controlled trials without randomization
Level 2-II	Evidence obtained from well-designed cohort or case-control analytic studies, preferably from more than one center or research group
Level 2-III	Evidence obtained from multiple time series with or without the intervention. Dramatic results in uncontrolled experiments (such as the results of the introduction of penicillin treatment in the 1940s) could also be regarded as this type of evidence
Level 3	Opinions of respected authorities, based on clinical experience; descriptive studies and case reports; or reports of expert committees

Source: US Task Force Guide to Clinical Preventive Services, 2nd edn.

A case-control study compares a group of individuals who have experienced an outcome of interest with a comparable group who have not, to determine the differences between their previous prognostic factors or other determinants of risk. A cohort study compares a group of individuals who have been exposed to an intervention or prognostic factor with a comparable group who have not, to determine the differences between their outcomes. The chief limitation of both of these study designs lies in insuring that the two groups are truly comparable in terms of all other prognostic factors. This can be accomplished to some degree by matching them according to known and measurable factors or by post-hoc statistical adjustment.

Example (*cont.*) Unfortunately, the evidence on the effectiveness of antiviral drugs for needle-stick injuries is limited. A case-control study of the use of zidovudine suggested that 81% of seroconversions to HIV could be prevented by prophylaxis. Less direct, but high-quality evidence comes from randomized trials of zidovudine and other antivirals to prevent vertical transmission of HIV, that is, transmission from mother to fetus. The first of these showed a 67% reduction. So we have some evidence of efficacy, but we do not precisely know how effective zidovudine alone is.

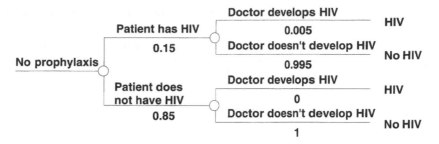

Figure 2.6   Chance tree for the needlestick example when no prophylaxis is given.

2.6 Combining probabilities

Many decision problems will involve more than one uncertainty. Decision analysis provides a means of weighing the competing benefits and harms for individuals or specific groups. We may need to combine the probabilities that represent diagnostic, prognostic, and treatment uncertainties. To combine these probabilities validly requires an understanding of a few important rules and ways of representing these probabilities in diagrams.

Recall the needlestick example, where there was both diagnostic uncertainty regarding the HIV status of the IV drug user, and prognostic uncertainty regarding the chance of developing HIV given a needlestick injury from an HIV-positive subject. Figure 2.6 shows the chance tree when no prophylactic treatment is given. In the bottom branch we have made explicit the assumption that, if the IV drug user was HIV-negative, then HIV cannot be transmitted to the health-care worker.

The overall probability of developing HIV is the sum of all the paths in the tree that result in HIV, that is: $(0.15 \times 0.005) + (0.85 \times 0) = 0.00075$. The final result could be more clearly presented in frequency terms: we can rewrite this probability and say that there is 1 chance in 1333 of developing HIV without prophylaxis $(1/0.00075 = 1333)$.

The chance tree here is quite simple, but the same process can be used to visualize far more complex sequences of probabilities, as we shall see in the chapters ahead.

2.6.1 Probability multiplication rules

To obtain the probability of HIV in the above example, we simply multiplied the two probabilities, diagnostic and prognostic. However, combining probabilities is sometimes less straightforward. Let us look at a second

Table 2.3. Observed distribution of human immunodeficiency virus (HIV) and hepatitis B virus (HBV) in 2202 intravenous drug users in Baltimore. Numbers in parentheses are the percentages of the total population in each cell

	HBV +	HBV −	Total
HIV +	500 (23%)	40 (2%)	540 (25%)
HIV −	1360 (61%)	302 (14%)	1662 (75%)
Total	1860 (84%)	342 (16%)	2202

Data from Levine et al. (1995).

example that incorporates the possibility of other blood-borne infections. Specifically, let us consider the chance of an IV drug user having both HIV and hepatitis B virus (HBV) together. It is not sufficient to multiply the separate probabilities, since the two infections are likely to occur together, that is, they are not independent events. Examine the data in Table 2.3 from a 1988–89 serological study of consecutive IV drug users at a street outreach clinic in Baltimore. The table shows the observed joint distribution of HIV and HBV results: the cells of this 2×2 table show the numbers (and percentages) of those with both, either one, or neither infection. Keep in mind that the percentages in the cells of the table are calculated in relation to the total population (2202) in the study.

2.6.2 Conditional probability

Does having one of these infections affect the chances of having the other? For example, what is the probability of having HIV, given that the person has HBV? How does this compare with the probability of HIV if he or she doesn't have HBV? These are the conditional probabilities, $P(\text{HIV}+|\text{HBV}+)$ and $P(\text{HIV}+|\text{HBV}-)$, and can be calculated from Table 2.3. To obtain $P(\text{HIV}+|\text{HBV}+)$ we look only at the HBV + column of the table, and note that 500 of the 1860 cases have HIV, or 27%. Similarly, to obtain $P(\text{HIV}+|\text{HBV}-)$ we look only at the HBV − column of the table and note that 40 of the 342 cases have HIV, or about 12%.

These are conditional probabilities because they express the probability of an outcome under the condition that the other outcome has occurred. You could also think of it as the probability within a particular subset. For example, $P(\text{HIV}+|\text{HBV}-)$ is the probability of HIV in the subset known to be negative for HBV. Since the probability of HIV depends on which subset we are referring to (the overall group (23%), the HBV + group

(27%), or the HBV− group (12%)), the HIV and HBV statuses are considered dependent events. Conversely, if these three probabilities turned out to be the same, then the events would be considered statistically independent.

2.6.3 Dependence and independence

DEFINITION

When the conditional probability of an event E, given another event F, is the same as the unconditional probability of event E, we say that events E and F are *probabilistically independent*. That is, if $P(E \mid F) = P(E)$, then E and F are independent events.

Generalizing the above example, we can formally define *probabilistic independence*.

Clearly, in any data set some difference may occur between the conditional and unconditional probabilities merely by chance. We will not develop the statistical methods to examine this issue in this book. You will encounter several methods that statisticians use to determine the probability that an observed difference in the data could have resulted from random chance. For example, in the data in Table 2.3 the difference in HIV probability between the HBV+ and HBV− groups is: 27% − 12% = 15%. Several methods may be used to calculate the probability that this difference could have resulted by chance if there were truly no difference in the underlying probabilities; in our example, this P-value is less than 0.0001, that is, a highly statistically significant difference. Another frequently used statistical method is to calculate a *confidence interval* for the difference; in this case, such a confidence interval may be calculated as 10–20%, which does not include zero. Thus, the difference in the conditional probabilities is not explained by chance. This is not surprising. Those IV drug users engaged in unsafe practices such as needle sharing are more likely to get both infections; those engaged in safe practices such as needle exchange and cleaning are more likely to avoid both infections. Statistical independence in a data set can be tested using the chi-squared test for independence, which can be found in any statistics book.

While commonly used, P-values and their close relatives, confidence intervals, have limitations as guides to decision making. Many statisticians and decision analysts object to the use of P-values because they do not tell us anything that would help us assess the probabilities of interest. In our example, a P-value of <0.0001 does *not* mean that the probability that HBV and HIV are independent is >0.9999! Similarly, a 95% confidence interval for a probability estimate does *not* imply that the true probability has a 95% chance of being inside the interval! The distinction we are drawing here is beyond the scope of this book, and it lies at the heart of the previously mentioned difference between the 'frequentists' and the

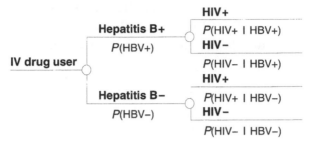

Figure 2.7   The chance tree for the human immunodeficiency virus (HIV) and hepatitis B virus (HBV) probabilities.

'subjectivists.' Even the authors of this book align themselves at different points along this philosophical spectrum! It is a testament to the power of decision analysis as a method that it can be couched comfortably within either outlook on chance and probability.

2.6.4 Multiplying probabilities

When we wish to combine probabilities, as when obtaining the chance of a sequence of events, the exact method used will depend on whether the events are dependent or independent. If the events are independent, we can multiply the probabilities of each of the events in the sequence. If the events are dependent, we need to know the probabilities for each event conditional on the previous events in the sequence. Figure 2.7 shows the chance tree for the HIV and HBV probabilities.

To obtain the probability of having both HBV and HIV requires multiplying the probability of having HBV, $P(\text{HBV}+)$, by the probability of HIV given HBV, $P(\text{HIV}+|\text{HBV}+)$.

DEFINITION

The probability of the concomitant occurrence of any number of events is called the *joint probability* of those events. The joint probability of two events, E and F, is written in probability notation as $P[E$ and $F]$ or as $P[E, F]$.

The calculation of the joint probability is performed as follows:

$$P(E \text{ and } F) = P(F) \times P(E|F) = P(E) \times P(F|E) \qquad (2.4)$$

Note that if E and F are independent this simplifies to $P(E \text{ and } F) = P(E) \times P(F)$. Verifying this relation is a test for independence.

Important conditional probabilities that we will consider in the next chapters are the probability of an outcome given different treatments and the probability of a test result given different diseases. These probabilities are crucial to rational diagnostic testing and treatment decisions.

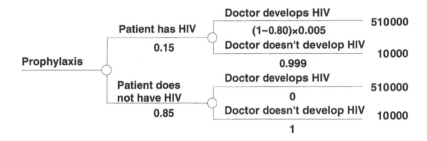

Figure 2.8   Chance tree of prophylaxis for the needlestick example with costs (in dollars) as outcome.

2.7 Expected value   *multiply each path and all then all together*

So far we have been concerned with situations where each outcome at a chance node can be represented as the probability of a single event, such as HIV infection. Events are combined by applying the basic laws of conditional and joint probability discussed in this chapter. This process is called *averaging out*. However, the concepts of expected value and averaging out can be generalized to outcomes which are not probabilities but are some other number, such as the number of seizures, migraine attacks, days of illness, years of life, or costs. In Chapter 4 we will show how a special scale, called a utility scale, can be constructed so that it is just as appropriate to apply averaging out to utilities as to probabilities. First, however, we shall look further at averaging out and describe its application to problems that involve expected fixed-term outcomes.

Example (*cont.*)   Suppose we are interested in the expected future health-care resource costs of needlestick injuries, including the cost of prophylaxis and later costs of treatment. Not all health-care workers will take prophylaxis, and whether they do or do not, only a few will develop an HIV infection. Given these uncertainties, how can we calculate the expected future costs? The chance tree for prophylaxis (Figure 2.8) outlines the uncertainties involved for that particular option.

Suppose that the cost of prophylaxis is $10 000 and the cost of treatment $500 000. Furthermore, assume that the effectiveness of prophylaxis in preventing HIV is 80%. To find the expected costs, we repeat the same averaging-out procedure as before, except now we multiply each path probability by the dollar values. The expected cost of prophylaxis is then:

$$0.15 \times [((1-0.80) \times 0.005 \times \$510\,000) + (0.999 \times \$10\,000)] + 0.85$$
$$\times[(0 \times \$510\,000) + (1 \times \$10\,000)] = 0.15 \times [(1-0.80) \times 0.005$$
$$\times \$500\,000] + \$10\,000 = 0.00015 \times \$500\,000 + \$10\,000 = \$10\,075$$

Thus, the expected cost is \$10 075. But note that no single case will have this particular cost. The expected value is a weighted average of costs representing our prediction of the average over a large series of similar cases.

DEFINITION

Suppose that an uncertain quantity X, such as cost or length of stay, may have different values denoted by $X_1, X_2 \ldots X_n$ with probabilities $P_1, P_2 \ldots P_n$. Then we define its *expected value* as:

$$E[X] = P_1 \cdot X_1 + P_2 \cdot X_2 + \ldots P_n \cdot X_n. \tag{2.5}$$

The notation $E[X]$ is read as 'the expected value of X.' The expected value is also called the mean of the distribution of the possible values of the quantity.

2.7.1 Averages, expected values, and the law of large numbers

The expected value is closely related to the usual notion of a weighted average, and the relationship is more than coincidental. Suppose that we observe 100 patients undergoing the same procedure as in our example and then compute the average number of days of hospitalization. Keep in mind that the average is simply the sum of all the days of hospitalization divided by the number of patients. You know intuitively that if you observe enough patients and the probabilities are correct, the average will tend to be very close to the expected value. Statisticians call this property the law of large numbers. As the number of independent, identical replications becomes very large, their empirical average is likely to get very close to the expected value. A more familiar example involves a coin-tossing game with a fair coin. If you win one dollar when heads come up but lose one dollar when tails comes up, your winnings on a single toss are values of one dollar (with a probability of 0.5) or minus one dollar (with a probability of 0.5). The expected value of this is:

$$[(1/2)\,(\$1)] + (1/2)\,(-\$1)] = \$0 \tag{2.6}$$

You will never get \$0, the expected value, on a single toss; you either get $-\$1$ or $+\$1$. However, the law of large numbers states that in the long run the average winnings per coin toss will be approximately zero.

2.8 Summary

Verbal expressions of uncertainties create two kinds of problems:

- There is wide variation in the interpretation of probabilistic terms. People can assign very different probability estimates to common verbal expressions such as 'likely,' 'possibly,' 'rarely,' and 'occasionally.' Hence, while it may seem that using these terms facilitates communication and understanding, we believe that their use can conceal important disagreements.
- If verbal expressions are assigned to different uncertainties in a complex problem, there is no agreed-upon, conventional, or normatively correct method for combining them into a single expression. This paves the way for still more misunderstanding and error.

Using probabilities and related numerical expressions to talk about uncertainty solves both problems: first, numbers are more precise than words and are therefore less likely to be misunderstood. Second, there are well-defined rules for combining probabilities mathematically. There are no rules for how verbal expressions should be combined, so there will be great variability in the conclusions drawn from a chain of verbal expressions.

We have identified three major types of uncertainties in health care:

- Diagnostic uncertainty is about the true underlying causes of illness. What is wrong with this patient?
- Prognostic uncertainty is about the future course of events. What may happen?
- Treatment uncertainty arises because for many diseases the effects of treatment are imperfect or incomplete. Many treatments offer some probability of both benefits and harms. These are best compared when the uncertainties are expressed numerically.

All of these uncertainties can be expressed as chance events in a balance sheet or chance nodes in a decision tree.

The probability of a sequence of events is calculated by multiplying the probability of each event, conditioned on the previous events in the sequence. A decision tree or probability tree is a convenient way of displaying the probabilities to be multiplied. These tools help the decision maker keep track of the relevant uncertainties and calculate the probability of clinically relevant outcomes.

Checklist A. *Assessing studies of diagnostic probabilities*

The ideal study of diagnostic probabilities examines a consecutive series (or random sample) of persons with the clinical presentation of interest and applies a comprehensive diagnostic workup with adequate follow-up of those initially undiagnosed. The specific design features to check are:

1. Did the study population represent the full spectrum of those who present with this problem?
   The patients should represent the full spectrum of presentations for your setting, including commonly confused disorders. This should usually be a consecutive series of persons who fulfill the presentation criteria.
2. Were the criteria for each final diagnosis explicit and credible?
   The workup of study subjects should be comprehensive and applied consistently to all of them. A reference standard needs to be defined and should be determined independently of the test under evaluation. Ideally all subjects undergo the reference standard. If this is ethically impossible, adjustments are made to the diagnostic probabilities.
3. For initially undiagnosed patients, was the follow-up sufficiently long and complete?
   For some subjects, the diagnosis will not be ascertainable on initial assessment. It is important that these persons be followed until either a diagnosis is made or the illness has resolved.
4. Was the diagnostic workup evaluated and described in sufficient detail?
   Procedures should be described in detail. Uninterpretable test results must be accounted for. The test's reproducibility should be addressed.

Source: Jaeschke et al. (1994a, 1994b).

Checklist B. *Assessing studies of prognosis*

In the ideal study of prognosis, a large representative sample of patients with the condition is followed to the end stage of the condition. The specific design features to check are:

1. Was an inception cohort of persons, all initially free of the outcome of interest, followed?
   Representative patients should be followed from a uniform point in the course of the disease. Inclusion criteria should be clearly stated.
2. Were at least 80% of patients followed until either a major study end point or completion of the study?
   To maintain the representativeness of the patients requires adequate follow-up of the initial inception cohort. This follow-up should continue for sufficient time to elucidate the major clinical changes in the illness. This may vary from days to weeks in acute illness, to years or decades for chronic illnesses.
3. Were all relevant outcomes reported and done so accurately?
   Objective criteria should be used to assess the outcome. The criteria should be reproducible and accurate. The analysis should be performed with adjustment for extraneous factors.

Source: Laupacis et al. (1994).

Checklist C: *Assessing studies of treatment or prevention*
In the ideal study of an intervention, the only difference between two groups of patients would be the use or nonuse of the intervention. All patient characteristics, co-interventions, follow-up, and outcome measurement methods should be similar in the groups. The specific design features to check are:

1. Was allocation of participants to the different interventions random and concealed?
   Check that comparable groups of patients have been created by random allocation. This random allocation should be concealed from the consenting patients and clinicians until registration and randomization are complete. This is known as allocation concealment or blinded randomization, and is best achieved by central telephone randomization; suspect methods include alternate days, alternate patients, open randomization lists, and envelopes (unless adequately policed).
2. Were outcomes measured for at least 80% of participants?
   Adequate follow-up is important to maintain the comparability created by the randomization process. Primary analysis should be by the treatment allocated to the patient (an intention-to-treat analysis), not by the treatment received.
3. Were all relevant outcomes reported and done so accurately?
   The outcomes measured should be those relevant to the patient rather than those relevant to the physician. Were objective criteria used to assess the outcome? Are the criteria reproducible and accurate?
4. Were outcomes measured blinded or were they objective, when feasible?
   The person assessing clinical outcome should be blinded to the treatment allocation of the patient. For outcomes where the patient provides the assessment, it is particularly desirable that the patient be blinded. When neither patient nor clinician can be blinded, then it is useful to substantiate the subjective outcomes with objective measures.

Source: Guyatt et al. (1993, 1994).

Exercises

Exercise 2.1

In a study by Kong et al., respondents (all in the medical profession) were asked to assist with research on probability expressions. The question was: 'One of the senior physicians in your hospital told you that a particular symptom was _____ in the disease you were discussing. What would be your estimate of the frequency of this symptom in this disease?'

The following probability expressions were used for the blank: 'certain,' 'unlikely,' 'frequent,' 'probable,' 'never,' and 'possible.'

(a) Ask yourself the above question for the six probability expressions and write down the probabilities (a number) that you associate with these expressions.

(b) Order the probability expressions from high to low.

(c) Compare you answers with other students.

(d) Compare your estimates and the order of the probability expressions with the table in the paper by Kong et al.

(e) Why do these figures differ from those presented in the chapter?

Reference: Kong, A., Barnett, G.O., Mosteller, F. & Youthz, C. (1986). How medical professionals evaluate expressions of probability. *N. Engl. J. Med.*, 315, 740–4.

Exercise 2.2

Pick a recent paper in your field of interest on diagnosis, one on prognosis, and one on therapy. For each paper do a critical appraisal using the checklists from this chapter.

Exercise 2.3

For the following exercise use Table 2.3.

(a) What is the probability that a patient with HIV has HBV infection?

(b) What is the probability that a patient without HIV has HBV infection?

(c) What is the probability that a patient has both HIV and HBV? Show that you can calculate this in two ways.

(d) Are HIV and HBV independent?

Exercise 2.4

In a hypothetical community, 50% of all people smoke and 40% are overweight. The percentage of people who are both overweight and smoke is 30%.

(a) What percentage of people smoke, are overweight or have both conditions? (Hint: construct a 2×2 table.)

(b) Use your calculation for the first question and verify the addition rule of probabilities: $P(A \text{ or } B) = P(A) + P(B) - P(A \text{ and } B)$

(c) You sample at random a person from this community and find that he or she smokes. What is the probability that he or she is overweight?

(d) Are smoking and overweight statistically independent?

Exercise 2.5

A 53-year-old man comes in for an influenza vaccine but during the consultation he asks about his risk of a heart attack because of the recent death of a friend. You note from his chart that his blood pressure is 160/95 mmHg; he has no diabetes; he smokes 20 cigarettes per day, and his total cholesterol is 5.2 mmol/l and his HDL is 0.9 mmol/l.

(a) Use the guideline for managing cardiovascular risk given in this chapter to calculate his 5-year risk of a cardiovascular event.

(b) What would his risk be if he were a nonsmoker?

REFERENCES

Armitage, P. & Berry, G. (1994). *Statistical Methods in Medical Research*, 3rd edn. Oxford: Blackwell.

Baker, S., Priest, P. & Jackson, R. (2000). Using thresholds based on risk of cardiovascular disease to target treatment for hypertension: modelling events averted and number treated. *B.M.J.*, **320**, 680–5.

Collette, D. (1994). *Modeling Survival Data in Medical Research*. London: Chapman & Hall.

Espehaug, B., Havelin, L.I. & Engesaeter, L.B. (1999). The effect of hospital-type and operating volume on the survival of hip replacements. A review of 39 505 primary total hip replacements reported to the Norwegian Arthroplasty Register, 1988–1996. *Acta Orthop. Scand.*, **70**, 12–18.

Fleming, K.A. (1997). Evidence-based pathology. *Evidence-Based Med.*, **2**, 132.

Guyatt, G.H., Sackett, D.L. & Cook, D.J. (1993). Users' guides to the medical literature II. How to use an article about therapy or prevention. A. Are the results of the study valid? *J.A.M.A.*, **270**, 2598–601.

Guyatt, G.H., Sackett, D.L. & Cook, D.J. (1994). Users' guides to the medical literature II. How to use an article about therapy or prevention. B. What were the results and will they help me in caring for my patients? *J.A.M.A.*, **271**, 59–63.

Jackson, R. (2000). Updated New Zealand cardiovascular disease risk–benefit prediction guide. *B.M.J.*, **320**, 709–10.

Jaeschke, R., Gordon, H., Guyatt, G. & Sackett, D.L. (1994a). Users' guides to the medical literature III. How to use an article about a diagnostic test. B. What are the results and will they help me in caring for my patients? *J.A.M.A.*, **271**, 703–7.

Jaeschke, R., Guyatt, G. & Sackett, D.L. (1994b). Users' guides to the medical literature. III. How to use an article about a diagnostic test. A. Are the results of the study valid? *J.A.M.A.*, **271**, 389–91.

Kannel, W.B. (2000). The Framingham Study: its 50-year legacy and future promise. *J. Atheroscler. Thromb.*, **6**, 60–6.

Laupacis, A., Wells, G., Richardson, S. & Tugwell, P. (1994). Users' guides to the medical literature. V. How to use an article about prognosis. *J.A.M.A.*, **272**, 234–7.

Levine, O.S., Viahov, D., Koehler, J. et al. (1995). Seroepidemiology of hepatitis B virus in a population of injecting drug users. *Am. J. Epidemiol.*, **142**, 331–41.

Shaw, N.J. & Dear, P.R. (1990). How do parents of babies interpret qualitative expressions of probability? *Arch. Dis. Child.*, **65**, 520–3.

Timmermans, D. (1994). The roles of experience and domain of expertise in using numerical and verbal probability terms in medical decisions. *Med. Decis. Making*, **14**, 146–56.

United States Preventive Services Task Force (USPSTF) (1996). *Guide to Clinical Preventive Services*, 2nd edn. Baltimore, MD: Williams & Wilkins.

Woloshin, K.K., Ruffin, M.T.Th. & Gorenflo, D.W. (1994). Patients' interpretation of qualitative probability statements. *Arch. Fam. Med.*, **3**, 961–6.

3

Choosing the best treatment

Firstly, do no (net) harm

(adapted from) Hippocrates

3.1 Introduction

Some treatment decisions are straightforward. For example, what should be done for an elderly patient with a fractured hip? Inserting a metal pin has dramatically altered the management: instead of lying in bed for weeks or months waiting for the fracture to heal while blood clots and pneumonia threatened, the patient is now ambulatory within days. The risks of morbidity and mortality are both greatly reduced. However, many treatment decisions are complex. They involve uncertainties and trade-offs that need to be carefully weighed before choosing. Tragic outcomes may occur no matter which choice is made, and the best that can be done is to minimize the overall risks. Such decisions can be difficult and uncomfortable to make. For example, consider the following historical dilemma.

3.1.1 Benjamin Franklin and smallpox

Benjamin Franklin argued implicitly in favor of the application to individual patients of probabilities based on previous experience with similar groups of patients. Before Edward Jenner's discovery in 1796 of cowpox vaccination for smallpox, it was known that immunity from smallpox could be achieved by a live smallpox inoculation, but the procedure entailed a risk of death. When a smallpox epidemic broke out in Boston in 1721, the physician Zabdiel Boylston consented, at the urging of the clergyman Cotton Mather, to inoculate several hundred citizens. Mather and Boylston reported their results (Schmidt, 1976):

Out of about ten thousand Bostonians, five thousand seven hundred fifty-nine took smallpox the natural way. Of these, eight hundred eighty-five died, or one in seven. Two hundred eighty-six took smallpox by inoculation. Of these, six died, or one in forty-seven.

Though at first skeptical, Franklin eventually saw the advantages of

61

inoculation and advocated the practice. After presenting statistics such as those just given, Franklin said (Schmidt, 1976):

> In 1736, I lost one of my sons, a fine boy of 4 years old, by the smallpox taken in the common way. I bitterly regretted that I had not given it to him by inoculation. This I mention for the sake of parents who omit that operation, on the supposition that they should never forgive themselves if a child died under it. My example shows that the regret may be the same either way, and that therefore the safer should be chosen.

Whichever strategy is chosen, there is a risk of dying from smallpox. That is unavoidable. So Franklin here urges the strategy with the low probability of death, having derived the probability for an individual patient from observed frequencies in other patients.

Clearly these probabilities depend on several factors, including risk of dying from smallpox inoculation and that from natural smallpox, as well as the risk of catching smallpox during an epidemic. If the risk of catching smallpox is sufficiently low, as during nonepidemic periods, then the inoculation would clearly not be worthwhile. At some critical level of risk, the inoculation becomes the better strategy. This risk is known as an *action threshold*. This chapter will focus on treatment decisions with trade-offs, and by explicitly describing and analyzing the complex risks and benefits, will provide insight into the central dilemmas of the problem. In particular we will look at the treatment threshold. This threshold provides a simple summary of a decision analysis which saves us from repeating the analysis for every new case. The treatment threshold can assist in providing rational guidelines for individual clinical decision making and for health policy.

3.2 Choosing the better risky option

Let us examine more closely the probabilities in Mather and Boylston's description. Of the 10 000 Bostonians, 286 chose inoculation; the remaining 9714 chose no inoculation. What were the consequences of these choices? Figure 3.1 shows the path probabilities emanating from each of the two choices. These paths contain two stages: first, the risk of smallpox, which in the case of inoculation is certain. Second, there is the risk of death given smallpox, with the risk being lower for smallpox from inoculation.

To calculate the expected rates of survival, we have given 'survive' a value of 1 and 'die' a value of 0 in the tree (Figure 3.1). The tree in Figure 3.2 shows the calculated overall chances of survival based on the path probabilities following each of the two options. For inoculation the survival is 0.979 and for no inoculation it is 0.909. The absolute risk difference is thus 0.07

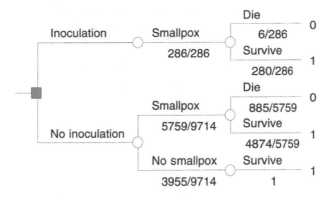

Figure 3.1   Decision tree for smallpox inoculation.

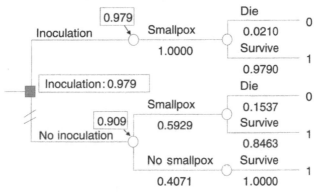

Figure 3.2   Calculating the expected rates of survival for the smallpox inoculation problem. Note that the probabilities for chance arms have been converted from fractions to proportions.

or 7%. We could also express this as the 'number-needed-to-inoculate,' which would be $1/0.07 = 14$, that is, for every 14 people inoculated, one smallpox death would be averted.

The proportions cited by Mather and Boylston overstate the advantage of inoculation, as they compared the risk of death from smallpox caused by inoculation with the risk of death from smallpox caught naturally. As drawing the tree makes clear, the correct comparison requires the additional consideration of the risk of catching smallpox during the epidemic. There are two further caveats on their analysis. First, the advantage of inoculation is not based on a randomized trial, so we cannot exclude another reason for the apparent difference, such as the relative ages or nutritional state of the groups, as an explanation for the apparent better survival of the inoculated group. Second, the risk of developing smallpox is based on the rates known *after* the epidemic was over, but you would have needed to make the decision about inoculation at the beginning of the epidemic. The appropriate choice of data might have been frequencies seen in previous epidemics. For example, figures from James Jurin indicated that over a period of 42 years before 1723, about one in 14 of London's population had died from smallpox, whereas from our decision tree we see that in the 1736 Boston epidemic the death rate was $1 - 0.909 = 0.091$ or about one in 11.

This decision problem is a variant of one that we will encounter frequently, a decision between treating now versus expectant management ('watchful waiting'). The recurring trade-off problem is this: if we treat now (in this case, give smallpox by inoculation), there is a small but measurable risk of harm that might be avoided by expectant management. If expectant management is selected (in this case, no inoculation), there is a chance (40%) that the patient will not become infected and will survive. Under these circumstances, the patient will be better off with watchful waiting. But watchful waiting has its own risks: if the patient contracts smallpox 'in the common way,' the mortality rate is much higher than with smallpox by inoculation. If that outcome occurs, we will wish that we had inoculated earlier, as Franklin expresses. The best action is determined by three factors: the chances of getting community-acquired smallpox, the associated death rate, and the death rate from smallpox after inoculation. Even in as simple a problem as this, it may not be immediately apparent whether a risky preventive measure is preferable to watchful waiting; a decision analysis clarifies the trade-offs. A moment's reflection will show that an increase in the mortality due to inoculation or a lower rate of community-acquired smallpox or a lower mortality from community-acquired smallpox would make the preventive strategy less attractive.

3.3 The best treatment option under diagnostic uncertainty

Sometimes treatment must be initiated before a clear diagnosis is reached. Of course, the usual order of medical management is to make a diagnosis, then select treatment based on this diagnosis. However, as we will discuss in detail later (Chapters 5–7), you will usually need to manage trade-offs in treatment options together with trade-offs due to the inaccuracy inherent in most diagnostic tests. In other words, despite our diagnostic efforts, a residual diagnostic uncertainty will often remain and we need to choose the best treatment option conditional on this uncertainty. There are some specific circumstances where this is a major problem.

1 Emergency conditions. In some urgent problems there may not be adequate time to obtain a firm diagnosis before starting treatment. For example, meningococcal meningitis (bacterial infection of the membranes that envelop the brain) can kill within hours, and hence we often need to treat, e.g., with intravenous penicillin, before the diagnosis can be confirmed. In acute abdominal pain, such as suspected acute appendicitis, operation will sometimes be needed without a clear diagnosis; this may mean removing a 'normal' appendix rather than delaying and risking perforation of the appendix. In these and other examples, the expected benefit to those with the disease needs to be weighed against the expected harm of 'unnecessary' procedures in those without the disease.

2 Invasive diagnostic procedures. Even if there is sufficient time, the toll of some diagnostic procedures may outweigh the potential benefit. For example, in a suspected blood clot of the lung (pulmonary embolism) confirming the diagnosis with pulmonary angiography (catheterization with X-ray imaging of the blood vessels of the lung) has a considerable risk of complications, including a fatality rate perhaps as high as one in 200 patients.

3 Residual uncertainty. Sometimes no cause of an illness will be found, even after thorough investigation. For example, no cause will be found for most cases of microscopic hematuria (blood in the urine); similarly, it is often difficult to find the cause of a chronic cough without use of empirical treatments for asthma or esophageal reflux (backflow of stomach contents into the esophagus).

The aim of diagnostic testing is to improve treatment decisions when the diagnosis is in doubt. Hence first understanding the treatment decision is important in devising a diagnostic strategy. This is the reverse order to practice: when seeing an individual patient, diagnosis precedes treatment; when analyzing diagnostic strategies, treatment precedes diagnosis. For example, when diagnosing a common cold, it does not help to identify the precise virus involved (there are over 200), because it does not affect the choice of treatment. An understanding of the treatment options thus guides the diagnostic process.

Let us begin by addressing the issue of when treatment is warranted despite an uncertain diagnosis. We then look at how and when the results of a diagnostic test should alter the treatment chosen and hence reduce the proportion of patients treated inappropriately.

Example	Suspected pulmonary embolism
	A 30-year-old, 7-month-pregnant woman presents at your clinic with right-sided chest pain that gradually increased overnight. She is breathing faster than usual (tachypneic) with 20 breaths/min and has a mildly increased pulse rate (88 beats/min). An electrocardiogram shows no signs of right heart strain (ventricular overload). She has no clinical signs of blood clot in the legs (deep venous thrombosis). You suspect that she has a blood clot in her lungs (pulmonary embolism (PE)). A special diagnostic test of her lungs – a ventilation–perfusion scan (V/Q scan) – has an indeterminate result, which implies that the V/Q scan gives no diagnostic information.

In discussing the problem we will use a proactive approach to decision-making, as introduced in Chapter 1.

3.3.1 Step 1: PROactive

P   Define the *problem*

R   *Reframe* from multiple perspectives

O   Focus on the *objective*

Given the patient's history, signs, and symptoms you are concerned that she may have had PE. PE is a life-threatening event. Treatment with anticoagulation is effective in preventing further PE and hence in reducing the fatality rate. Anticoagulation, however, has a risk of major bleeding which can be fatal and therefore one would like to avoid anticoagulation if it is unnecessary. A pulmonary angiogram (a catheterization and X-ray examination in which the vessels of the lungs are opacified) would provide accurate diagnostic information about whether she has had a PE, but because the patient is pregnant you would like to avoid any examination associated with X-rays.

Thus, you need to make a decision whether or not to treat the patient with anticoagulation. Anticoagulation for her would mean subcutaneous injections of heparin, temporarily stopping anticoagulation during delivery and postpartum, and oral anticoagulation thereafter.

The main objective of management is to avoid a recurrent PE which may be fatal. From the perspective of the physician, he or she should try to maximize the survival chances for both the patient and her unborn child. Clearly the fetus's chances of survival are directly related to the woman's chances of survival. By optimizing the patient's survival chances we will concurrently be optimizing the chances of survival of the unborn child and both their chances of living without morbidity. In this example we will

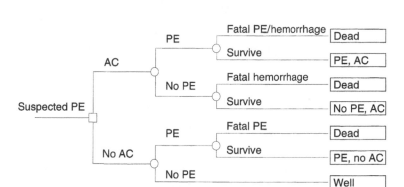

Figure 3.3 Decision tree comparing two strategies for suspected pulmonary embolism (PE). AC, anticoagulate.

therefore focus on survival of the pregnant woman.

The problem then is whether or not to anticoagulate this pregnant woman in order to avoid the possible mortality of recurrent PE. In deciding, we need to take into account that we are uncertain whether PE is present and that anticoagulation has a small risk of fatal hemorrhage.

3.3.2 Step 2: ProACTive

A Consider all relevant *alternatives*
C Model the *consequences* and estimate the *chances*
T Identify and estimate the value *trade-offs*

As we indicated in Chapter 1, the management alternatives are intervention (treatment with anticoagulation), wait-and-see (withholding anticoagulation), or getting more diagnostic information. At this point we have decided that obtaining more information is too risky because it would entail performing angiography, which is considered contraindicated because of the pregnancy. Although this contraindication may be debatable, for this example we would like to focus solely on the choice between anticoagulation and no anticoagulation.

In considering the consequences it is convenient to structure the problem in the form of a decision tree (Figure 3.3). The decision tree starts on the left with the decision node and decision options. For our example these are 'anticoagulate' (AC) or 'do not anticoagulate' (no AC). Following each

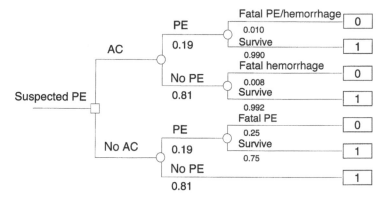

Figure 3.4   Decision tree comparing two strategies for suspected pulmonary embolism (PE) with the event probabilities and outcome values filled in. AC, anticoagulate.

option the consequences are modeled to represent all the possible states (e.g., diagnoses) that may exist and events that may occur. Under both treatment options PE may or may not be present. The chance node is used to represent the uncertainty of the underlying true disease status and this probability reflects one of the unknowns for this particular decision problem. If PE is present, it may be fatal. The probability of death is conditional on whether PE is present and on whether anticoagulation is given. With anticoagulation the risk of death from PE is reduced. Anticoagulation, however, has a risk of fatal hemorrhage which may occur whether PE is present or not.

The decision tree represents the chronological order of events from left to right: first the management options leading from the decision node (the square) and subsequently the chance events leading from the chance nodes (the circles). At the end of each path of events in the tree we visualize the outcome of that path. For example, at the end of the path 'AC → PE → fatal PE/hemorrhage,' the outcome is 'dead.' In this tree we combined the events fatal PE conditional on PE and fatal hemorrhage conditional on AC because both would result in death and because we do not have estimates of the probabilities of these events separately.

After formulating the problem, considering all the possible alternatives, and structuring the consequences in the form of a decision tree, we need to assign probabilities to the events and values to the outcomes (Figure 3.4). The probabilities related to this problem are tabulated in Table 3.1. An important point to keep in mind when filling in the event probabilities is that each probability should be determined conditional on all the events that preceded it, i.e., on the events to the left of the index event in the

Table 3.1. Balance sheet for treatment options for a patient with suspected pulmonary embolism (PE)

	Anticoagulate (AC)	Do not anticoagulate (no AC)
Risk of death from PE or hemorrhage	1% if PE 0.8% if no PE	25% if PE 0% if no PE
Other benefits/downsides	Medication for 6 months: subcutaneous heparin injections followed by oral AC	No medication
Costs	Costs of AC	Avoid cost of AC

Data from van Erkel and Pattynama (1998).

decision tree. For example, the probability of a fatal PE or fatal hemorrhage in our decision tree is conditional on whether PE is present and whether anticoagulation is given or not.

From the balance sheet in Table 3.1 we see that there are risks and benefits to both options. The main trade-off is between the risk of death due to untreated PE and the risk of death due to hemorrhage caused by anticoagulation. The risk of a fatal bleed with anticoagulation is 0.008. Withholding anticoagulation, we assume that the risk of a fatal bleed is practically zero. The mortality risk (combined fatal PE or fatal hemorrhage) if PE is present is 0.25 if anticoagulation is withheld and is reduced to 0.01 if anticoagulation is given.

In this example the value trade-offs in the outcomes are fairly straightforward because we have chosen to optimize survival and not to include morbidity or costs explicitly in our decision model, even though we did consider them in our balance sheet. Therefore we use a very straightforward outcome value, namely alive or dead, alive being assigned a value of 1.0 and dead a value of 0.0. Alternatively we could value the outcomes with life expectancy, quality-adjusted life years, costs, or some other values that reflect our preferences. Whatever we use, the unit of outcome should represent the outcome we wish to optimize and should include any trade-offs we wish to capture in the outcomes. This will in turn be determined by the perspective we are taking in analyzing the decision problem and our objective. We will return to the subject of valuing outcomes in Chapter 4.

3.3.3 Step 3: ProactIVE

I *Integrate* the evidence and values

V Optimize expected *value*

E *Explore* the assumptions and *evaluate* uncertainty

The next step in the decision-making process is to integrate the evidence and the values. Based on the decision tree we calculate the average outcome value that we can expect (the expected value) for each option by integrating the evidence of the event probabilities and the value of the outcomes. As we did in the previous chapter, to find the expected value we work backwards from the right-hand side of the tree successively averaging out at each chance node until we have folded back the entire tree to the decision node. *Averaging out* refers to this process of multiplying the probability by the outcome value for each of the events leading from a chance node and doing this successively from right to left. Averaging out in fact calculates the weighted average of the outcome values (the numbers at the tips of the branches) with each outcome value weighed for the probability that it will occur (the path probability of that branch). In this example the outcome values are simply 0 or 1, 0 being equivalent to dead and 1 being alive. Thus, multiplying the outcome values by probabilities will yield the probability of being alive.

After repeating the above procedure for all the possible options at the decision node, we need to decide which option is best. If we have used a positive (desirable) outcome value such as survival or life expectancy, we will want to maximize the expected value. If we have used a negative (undesirable) outcome value, such as mortality or costs, we will want to minimize the expected value. This process of removing less optimal alternatives from further consideration is called *folding back*. Averaging out and folding back are together referred to as *rolling back*.

In our example, the overall expected survival chances are 99% with anticoagulation and 95% without anticoagulation (Figure 3.5). Therefore, given the case as presented and given the problem as we have defined it, and given all the assumptions we have made, and given the simplifications we have used, and assuming we want to optimize survival, we would, on average, choose to anticoagulate. But notice all the caveats we made: to be really confident about our decision we need first to explore how our assumptions will affect the decision in a 'what-if' analysis – a *sensitivity analysis*.

We may justifiably doubt the validity and generalizability of our analysis for several reasons. We may, for example, be unsure of the accuracy of the

DEFINITION

A *sensitivity analysis* is any test of the stability of the conclusions of an analysis over a range of structural assumptions, probability estimates, or outcome values.

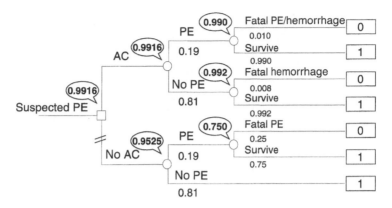

Figure 3.5   Rolled back decision tree comparing two strategies for suspected pulmonary embolism (PE). AC, anticoagulate.

probability estimates or the applicability of the outcome values. To evaluate whether our results apply under other assumptions, we can repeat the analysis substituting a range of estimates for the probabilities or outcome values in question to see whether this alters the conclusion of the analysis. This is called a 'what-if' or sensitivity analysis. If the conclusion does not change over a range of estimates around the initial estimate, this should reassure us. If, on the other hand, the conclusion is sensitive to small alterations in a key probability, this may lead us back to the literature or to experts in search of a more refined estimate.

For example, we might ask how the results of our analysis would change if the probability of PE were higher or lower than initially estimated. In Figure 3.6 we have plotted the survival probability for both the 'anticoagulate' and 'do not anticoagulate' options over the full range of probabilities of PE from 0 to 1. Both options demonstrate a decrease in expected value with an increasing probability of PE; however the 'do not anticoagulate' strategy is far more sensitive to this probability because the mortality risk given PE is far larger without anticoagulation. For extremely low probabilities of PE, withholding anticoagulation yields a higher expected value because the harm of anticoagulation outweighs the benefit. For high probabilities of PE anticoagulation yields a higher expected value because the benefit of anticoagulation outweighs the harm. Hence there must be a probability where we switch between the two options. This is the *treatment threshold (treat–do not treat threshold)*. Below this threshold, withholding treatment is better; above the threshold treatment is better, and at the threshold, treatment and no treatment are exactly equal (Pauker and Kassirer, 1975, 1980).

DEFINITION

The *treatment (treat–do not treat) threshold for diagnostic uncertainty* is the probability of disease at which the expected value of treatment and no treatment are exactly equal, and neither option is clearly preferable.

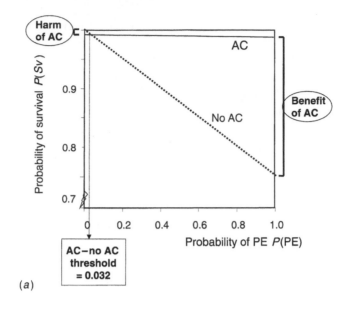

(a)

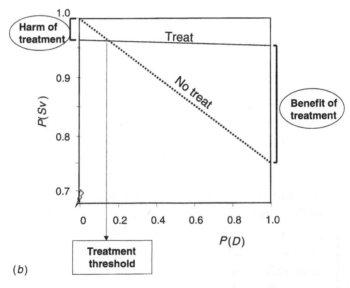

(b)

Figure 3.6   Graphical presentation of the ratio of harms to benefits of treatment and how this affects the associated treatment (treat–do not treat) threshold (*a*) for a young pregnant woman with suspected pulmonary embolism (PE: labeled specifically for this problem) and (*b*) for an elderly woman postsurgery with suspected PE (labeled generically for the treatment decision (*D*)). Notice how the treatment threshold increases as the ratio of harm to benefit increases. AC, anticoagulate; no AC, do not anticoagulate.

Table 3.2A. Sensitivity analysis on the probability of disease (PPE) for the range 0 to 0.10

PPE	AC	No AC	Optimal decision
0	0.9920	1.0000	No AC
0.01	0.9920	0.9975	No AC
0.02	0.9920	0.9950	No AC
0.03	0.9919	0.9925	No AC
0.04	0.9919	0.9900	AC
0.05	0.9919	0.9875	AC
0.06	0.9919	0.9850	AC
0.07	0.9919	0.9825	AC
0.08	0.9918	0.9800	AC
0.09	0.9918	0.9775	AC
0.10	0.9918	0.9750	AC

AC, anticoagulate; no AC, do not anticoagulate.

There are several different ways to perform sensitivity analysis and find the treatment threshold. We can use a numerical, algebraic, or graphical method. All these methods are useful to have in your decision analysis toolkit, as they will each be useful in different circumstances. We will look at each in turn.

3.3.3.1 Numerical sensitivity and threshold analysis

Sensitivity analysis can be performed numerically by constructing a decision tree and inserting the uncertain variable, in this case the disease probability, as a variable (e.g., call it PPE). We then either plot or tabulate the expected value for all values of this probability. For example, in Figure 3.4 we could replace the disease probability with a variable name PPE and subsequently we can calculate the expected value over a range of values of this probability (Table 3.2). For obvious reasons this is preferably done using computer programs.

From Table 3.2A we can conclude that for probabilities of PE of 0.03 or lower, withholding anticoagulation is best whereas for probabilities of PE of 0.04 or higher, anticoagulation is best. The treatment threshold is therefore somewhere between 0.03 and 0.04. Rerunning the analysis for the range of values between 0.03 and 0.04 (Table 3.2B) we find a more precise estimate of the threshold variable which is (rounded-off) 0.032. Clearly these repeated calculations are tedious (and best done by computer), but for many problems there are some simple formulas for finding thresholds, which we will now examine.

Table 3.2B. Sensitivity analysis on the probability of disease (PPE) for the range 0.03 to 0.04

PPE	AC	No AC	Optimal decision
0.030	0.9919	0.9925	No AC
0.031	0.9919	0.9923	No AC
0.032	0.9919	0.9920	No AC
0.033	0.9919	0.9918	AC
0.034	0.9919	0.9915	AC
0.035	0.9919	0.9913	AC
0.036	0.9919	0.9910	AC
0.037	0.9919	0.9908	AC
0.038	0.9919	0.9905	AC
0.039	0.9919	0.9903	AC
0.040	0.9919	0.9900	AC

AC, anticoagulate; no AC, do not anticoagulate.

3.3.3.2 Algebraic sensitivity and threshold analysis

To perform sensitivity analysis algebraically, we construct the decision tree and insert the disease probability as a variable (e.g., call it PPE). Subsequently we average out algebraically. For example, for the young pregnant woman the option 'anticoagulation' has an expected value of (Figure 3.5):

$$\text{Expected value (AC)} = 0.990 \times PPE + 0.992 \times (1 - PPE) \tag{3.1}$$

For the option withholding anticoagulation the expected value is:

$$\text{Expected value (no AC)} = 0.750 \times PPE + 1.0 \times (1 - PPE) \tag{3.2}$$

Setting the expected values of the options to be equal we can solve for the unknown threshold probability of PPE:

$$0.990 \times PPE + 0.992 \times (1 - PPE) = 0.750 \times PPE + 1.0 \times (1 - PPE)$$
$$0.240 \times PPE = 0.008 \times (1 - PPE)$$
$$PPE/(1 - PPE) = 0.008/0.240$$
$$PPE = 0.008/(0.240 + 0.008)$$
$$PPE = 0.0323$$

3.3.3.3 Graphical sensitivity and threshold analysis

A simple and helpful method for determining the treatment threshold is to compare the benefits and harms of treatment directly and visualize them graphically. The smaller the harm relative to the benefit, the lower the treatment threshold should be. Conversely, the larger the harm relative to the benefit, the higher the treatment threshold should be. To illustrate this, Figure 3.6*a* presents the results of our analysis for the presented example. In our example the harm of anticoagulation is relatively small compared with the benefit and the treatment threshold is therefore low.

Now consider another similar case of suspected PE. A 67-year-old woman who 2 days ago underwent hysterectomy and lymph node dissection for sarcoma presents with a similar picture of chest pain, faster breathing, increased pulse rate, no clinical signs of blood clot in the legs (deep venous thrombosis), and an indeterminate result on the V/Q scan. This lady has a different ratio of benefit to harm because her chances of a fatal bleed are much higher given that she has just undergone major abdominal surgery. In fact, we would expect her chances of a fatal bleed to be approximately 0.04. The combined mortality rate from a bleed or fatal PE if she has PE and receives anticoagulation will be approximately 0.05. If she has PE but anticoagulation is withheld, we would expect a similar mortality rate as before of 0.25. The net harm of treatment is thus larger and the net benefit of treatment with anticoagulation is less than for the young pregnant woman. The treatment threshold therefore shifts to higher values (Figure 3.6*b*).

Figure 3.6 can be seen as analogous to a scale where the harms and benefits are weighed. The harms are indicated on the left axis, the benefits on the right axis, and the treatment threshold is the pivot point. As the ratio of harms to benefits increases, the scale becomes heavier on the left in comparison to the right, and in so doing the pivot point representing the treatment threshold increases.

To quantify the harms, benefits, and treatment threshold precisely, we define both benefit and harm.

DEFINITION

The *benefit* of a treatment is the difference in outcome in patients with the disease who receive treatment and similar patients who do not receive treatment. That is,

Benefit = utility(treatment | disease) − utility (no treatment | disease) (3.3)

We shall formally define *utility* in the next chapter, but for now we just need to interpret it as the value of the outcomes to the patient. A utility with a positive sign implies the outcome is desirable and a utility with a negative sign implies it is an undesirable outcome. For example, in our patients with suspected PE the benefit of treatment is the difference in outcome between anticoagulation vs. withholding anticoagulation in those with PE. For the young pregnant woman this is $(1-0.01)-(1-0.25)=0.99-0.75=0.24$, that is, an increase in survival chances of 0.24. Alternatively, we may express the results in terms of a disutility (i.e., an outcome that is undesirable to the patient, in this case mortality) but to be consistent we would then need to calculate the harm also in terms of a disutility. In terms of disutility, the benefit is $0.01-0.25=-0.24$, that is a reduction (indicated by the negative sign) in mortality risk of 0.24. For the elderly woman the benefit is $(1-0.05)-(1-0.25)$ or a gain in survival of 0.20.

DEFINITION

The *harm* of a treatment is the difference in outcome between patients without a disease who do not receive treatment and similar patients who do receive that treatment. That is:

Harm = utility(no treatment | no disease) − utility(treatment | no disease)   (3.4)

For example, in our patients the harm of treatment is the difference in outcome between withholding anticoagulation vs. anticoagulation in those without PE. For the young woman this is $(1-0)-(1-0.008)=0.008$, i.e., no treatment increases survival by 0.008 compared to treatment. For the elderly woman the harm is $(1-0)-(1-0.04)=0.04$.

The benefit and harm can be marked on the vertical axes of the sensitivity analysis figure (Figure 3.6). Benefit is marked on the right-hand axis by indicating the expected outcomes with and without treatment in a group with the disease (that is, $PPE=1$). Similarly, harm is marked on the left-hand vertical axis by indicating the expected outcomes with and without the treatment in those without the disease (that is, $PPE=0$). The line joining the value of treating the nondiseased (at probability 0) and the value of treating the diseased (at probability 1) represents the expected value of treatment over the range of values from 0 to 1. Similarly, the expected value of no treatment is the line joining the value of withholding treatment from the nondiseased (at probability 0) and the value of withholding treatment from the diseased (at probability 1). These two lines cross at the treatment threshold where the expected value of the two options is equal. This threshold point may be found by direct comparison of the harm and benefit, that is:

Treatment threshold = harm/(harm + benefit)   (3.5)

Our intuition, the graphical presentation of Figure 3.6, and this formula all tell us that if the harm is much smaller than the benefit, the treatment threshold should be low. Conversely, if the harm is large compared with the benefit, then the treatment threshold should be high. And if benefits and harms are equal, the treatment threshold is 0.5.

3.3.3.4 Geometric proof of the threshold formula

A simple geometric proof of the threshold formula can be seen from Figures 3.6 and 3.7. Observe that the bases on the y-axes of the benefit and harm are the bases of similar triangles. Figure 3.7 illustrates that the ratio b/d equals the ratio $P/(1-P)$. Also, the ratio a/b equals the ratio c/d. Thus, $a/c = b/d$ and therefore $P/(1-P) = a/c$. Hence the harm and benefit are in the same ratio as the threshold probability P and its complement $(1-P)$, that is, $P/(1-P) = \text{harm/benefit}$. Adding the numerator to the denominator on both sides, which is equivalent to converting from odds to probabilities on both sides, gives $P = \text{harm}/(\text{harm} + \text{benefit})$. For our example cases, we can now calculate the treatment thresholds using the formula developed above. For the young pregnant woman the ratio of harm to benefit is 0.008:0.24, or 1:30, and the treatment threshold is therefore low:

$$\text{Treatment threshold} = \text{harm}/(\text{harm} + \text{benefit}) = 0.008/(0.240 + 0.008)$$
$$= 1/31 = 0.032 \tag{3.6}$$

Notice that this is exactly the same formula we derived algebraically. For the elderly woman the ratio of harm to benefit is 0.04:0.20, or 1:5, and the treatment threshold therefore shifts to higher values, as can be seen graphically in Figure 3.6:

$$\text{Treatment threshold} = \text{harm}/(\text{harm} + \text{benefit}) = 0.04/(0.04 + 0.20)$$
$$= 1/6 = 0.167 \tag{3.7}$$

Hence, we would prefer to anticoagulate the young pregnant woman if the probability of PE is higher than 0.032 and withhold anticoagulation if it is lower. If the probability is exactly 0.032 we are indifferent as to whether we anticoagulate or not. For the elderly woman the threshold probability is 0.167.

3.3.4 Subjective treatment threshold estimates

When there is insufficient time for the type of formal analysis described above, a quick approximate and subjective alternative would be to ask: 'How many times worse is not treating a case of true disease compared to unnecessarily treating a case without the disease?' If your answer is N times,

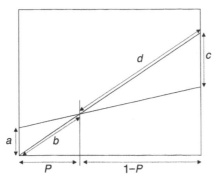

Figure 3.7   Geometric proof of the formula for the treatment threshold: the ratio of P to $1-P$ is the same as the ratio of a (harm) to c (benefit).

then the corresponding treatment threshold is $1/(N+1)$. For example, you might ask for treatment of suspected meningococcal meningitis (an infection that is often rapidly fatal if not treated): 'How many times worse is failing to treat a case of meningococcal meningitis compared to the harm of giving parenteral penicillin to a child who does not have meningococcal meningitis?' The treatment threshold here is clearly very low. You might consider it 100 times worse, in which case the treatment threshold is $1/(100+1) = 1\%$. This does not mean that only $1:100$ patients you might treat will turn out to have meningitis. The actual patients will have a range of presenting features and hence a range of chances of meningitis. Among these may be a few near the $100:1$ threshold while others may have much higher probabilities.

3.3.5 One-way, two-way, three-way, and n-way sensitivity analysis

Thus far we performed one-way sensitivity analysis: the value of one probability was varied while the other probability and outcome values remained constant. After exploring the effect of a change in the variable values one at a time, one may question the effect of simultaneous changes in the variables. In two-way sensitivity analysis the effect of simultaneous changes in two variable values is evaluated. For example, for our case example we could question what the threshold probability of PE would be if the risk of a fatal recurrent PE without anticoagulation were to be lower than the initially estimated value of 0.25. Varying the two variables simultaneously yields a graph that shows for which combinations of values of the two variables treatment with anticoagulation is preferred and for which values withholding anticoagulation is preferred (Figure 3.8). If we repeat

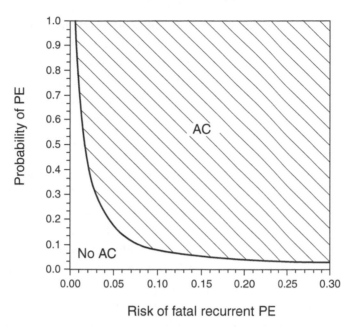

Risk of fatal recurrent PE

Figure 3.8 — Two-way sensitivity analysis determining the threshold probability of pulmonary embolism (PE) for different values of the risk of a fatal recurrent PE without anticoagulation (AC). AC indicates the combinations of the two variable values for which anticoagulation has the highest expected value and no AC indicates the combinations of the two variable values for which withholding anticoagulation has the highest expected value.

the two-way sensitivity analysis for various values of a third variable we get a three-way sensitivity analysis.

In n-way sensitivity analysis we vary multiple variable values at the same time. An n-way sensitivity analysis is useful to evaluate the results for a different setting, for different types of patients, and for best- and worst-case scenarios. In best- and worst-case scenarios we would pick extreme values for the variables, biasing towards and subsequently against the program under consideration. Evaluating variability and uncertainty is discussed in more detail in Chapter 11.

3.4 The decision to obtain diagnostic information and the do's and don'ts of tree building

Whereas we felt that a pulmonary angiogram was contraindicated in the case of the young pregnant woman, in the elderly woman we may want to consider obtaining more diagnostic information by performing an angiogram. The aim of obtaining more diagnostic information would be to shift our probability assessment across the treatment threshold. In other words, performing a diagnostic test to obtain additional information is worthwhile only if at least one decision would change by the test results and if the risk to the patient associated with the test is less than the expected benefit that would be gained from the subsequent change in the decision.

We can model the decision to obtain diagnostic information by adding this option in the decision tree (Figure 3.9). Strictly speaking, after performing the pulmonary angiogram we are again faced with the choice of whether or not to give anticoagulation (AC vs. no AC) and thus the decision tree contains embedded decision nodes. After performing a pulmonary angiogram, however, we will know whether or not the patient actually has a PE. If she has a PE, anticoagulation is clearly the better option. If she does not have a PE, withholding anticoagulation is clearly better. It would be perfectly permissible at this point to *prune* the tree by eliminating the branches that would never apply anyway. The branches that can be pruned even before calculating the expected value are withholding anticoagulation if PE is definitely present and giving anticoagulation if PE is definitely absent. In this simple case, pruning the tree has changed it from a decision tree in *extensive form* (Figure 3.9*a*) to one in *strategic form* (Figure 3.9*b*).

The options are expressed as strategies in terms of 'do *A*. If *X*, then do *B*. If *Y*, then do *C*.' In the strategic form of a decision tree that models diagnostic strategies, for example, the next management decision given the test result would be included in defining the overall diagnostic strategy. To illustrate the difference between the extensive and strategic form of a decision tree modeling diagnostic workup, consider the first case example (the young pregnant woman) but now prior to performing the *V/Q* scan. Figure 3.10*a* presents the decision tree in extensive form. It has been pruned to eliminate the branches that are clearly irrelevant but it still contains embedded decision nodes. We can redraw the tree in strategic form (Figure 3.10*b*) by bringing all the decision nodes up front and, instead of only letting the immediate decision lead from the initial decision node, we define the entire set of diagnostic strategies up front. This can be useful for several reasons. In particular, it is necessary for sensitivity analysis and for determining the thresholds between strategies.

In building decision trees one needs to be careful about sequencing decision nodes and chance nodes in the correct order. Going from left to right, a decision tree generally depicts the sequence of events as they may occur over time, i.e., in chronological order. For example, one would first

DEFINITION

A decision tree in *strategic form* contains no embedded decision nodes but instead all options are strategies.

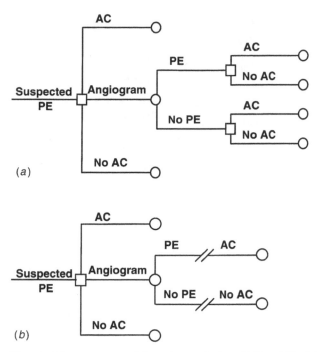

Figure 3.9   The decision to treat with anticoagulation (AC), withhold anticoagulation (no AC), or perform a pulmonary angiogram in suspected pulmonary embolism (PE). (*a*) Extensive form of the tree with embedded decision nodes and (*b*) strategic form of the decision tree.

do the noninvasive test (such as the V/Q scan for suspected PE) and only after doing the reference test (the pulmonary angiogram in this case) will we know whether the disease is present or not. To model this chronologically we would model the test result first and then the true disease status (Figure 3.10*a*).

Sometimes, however, it can be convenient to model it the other way around, that is, model disease status first followed by the test result. But watch out when you do this! Modeling disease status first and then the test result is only permissible if there are no intervening decisions or events that may influence the course of the disease or affect probabilities thereafter. Most important is that you need to remember to let the next management decision depend on the test result, which you observe, and not on the true disease status, which is the underlying truth but unknown to the decision maker as long as a reference test has not (yet) been performed. You can think of it as follows: there are two worlds. The one is the observable perceived reality, and the other is the underlying truth which you will never

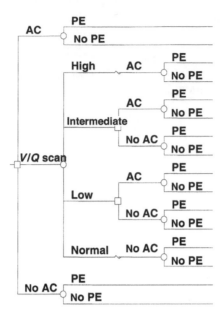

(a)

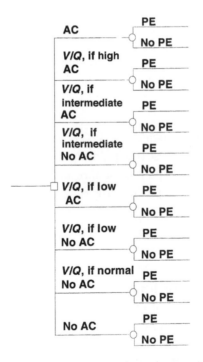

(b)

Figure 3.10   The decision to treat with anticoagulation (AC), withhold anticoagulation (no AC), or perform a ventilation–perfusion (V/Q) scan in the young pregnant woman with suspected pulmonary embolism (PE). (a) Extensive form of the tree with embedded decision nodes and (b) strategic form of the decision tree.

know with absolute certainty unless you have performed the reference test (if there is such a test for the disease). We model both the observable reality and the underlying truth but our decisions can only be based on the observable world. We will return to the sequencing of events in the decision tree in the context of interpreting diagnostic test information when we invert diagnostic decision trees in Chapter 5. In Chapter 6 we will discuss the threshold probabilities for the choice between no treatment and performing a test and between performing a test and treatment.

3.5 Summary

Every decision problem should first be defined from the relevant perspective and the objective should be formulated. A decision tree is useful to visualize and structure the alternatives, the consequences of each alternative and the associated chances, and the value trade-offs for a decision problem. The evidence and values are integrated by calculating the expected value of each option which equals the sum of the outcome values of that option, each outcome value weighed for the probability that it will occur. We choose the option that maximizes the expected value if value is expressed as a desirable outcome and minimizes expected value if it is expressed as an undesirable outcome. Finally, we explore our assumptions and evaluate the uncertainty of our probability and value estimates through sensitivity analysis.

In choosing whether or not to treat a patient in the face of diagnostic uncertainty, a threshold probability exists for the probability of disease below which withholding treatment is better and above which treatment is better. At the treatment threshold the expected value of treatment and withholding treatment are exactly equal. The treatment threshold is determined by the ratio of net harm incurred by treating patients without the disease and the net benefit incurred by treating patients with the disease. The smaller the harm relative to the benefit, the lower the treatment threshold should be. Conversely, the larger the harm relative to the benefit, the higher the treatment threshold should be.

Exercises

Exercise 3.1

Consider patients in the emergency room that are being observed for abdominal pain. The probability that a patient with abdominal pain has appendicitis (inflamed appendix) is 0.16. If the patient does have appendicitis, there is a 0.1875 chance that the appendix has already perforated; if you wait 6 h, this probability increases to 0.24.

If the appendix has perforated at the time the patient entered the hospital or by the end of 6 h, there is a 0.84 chance that the symptoms will have become worse and a 0.16 chance that they will have stayed the same. If the appendix is inflamed but has not perforated by the end of 6 h, there is a 0.8 chance that the symptoms will have become worse and a 0.2 chance that they will have stayed the same. If the appendix is not diseased, there is a 0.39 chance that the symptoms will remain the same for 6 h and a 0.61 chance that they will improve.

(a) Calculate the probability that a patient has a perforated appendix by the end of 6 h given that the appendix was inflamed but not perforated at the time the patient entered the hospital.

(b) Draw a chance tree to calculate the probabilities asked in question c–g.

(c) Calculate the probability that the patient has a perforated appendix at the beginning of the 6 h.

(d) Calculate the probability that the patient will have a perforated appendix if you wait 6 h.

(e) Calculate the probability that the patient's symptoms will (i) get worse; (ii) stay the same; (iii) improve.

(f) Calculate the conditional probability that the patient has a perforated appendix if the symptoms (i) get worse; (ii) stay the same; (iii) improve.

(g) Calculate the conditional probability that the patient has appendicitis if the symptoms (i) get worse; (ii) stay the same; (iii) improve.

Exercise 3.2

Consider the following clinical problem: a 45-year-old man presents to the Accident & Emergency department with 3 h of severe central chest pain. Patients presenting with central chest pain may have one of several conditions requiring different treatments, the most serious common condition being acute myocardial infarction (a 'heart attack'). Acute myocardial infarction is caused by a clot in one of the coronary arteries which supply the heart muscle with blood. Dissolving the clot with thrombolytic agents (such as streptokinase or recombinant tissue plasminogen activator) has been demonstrated to reduce mortality, provided that the thrombolytic therapy is given sufficiently early. If the patient has another cause of chest pain, which may be clinically indistinguishable from acute myocardial infarction, thrombolytic therapy will do no good at all and may even occasionally induce major bleeding. If we are uncertain about whether a patient has a myocardial infarction, should we treat early (and risk bleeding), or wait for several hours until serial electrocardiograms (EKGs) and blood tests will give a definite diagnosis but thrombolytic therapy will be less effective?

There are two possible management strategies: first, wait-and-see, and give delayed treatment with thrombolytic agents if the diagnosis of acute myocardial infarction is definite; second, immediate thrombolytic treatment, irrespective of knowing if the patient suffered from an acute myocardial infarction.

The probability that this patient has an acute myocardial infarction equals 0.20. A 45-year-old man with a myocardial infarction who is not treated with thrombolytic agents has an estimated short-term mortality risk of 11%. A combined analysis of the major randomized trials (Fibrinolytic Therapy Trialists' Collaborative Group, 1994) showed that giving thrombolytics between 0 and 6 h after the start of chest pain prevents 30 deaths per 1000 patients; between 7 and 12 h it prevents only 20 deaths per 1000 patients treated. Thus, with delayed thrombolysis the mortality risk is reduced to 9%, and with immediate thrombolysis it is reduced to 8%. These estimated risks include the risk of complications due to thrombolytic therapy, which may be gastrointestinal bleeding but, more importantly, include four intracerebral bleedings per 1000 patients treated. Assume that these intracerebral bleedings are fatal.

(a) Make a decision tree for this scenario.
(b) What is the probability that a patient will die if you start thrombolytic treatment immediately?
(c) What is the probability that a patient will die if you follow the wait-and-see strategy?
(d) Which strategy would you prefer?

Now assume that the life expectancy of this patient after having a myocardial infarction would be 10 years. If he did not suffer from a myocardial infarction his life expectancy would be 25 years.

(e) Which strategy would be the preferred one if you consider life expectancy?

Reference: Fibrinolytic Therapy Trialists' (FTT) Collaborative Group (1994). Indications for fibrinolytic therapy in suspected acute myocardial infarction: collaborative overview of early mortality and major morbidity results from all randomised trials of more than 1000 patients. *Lancet*, **343**, 311–22.

Exercise 3.3

An elderly patient is found to have an abdominal aortic aneurysm 5 cm in size. If you operate and he survives the elective operation, he will have a life expectancy of 10 years. In a series of 100 similar patients from your hospital, five died perioperatively. If you choose not to operate electively, 30% of such patients will rupture their aneurysm (assume this happens on average after 5 years), only 50% of whom will survive the emergency operation. If the patient survives the emergency operation, he will have on average another 5 years to live.

(a) Draw a decision tree for the problem of choosing whether or not to operate electively. Calculate the life expectancies for each choice. Which choice do you prefer?

(b) A 95% confidence interval for the mortality rate from the elective operation based on your hospital's data ranges from 1.6% to 11.3%. Do you think gathering more data on the mortality rate would be helpful? Explain.

Exercise 3.4

Consider the second patient with suspected PE (the 67-year old woman who underwent hysterectomy and lymph node dissection for sarcoma) discussed in this chapter.

(a) Reconstruct the decision tree that was presented, preferably using decision analytical software and check that the treatment threshold presented is correct.

(b) Redo the analysis using life expectancy as outcome value. Assume the patient has a life expectancy of 5 years if she truly has a PE and survives without recurrence and without a bleed and that she has a life expectancy of 7 years if she has no PE.

(c) Now add the option of performing an angiogram which will give you perfect diagnostic information but has a mortality risk of 1%. Calculate the threshold probability of PE for the choice between no anticoagulation and performing an angiogram and the threshold for the choice between performing an angiogram and anticoagulation.

REFERENCES

Pauker, S.G. & Kassirer, J.P. (1975). Therapeutic decision making: a cost–benefit analysis. *N. Engl. J. Med.*, **293**, 229–34.

Pauker, S.G. & Kassirer, J.P. (1980). The threshold approach to clinical decision making. *N. Engl. J. Med.*, **302**, 1109–17.

Schmidt, W.M. (1976). Health and welfare of colonial American children. *Am. J. Dis. Child.*, **130**, 694–701.

van Erkel, A.R. & Pattynama, P.M. (1998). Cost-effective diagnostic algorithms in pulmonary embolism: an updated analysis. *Acad. Radiol.*, **5**, S321–7.

4

Valuing outcomes

Values are what we care about. As such, values should be the driving force for our decision making. They should be the basis for the time and effort we spend thinking about decisions. But this is not the way it is. It is not even close to the way it is.

Ralph Keeney

4.1 Introduction

Value judgments underlie virtually all clinical decisions. Sometimes the decision rests on a comparison of probability alone, such as the probability of surviving an acute episode of illness. In such cases, there is a single outcome measure – the probability of immediate survival – that can be averaged out to arrive at an optimal decision. In most cases, however, decisions between alternative strategies require not only estimates of the probabilities of the associated outcomes, but also value judgments about how to weigh the benefits versus the harms. Consider the following examples.

Example 1 | Genetic susceptibility for breast cancer
A 28-year-old woman has a strong family history of breast cancer, including a sister who developed the disease at age 35. Her sister has undergone genetic testing for cancer predisposition and has been found to carry a mutation in the BRCA1 breast cancer gene. The woman is concerned about her own risk of breast cancer and chooses to be tested. She is found to have the same mutation, and is told that her lifetime risk of developing breast cancer is approximately 50%. With careful surveillance, including mammography, it is likely that if she develops breast cancer, it will be detected early (80% probability of Stage 1 disease). With treatment, including surgery, radiation therapy, and chemotherapy, the probability that a woman with Stage 1 breast cancer will develop a subsequent recurrence is 30% over 10 years, and 1% per year thereafter. Three-fourths of women with recurrence will have metastatic disease, with an annual mortality of 40%. Alternatively, she might choose prophylactic mastectomy – surgical removal of both breasts – which has been shown to reduce the risk of breast cancer in women at elevated risk by approximately 90%.

Does the benefit of risk reduction associated with prophylactic mastectomy outweigh the impact of prophylactic mastectomy on sexual function, body image, and the ability to nurse one's children?

Example 2	Atrial fibrillation
	A 58-year-old man with stable angina is noted on a routine physical examination to have atrial fibrillation – an irregular heart rhythm. Patients with atrial fibrillation have an increased risk of stroke due to emboli. Anticoagulation with warfarin can reduce that risk by about 70%, while aspirin reduces the risk by about 20%. However, warfarin is associated with an increased risk of major bleeding, including hemorrhagic stroke. Furthermore, patients taking warfarin require regular blood testing, must avoid activities that increase the chance of head injury, and are advised to restrict their intake of alcohol.
	Is a reduction in the risk of stroke enough of a benefit to outweigh an increased risk of major bleeding and the need to restrict one's activities?

In both these examples, choosing a treatment strategy requires value judgments. In both cases, we are concerned not only with the probabilities of surviving or dying from either the treatment or the disease. We are concerned too with the impact of treatment on the life of the patient. All of the treatments under consideration carry a chance of nonfatal harms that may reduce the quality of the patient's life. Clearly the choice of treatment will vary depending on one's values. Value judgments about the quality of life are especially important when a disease cannot be definitively cured and a patient may live many years in a state of considerably less than perfect health, or when a treatment, even if ordinarily quite effective, carries some risk of severe side-effects. In such cases, are explicit, quantitative valuations of each of the possible outcomes required for optimal decision making? The answer depends on how the benefits and harms are valued, and by whom (Tsevat et al., 1994).

In this chapter we will first describe two decision-making perspectives, the individual and the societal, then discuss how these require different styles of valuation. We will then look at the methods and validity of several ways of measuring patient values, and how and when they may be used in different decision-making settings.

4.2 Decision-making paradigms

In considering each of the following decision-making paradigms, it may be helpful to ask yourself the following questions. First, who is the decision maker? Is it the doctor, the patient, the insurer, the policy maker? Second, what information does the decision maker need? And third, how can the decision maker be helped to clarify his or her values? The answers to these questions provide a qualitative framework for value clarification in each setting.

4.2.1 The clinical encounter

In this decision-making setting, a doctor and patient face choices among alternative treatment strategies. Their goal is to choose the best treatment for that particular patient. It has been well documented that most patients in this situation want to be provided with information about their medical condition and options for managing it. However, they vary widely in the degree of decision-making autonomy they wish to exercise (Degner and Sloan, 1992). Some patients, especially those who are young and healthy, prefer to assume the primary responsibility for making decisions about their own care. Others, especially those who are older or more seriously ill, would rather cede some or all of the decision-making responsibility. They prefer that the physician make a recommendation to them, which they can choose to accept or reject (Degner and Sloan, 1992).

What are the information and decision support needs of patients who choose to be 'active decision makers'? In other words, what are patients' needs when they assume decision-making autonomy? Like all decision makers, they need to know the list of the possible outcomes associated with each strategy under consideration, the probability that each outcome will occur, and the likely impact of those outcomes on their lives. They can then apply their own values in weighing the benefits and harms of each strategy, and choose the option that maximizes the outcomes that matter most to them.

Let's return to the example of the woman considering alternative strategies for managing her elevated breast cancer risk. One option, careful surveillance, is associated with a 50% risk of breast cancer. The other option, prophylactic mastectomy, would reduce her risk of breast cancer by 90%, but would require that she undergo the drastic and irrevocable step of having both breasts surgically removed. What information does she need to make this very difficult decision? The list of possible outcomes, and the probabilities with which they occur, are well described in the scenario. However, the way the information is presented reflects the nature of the clinical studies that have been done addressing this question, rather than the information needs of patients.

Table 4.1. Life expectancy (LE) gains in years for prophylactic mastectomy (PM)
compared with breast preservation for BRCA1-positive and usual risk women

Clinical strategies[a]	BrCa1 +	Usual risk
Age 20		
LE with breast preservation	46.52	58.99
LE gain with PM	6.44	0.56
LE gain with PM delayed for 10 years	5.88	0.55
Age 30		
LE with breast preservation	37.14	49.20
LE gain with PM	6.05	0.56
LE gain with PM delayed for 10 years	4.11	0.49
Age 40		
LE with breast preservation	28.96	39.65
LE gain with PM	4.80	0.50
LE gain with PM delayed for 10 years	1.80	0.34
Age 50		
LE with breast preservation	25.04	30.63
LE gain with PM	3.04	0.35
LE gain with PM delayed for 10 ycars	1.12	0.22
Age 60		
LE with breast preservation	19.38	22.33
LE gain with PM	1.69	0.24
LE gain with PM delayed for 10 years	0.17	0.01

Adapted from Schrag et al. (1997).
[a]Values are in years.

Most women considering this choice would want to know whether and by how much their lives could be extended by opting for surgery. Because there have not been (and probably never will be) any randomized trials of prophylactic mastectomy, this information is not available from a single source. However, a formal decision analysis has been done in which the best available data on the natural history of breast cancer in women who carry BRCA1 and 2 cancer predisposition genes, and the effectiveness of prophylactic mastectomy, have been used to estimate the life expectancy benefits associated with surgery (Schrag et al., 1997). The results of that decision analysis are shown in Table 4.1.

As shown in the table, younger women gain larger increments in life expectancy from prophylactic surgery than older ones, and at any given age, a decision to delay surgery results in some compromise in the life expectancy gain. An individual woman considering prophylactic mastectomy could turn to the results of this decision analysis to obtain estimates about one of the potential benefits of the intervention, gain in life expectancy. She is then in a better position to apply her own values in deciding whether that benefit outweighs the harm, in impact on body image, sexuality, and reproductive function, for her.

Presented with all the requisite information, active decision makers are in a position to apply their own values to choose the best treatment for them. This process can be facilitated with decision aids, that clearly present the trade-offs involved in choosing between treatments. Consider the example above of whether to opt for aspirin or warfarin anticoagulation in atrial fibrillation. Figure 4.1 depicts two panels from a decision aid developed to assist patients in making this choice (Man-Son-Hing et al., 1999). Decision aids have also been developed using decision boards, interactive videodiscs, and websites.

Whether or not the decision-making process is facilitated by decision aids, in this paradigm the choice is essentially made in a 'black box.' Information on the nature and probabilities of various outcomes is supplied by the physician or other sources, and the patient applies his or her own values to weight those outcomes to generate a decision about which choice is best for him or her. In this decision-making model, the process of combining the relevant probabilities and values is intuitive (in the black box), not explicit.

Not all patients want to be active decision makers. It is not at all uncommon for patients presented with a choice between two treatment options to turn to the physician and ask, 'What would you do if you were me, Doc?' This is often not a simple question to answer. To generate a recommendation, the physician must not only know the probabilities of various outcomes, but also weight them according to someone's values. Only by applying value judgments can the physician determine whether the morbidity of a toxic therapy is justified by a small resulting increase in life expectancy, or whether it is worth accepting a particular side-effect, such as nausea, to be relieved of a symptom, such as pain.

Whose values should apply in making these choices? Obviously, the physician's goal in counseling the patient wanting guidance should be to identify the best option for that patient. The relevant values are the patient's, not the physician's. Often, qualitative techniques are sufficient to guide this process. Several directed questions to patients to elicit their

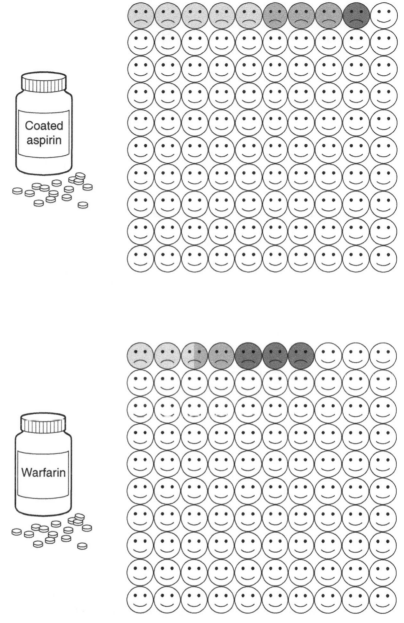

Figure 4.1   Panel from a patient decision aid to illustrate the risk of antithrombotic therapy for stroke prevention in atrial fibrillation. The light unhappy faces indicate minor stroke, middle shaded unhappy faces indicate major stroke, and dark unhappy faces indicate severe bleeding. Reproduced from Man-Son-Hing, M., Laupacis, A., O'Connor, A.M. et al. (1999). A patient decision aid regarding antithrombotic therapy for stroke prevention in atrial fibrillation: a randomized controlled trial. *J.A.M.A.*, **282**, 737–43, with permission. Copyrighted (1999), American Medical Association.

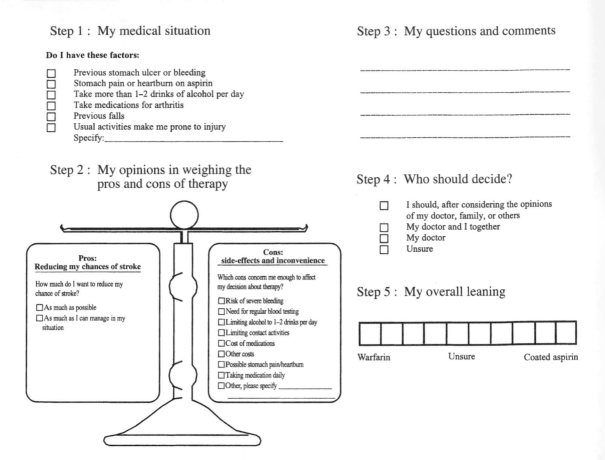

Step 1 : My medical situation

Do I have these factors:

- ☐ Previous stomach ulcer or bleeding
- ☐ Stomach pain or heartburn on aspirin
- ☐ Take more than 1–2 drinks of alcohol per day
- ☐ Take medications for arthritis
- ☐ Previous falls
- ☐ Usual activities make me prone to injury
  Specify:_____

Step 2 : My opinions in weighing the pros and cons of therapy

Pros:
Reducing my chances of stroke

How much do I want to reduce my chance of stroke?

- ☐ As much as possible
- ☐ As much as I can manage in my situation

Cons:
side-effects and inconvenience

Which cons concern me enough to affect my decision about therapy?

- ☐ Risk of severe bleeding
- ☐ Need for regular blood testing
- ☐ Limiting alcohol to 1–2 drinks per day
- ☐ Limiting contact activities
- ☐ Cost of medications
- ☐ Other costs
- ☐ Possible stomach pain/heartburn
- ☐ Taking medication daily
- ☐ Other, please specify _____

Step 3 : My questions and comments

Step 4 : Who should decide?

- ☐ I should, after considering the opinions of my doctor, family, or others
- ☐ My doctor and I together
- ☐ My doctor
- ☐ Unsure

Step 5 : My overall leaning

Warfarin   Unsure   Coated aspirin

Figure 4.2	Panel from a patient decision aid regarding antithrombotic therapy for stroke prevention in atrial fibrillation. From http://www.lri.ca/programs/clinical_epidemiology/ohdec/ decision_aids. asp.

feelings about the key outcomes affected by the choice may be enough to allow the physician to make a tailored recommendation. Figure 4.2, another panel from the decision aid for atrial fibrillation (Man-Son-Hing et al., 1999), provides an example of how written materials can help structure such an interaction. Decision analysis can play a key role in focusing these discussions by identifying, through sensitivity analysis, the one or two critical values that are needed to determine the optimal treatment for an individual. For more complex decisions, it may occasionally be helpful to go one step further, and actually elicit quantitative values from the patient, using one of the methods described later in this chapter.

4.2.2 Societal decision making

Many health-care decisions must be made at the level of populations. Examples include immunization programs, food and transportation safety regulations, and health education activities. Increasingly, in addition, medical decisions are made for classes or groups of patients, at a level removed from the encounter between the individual patient and physician. For example, clinical practice guidelines specify how patients in particular clinical circumstances should be treated. Guidelines are designed to eliminate variation in patterns of care that represent deviations from what is believed to be the most effective therapy for a given disease. Insurers and policy makers allocating limited health-care resources face the even more difficult task of determining not only whether an intervention is effective, but also whether they can afford to offer it to their constituents. Medical decisions are made in the formulation of both guidelines and resource allocation decisions, but they are made on behalf of groups of people, such as members of a particular health plan, or members of society.

Whose values should be reflected in these decisions? Framed in this way, the answer seems obvious. The relevant values are those of the group whom the decision makers are charged to represent. For insurers, the goal should be to write guidelines and set coverage policies that reflect the values of their subscribers. For governmental policy makers, charged with making decisions about how to allocate tax dollars, the relevant values are societal. But it is also clear that this type of decision making cannot rely on the 'black box' model that is both useful and appropriate for the clinical encounter with a single patient. A strategy is needed that weighs the harms and benefits of competing alternatives explicitly in accordance with the values of the population to whom the decisions will apply, and facilitates comparisons of the net benefits generated by alternative uses of health-care resources across a variety of medical conditions. Values must be explicit, and must be elicited from others. Methods to accomplish this task are the subject of the remainder of this chapter.

4.3 Attributes of outcomes

The first step in valuing outcomes is to recognize that some decisions involve more complicated outcomes than others. Consider the following taxonomy of outcome measures.

4.3.1 Two possible outcomes

The first and simplest kind of value problem is one in which there are only two possible outcomes. Examples might be such dichotomies as survive or die, cure or no cure, success or failure, or patient satisfaction or dissatisfaction. The pulmonary embolism problem in Chapter 3 is an example of a value problem with two outcomes, survival or death. In such cases the need for explicit value assessment does not arise. The criterion for decision making is simply to choose the strategy that gives the highest probability of the better outcome or, equivalently, the lowest probability of the worse outcome. In these cases, the method of averaging out is equivalent to the process of combining probabilities according to the principles developed in Chapter 2, to arrive at the overall probability of the outcome of interest for each strategy.

4.3.2 Many possible outcomes: the single-attribute case

The second and more complex type of value problem occurs when there is a spectrum of possible outcomes, ranging on a scale from least preferred through somewhat preferred up to most preferred. Often in this class of problems there is an underlying scale associated with the outcomes, which might naturally serve as the values we are seeking. The most commonly used single-attribute outcome is survival time. For example, if one were willing to accept that the only important outcome to consider in the genetic breast cancer susceptibility example was survival, then the optimal treatment at any age might be identified from Table 4.1 by choosing the option that maximizes life expectancy. But perhaps it wouldn't. A simple averaging of survival times could fail to reflect a patient's preferences about risk or the timing of benefits. For example, a patient might prefer 9 years of survival over a 50–50 chance between 20 years of survival and immediate death. Notice that the expected value of the latter gamble is 10 years, but the patient might still prefer to have 9 years for certain. We might, therefore, wish to modify this underlying scale to account for the possibility that a person might be risk-averse, and/or place greater importance on outcomes occurring in the near term than later in the future. We will return to the topics of risk aversion and time preference in Section 4.12.

4.3.3 Many possible outcomes: the multiattribute case

In the third and most complex class of value problems, there are two or more dimensions or values. In the breast cancer susceptibility case, for

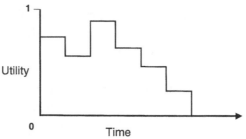

Figure 4.3   Quality-of-life score for a patient with a symptomatic disease, showing transient remission due to toxic therapy, subsequent progressive worsening of disease and symptoms, and eventually death.

example, the outcomes of both therapeutic alternatives (surveillance vs. prophylactic mastectomy) have two basic components: life expectancy and quality of life. The decision is challenging because one must decide how to make trade-offs between the competing values associated with the two dimensions, or attributes. For example, one must decide whether a life that is 5 years longer, but spent without breasts, is better or worse than a life that is somewhat shorter but in which the breasts have not been removed prophylactically. Decisions about such trade-offs are made much easier if the outcomes can be measured on a single scale that reflects the importance of both attributes. And if this scale is generic rather than disease-specific, it could serve as the basis for comparisons of benefits across conditions.

4.4 Quality-adjusted survival

How might one go about constructing a scale that measures both length and quality of life? Consider the plot in Figure 4.3. This figure represents quality-of-life scores for a patient presenting with a symptomatic disease, who then receives toxic therapy, enjoys a transient remission, goes on to have progressively worsening disease and symptoms, and eventually dies.

What's interesting about this figure is that the area under the curve is a function of both the length and quality of life of this patient. Therefore, the area under the curve might function as a metric for valuing the two attributes of length and quality of life on a single scale, and maybe even in units that are generic, rather than disease-specific, depending on how quality of life is measured. But there's a catch. This only works if quality of life is measured in such a way that the product of length of life and quality of life is meaningful. For example, 1 year of life at a quality of life 'x' must be exactly as desirable as 6 months of life at a quality of life of '$2x$.'

What are the characteristics of a quality-of-life measure that satisfies this condition? First, it must be a global evaluation of a state of health. This global measure should reflect all aspects of the state of health being assessed. A more focused measure, that only considers some of the attributes of quality of life and leaves others unspecified, will not fully capture the nature of the trade-off between length and quality of life involved in taking the area under this curve. Second, it must be measured on a ratio scale, between extremes of perfect health and death. This means that if perfect health is 1 and death is 0, then a value of 0.5 is exactly half as desirable as perfect health, and a value of 0.25 is exactly half as desirable as that. And finally, it must use length of life as the metric for measuring the subject's preference for the quality of life in a given health state. This last condition is the most difficult, but follows directly from the way in which we are using this quality-of-life measure as a factor for weighting length of life.

It is no coincidence that we have just described a *utility*, defined as the quantitative measure of the strength of a person's preference for an outcome. This concept has its origins in expected-utility theory (Von Neumann and Morgenstern, 1944; Raiffa, 1968). The notion of quality-adjusted survival, measured in quality-adjusted life years (QALYs), was later developed from this theoretical groundwork, rather than the reverse. None the less, we have introduced utilities by using quality-adjusted survival to provide a more intuitive context for understanding what utilities are, as well as a motivation for trying to measure them.

4.5 Techniques for valuing outcomes

Utilities are clearly different from more familiar, descriptive quality-of-life measures. Generic quality-of-life instruments such as the 36-Item Short Form developed in the Medical Outcomes Study (SF-36) (Ware and Sherbourne, 1992; McHorney et al., 1993) or disease-specific instruments such as the Beck Depression Scale (Beck et al., 1961) capture information on the nature of the quality-of-life impairments of respondents. These scales are often summarized into scores for several different domains, like physical functioning, emotional functioning, pain, and others. Most do not measure global quality of life directly or indirectly, and when they do, they do not capture preferences for a given state of health on a scale that lends itself to being averaged out. Utility measures are fundamentally different; they reflect how a respondent *values* a state of health, not just the characteristics of that health state.

This difference is best illustrated with an example. Imagine that you and your best friend both injure your right knees in a car accident. You are both left with some chronic discomfort in the knee, and this is relieved by nonsteroidal antiinflammatory medications. Both of you are able to run 1 km, but not longer distances. You are both avid distance runners and are very distressed by this limitation. However, you believe that it will be possible for you to find other athletic pursuits that you will enjoy, while your friend does not. It is likely that you and your friend would score nearly identically on quality-of-life instruments measuring physical functioning, pain, and even distress. However, your utilities for this health state would likely differ. Your friend might consider a somewhat shorter life without this disability to be as desirable as a longer one with it, while you would probably not be willing to make this trade-off. Simply put, your preferences for this health state are different.

Utilities can also be defined functionally. A true utility scale is one that can be averaged out in a decision tree without distorting the preferences of the individual whose preferences are represented. In the example of life span, if each duration of survival were assigned a utility equal to its duration (20 years = 20, 10 years = 10, 0 years = 0), then the expected utility of a 50–50 gamble between 20 years and 0 years would be 10. Since the patient in the example used earlier prefers 9 years over the gamble, this cannot be a utility scale for this patient. But other functions could serve as utility scales for this patient. For example, a utility scale which assigns to each life span the square root of the length of life would be consistent with this ranking of options, because:

$$0.5 \cdot \mathrm{sqrt}(20) + 0.5 \cdot \mathrm{sqrt}(0) < \mathrm{sqrt}(9) \tag{4.1}$$

A scale of QALYs is frequently used in decision analysis and in economic evaluations as a utility measure. But it is not guaranteed that quality-adjusted life expectancy (i.e., averaged-out quality-adjusted survival) will reflect a decision maker's preferences regarding decisions under uncertainty, unless particular conditions apply. We will return to these conditions later in this chapter.

There are several different strategies for capturing such preference-based measures of quality of life. They vary in their theoretical underpinnings, conceptual difficulty, and practical feasibility. It's important to be familiar with all the techniques. The best one to use for a particular application may depend on the goals and nature of the study being done (Stiggelbout, 2000).

> **DEFINITION**
>
> A *utility* scale (or *utility function*) is an assignment of numerical values to each member of a set of outcomes, such that if the expected value of the utilities assigned to the outcomes in one chance tree is greater than the expected value of the utilities assigned to the outcomes in another chance tree, then the first chance tree is preferred to the second chance tree, and vice versa.

4.5.1 Rating scale

The simplest approach to measuring a subject's preference for a given state of health, whether it's the subject's own state of health or a hypothetical one, is a *rating scale*. An example of a verbal rating scale is:

'On a scale where 0 represents death and 100 represents excellent health, what number would you say best describes your current state of health over just the past 2 weeks?'

Very similar results are obtained with visual stimuli such as 'feeling thermometers,' as shown in Figure 4.4, and visual analog scales (oriented horizontally).

The rating scale is a global measure that captures a subject's valuation of a particular state of health. This approach is easily explained to most people and it is easy to administer. However, it is not a true utility because it isn't a ratio scale between perfect health and death. There is no reason to think that a subject who rates an impaired state of health at '50' would be willing to trade away half of his or her life expectancy to be relieved of that impairment, in other words, to improve that state of health to '100.' As a result, the rating scale does not necessarily satisfy the criterion of expected value. A certain life span of 20 years in a health state whose rating is 40 is not necessarily less desirable than a 50–50 chance of living those 20 years in perfect health (rating = 100), with the alternative of death (rating = 0). Several 'transformations' of rating scale scores have been proposed to try to approximate true utilities, however, and will be discussed in Section 4.8.

4.5.2 Standard (reference) gamble

The approach to utility assessment most firmly grounded in expected-utility theory is the *standard gamble* (or *reference gamble*). The essence of the standard gamble is that it assesses the utility for a health state by asking how high a risk of death one would accept to improve it. This is done by asking a respondent to choose between life in a given clinical state and a gamble between death and perfect health. The utility of the health state is then given by the probability of perfect health in the gamble such that the respondent is indifferent between the gamble and the certain intermediate outcome.

Let's illustrate this process with an example. Consider the following health state.

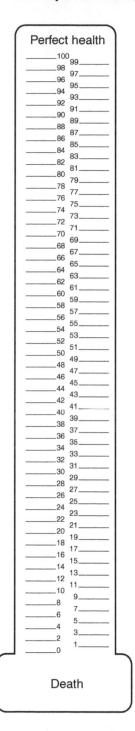

Figure 4.4   Feeling thermometer: a visual aid used to elicit a score for the current state of health.

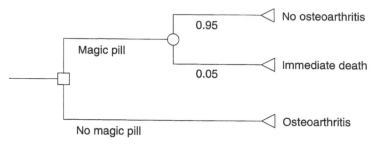

Figure 4.5 Chance tree to illustrate the standard (reference) gamble.

Imagine that you have osteoarthritis that affects your hips. You need a walker when you are out of your home, and you cannot run at all. You have moderate pain that is partially relieved by daily nonsteroidal medications. Now imagine that a genie offers you a magic pill. If you take this pill, there is a 50% probability that you will be completely relieved of your arthritis forever and will live out your natural life expectancy. However, the pill has one side-effect. There is a 50% probability that it will cause immediate painless death. Would you take the pill? If the answer is no, would you consider taking the magic pill if there were a 99% probability that you would be relieved of your arthritis and a 1% probability of immediate painless death? If the answer to this question is yes, would you consider taking the magic pill if there were a 75% probability that you would be relieved of your arthritis and a 25% probability of immediate painless death?

In the standard gamble, this iterative process is repeated, varying the probabilities in the gamble, until the respondent feels that the two options, taking the magic pill and not taking the pill, are equally desirable. This is called the 'point of indifference' (although many individuals experience increasing discomfort as this point is approached), because at that point the subject no longer expresses a preference between the two options. At the point of indifference, the respondent's utility for the health state, osteoarthritis in this example, is given by the probability that the magic pill will work. So if you reached the point of indifference when offered a magic pill associated with a 95% probability of permanent relief of arthritis and a 5% probability of immediate death (as shown in Figure 4.5), your utility for the health state would be 0.95. The disutility of this health state, defined as 1 minus the utility, would therefore be 0.05.

Now let's describe the process we just went through a bit more rigorously. Consider a choice between life in a given clinical state H and a gamble between death (with probability $= 1 - P$) and perfect health (with probability P). Suppose that we arbitrarily assign a value of 1.0 to perfect health and of 0.0 to death. Then the expected value of this gamble $= [P \times 1.0 + (1 - P) \times 0] = P$. We recognize this expected value as the probability of getting perfect health in the gamble. If the respondent considers the gamble equally desirable as a health state H, then the utility of that health state must be P. We denote this by $u(H) = P$. By varying the probability P in the standard gamble until the respondent declares himself or herself indifferent between the gamble and the health state, we can find the utility of any health state between perfect health and death by a series of choices between gambles.

In order to avoid having patients deal repeatedly with lotteries involving a risk of death, a variant of the standard gamble has been introduced – a chained gamble. The chained procedure requires that an anchor health state be evaluated in relation to a lottery between perfect health and death; then all other health states can be evaluated in relation to perfect health and the anchor health state (Jansen et al., 1998).

At this point, two comments on terminology are in order. First, it is customary in decision analysis to use the word 'indifferent' to reflect a situation in which an individual is equally happy (or unhappy) with two outcomes or gambles. It does not mean that the person doesn't care about the choice; it does mean that the person has no preference one way or the other.

Second, we use the term 'gamble,' despite its frivolous connotations, to refer to any chance tree involving outcomes of interest. The use of this word in decision theory has a long history, and we apologize to any readers who take our use of this word to imply anything less than the greatest respect for the seriousness of life-and-death choices.

A critical feature of the standard gamble is that it reflects decision making under uncertainty. You do not know for sure which of the two outcomes in the gamble you will experience, only the probability that each will occur. As a result, your utility measured with a standard gamble reflects not only your preferences about life in that state of health, but also your attitudes toward risk.

4.5.3 Time trade-off

The third approach to direct measurement of preference for states of health is the *time trade-off*. In this case, the utility for a health state is assessed by asking how much time one would give up to improve it. This is done by asking a respondent to choose between a set length of life in a given compromised health state and a shorter length of life in perfect health. The

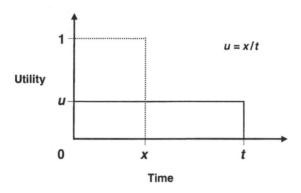

Figure 4.6   Illustration of the time trade-off. See text for details.

respondent's utility for the compromised health state is given by the ratio of the shorter to the longer life expectancy at which the respondent finds the two health states equally desirable.

Consider the osteoarthritis health state once again.

Assume that your natural life expectancy is 40 years with osteoarthritis. Now imagine that another genie offers you a different magic pill. If you take this pill, you will be relieved of your arthritis forever, but you will live only 20 more years, instead of 40. Would you take this pill? If the answer is no, would you take the pill if it would relieve your arthritis and you would live 39 more years? If the answer is yes, would you take the pill if it would relieve your arthritis and you would live 30 more years?

In the time trade-off, this iterative process is repeated, varying the length of life in perfect health, until the respondent feels that the two options, taking the magic pill and not taking the pill, are equally desirable. As in the standard gamble, this is called the 'point of indifference.' At this point, the respondent's utility for the health state, osteoarthritis in this example, is given by the ratio of the length of life in perfect health to the length of life in the compromised health state. This concept is illustrated graphically in Figure 4.6.

At the point of indifference, the subject believes that the life characterized by time t spent in health state with utility u is equivalent to the life with length x, spent in perfect health with utility '1'. Assuming this subject does not have a time preference (as will be discussed in Section 4.12), then the area under the curve for the longer life, t times u, is equal to the area under the curve of the shorter life, x times 1. Hence, u equals x/t. So if you reached this point of indifference when offered a magic pill associated with a reduction in your life expectancy from 40 to 38 years, your utility for the health state would be 0.95.

In contrast to the standard gamble, the time trade-off represents decision making under certainty. Whether you choose to take the magic pill or not, you know exactly what your outcome will be. Therefore, the utility it generates is unaffected by your attitude toward risk.

4.5.4 Other techniques for valuing outcomes

It's worth noting briefly that several other techniques are sometimes used to quantify values for states of health. Assessments of the *willingness to pay* (WTP) ask how much the respondent would be willing to pay in financial terms to improve a state of health, avoid a particular outcome, or reduce the chance of death (Gafni, 1991; O'Brien and Viramontes, 1994; O'Brien and Gafni, 1996). Alternatively, the question can be framed to ask how much the respondent would want to receive to remain in an impaired state of health. The result puts a monetary value on a health outcome, and is used largely for cost–benefit analyses. Cost–benefit analyses are economic evaluations in which all outcomes are expressed in monetary terms, in contrast to cost-effectiveness (or cost–utility) analyses, in which health outcomes are expressed in terms of (quality-adjusted) life years, and results are expressed in terms of cost per (quality-adjusted) life year. We will return to cost–benefit analysis in Chapter 9, although most of the attention will be devoted to cost-effectiveness analysis. WTP has been little used in decision making for individual patients.

Magnitude estimation asks the respondent how many times better or worse one health state is than another. This method has its roots in psychophysics and has not been widely used in medical decision making. The meaning of the scores is not clearly linked to a choice process, as utilities derived by standard gamble and time trade-off, nor is the method especially convenient and easy to administer, unlike a visual analog scale.

Equivalence measures (also called *person trade-off*) ask the respondent to indicate how many people would have to be cured of one health state to be equivalent to curing 100 people in another impaired health state. It asks about the social worth of alternative health-care interventions, and is generally viewed as better suited for policy making than for clinical decision making (Richardson and Nord, 1997). Even in that context, it has been criticized as paternalistically reflecting preferences for 'other people.'

4.6 Comment on nomenclature

Often the terms 'preferences,' 'values,' 'utilities' are used interchangeably. However, there are subtle but important differences among them. The most generic of the three terms is *preferences*. All of the techniques described in the previous section measure preferences for different states of health. Purists would limit use of the term *utility* to describe the results of a standard gamble, arguing that a true utility must reflect decision making under uncertainty (Torrance, 1986). They would argue that the term *values* should be used to describe the results of measurements done under conditions of certainty, including rating scales and time trade-offs. However, most experts in the field are willing to grant the status of 'utility' to the results of a time trade-off (particularly if adjusted for the time preference rate: see Section 4.12), a convention we follow throughout this text.

4.7 Relationships among techniques for valuing outcomes

Ideally, the three major techniques for valuing outcomes – the rating scale, the standard gamble, and the time trade-off – would yield the same numbers, or at worst, would yield scores that are easily transformable from one scale to another, as we can do with the fahrenheit and centigrade scales. As our discussion should have made clear, reality is more complex. The techniques measure somewhat different but related concepts. Not surprisingly, when the same subjects are asked to evaluate health status using each of the measures, the results are not identical. In general, the utilities elicited with the standard gamble are the highest. Most subjects are unwilling to accept much risk of immediate death, even if the impaired health state involves serious compromise in quality of life. Utilities elicited with the time trade-off tend to be somewhat lower, suggesting that a known, limited decrease in life expectancy is a more acceptable 'price' to pay for being relieved of a quality-of-life impairment than a low probability of immediate death, even if the overall life expectancies are equivalent. Given errors of measurement and the psychological differences between risky and riskless choices, the scores or utilities elicited are not easily transformable. None the less, standard gamble and time trade-off utilities are often used interchangeably.

Rating scale values tend to be considerably lower than utilities generated by either of the other two techniques. This makes sense, because there is no 'penalty' associated with assigning a health state a rating scale value lower than that of perfect health. Respondents who would not be willing to accept any risk of death, or decrease in the length of their life, to be relieved of a mild impairment in quality of life, might well assign it a less than perfect score on a rating scale. But because rating scales are considerably easier to administer than either of the other two techniques, there has been a long-standing interest in finding a way to 'transform' the values they generate into utility scores. One commonly used strategy is to increase the rating scale value according to an empirically derived statistical relationship. One such relationship that has been found to fit the data rather well is a power function. For example, Torrance et al. (1996) observed the following relationship between the rating scale values and standard gamble utilities for the same states of health:

$$\text{utility} = 1 - (1 - \text{value})^r \qquad\qquad (4.2)$$

where the exponent r has been estimated consistently in the range from about 1.6 to 2.3.

A number of comparisons have also been done between the results of preference measures and conventional quality-of-life or health status measures. This literature demonstrates that the correlations are usually poor, and there is no simple relationship that might serve as the basis for transformations between them (Bosch and Hunink, 1996). Because scales like the SF-36 are so widely used, the search continues for functions that can conveniently transform these quality-of-life scales to utilities for decision making (e.g., Fryback et al., 1997). None the less, as discussed earlier, preferences and descriptive quality of life are different concepts.

4.8 Health indexes

There is, however, an important approach to assessment of utilities that is in some ways a hybrid between descriptive quality-of-life measurement and utility assessment. The Health Utilities Index (HUI) and the EuroQol with five dimensions (EQ-5D) are two widely used examples of these so-called health indexes or multiattribute utility measures (Torrance et al., 1995, 1996; Feeney et al., 1996; Dolan, 1997). As shown in Figure 4.7, health indexes include two components: a health state classification instrument, and a formula for assigning a utility to any unique set of responses to that instrument.

The health state classification instrument measures health-related quality of life and, as a result, generates descriptive data regarding the quality of life of the patient who completes it. The HUI questionnaire leads to a classification of a health state along eight domains, or dimensions, or attributes: ambulation, dexterity, cognition, emotion, pain and discomfort, vision, hearing, and speech (Torrance et al., 1995; Feeney et al., 1996).

The special feature of a health index is the mapping rule. This is developed by polling members of a 'reference population' to elicit their

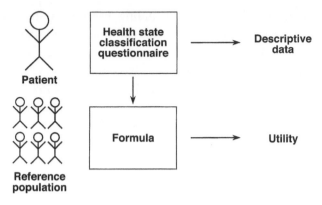

Figure 4.7   Health indexes and their components.

utilities for all of the states of health that can be described by possible combinations of responses to the health state classification instrument. The reference population is often comprised of members of the general public from which the subject originates. In the case of the HUI, the mapping rule is based on utilities assessed by a combination of standard gambles and adjusted (by a power function transformation) rating scales. The two principal advantages of health indexes are that they are easily completed by patients in a clinical trial or other clinical study, and the utilities they generate represent community or societal preferences.

4.9 Off-the-shelf utilities

For decision analyses in which the analyst has neither the time nor resources to administer a utility survey, or even to administer a preference-weightable health index such as the HUI or EQ-5D, it is possible to turn to any number of utilities previously obtained from surveys. While the health states are necessarily described in very general terms, such as 'asthma' or 'hip fracture,' these sources may be serviceable approximations. Examples of such 'off-the-shelf' utilities are available from the Beaver Dam Health Outcomes Study (Fryback et al., 1997), from preference-weighted items from the National Health Interview Survey (Gold et al., 1998), and from a catalog of published analyses (Bell et al., 2001).

4.10 Health states worse than death

Thoughtful readers may have been asking whether it is possible to accommodate a preference that a particular health state is worse than being dead.

While this possibility raises difficult ethical questions, such as the some-times conflicting responsibilities of the physician to respect a patient's wishes and to preserve life, the technical answer to the question is 'yes,' it is possible to have utilities less than zero. The elicitation procedures, using the rating scale, time trade-off, and standard gamble, all require modifica-tion, but it can be done (Patrick et al., 1994). In the HUI mapping function, several health states have utilities less than zero, the minimum being -0.34 for the health state corresponding to the worst level of all eight attributes.

4.11 Practical considerations in utility measurement

Perhaps because utility techniques are grounded in theoretical rather than empirical considerations, they are challenging to administer. Utility elicita-tion requires that respondents consider hypothetical situations, grasp the nature of probabilities, and imagine experiencing some rather dreadful outcomes, including immediate death. There is general consensus that, while rating scale values can be elicited reliably in self-administered sur-veys, utility measurement with standard gambles and time trade-offs is best done in an interactive format. A major advantage of these methods is that they allow the questions to be administered as a series of dichotomous choices. So, instead of asking a single open-ended question about what risk of death the subject might accept to be relieved of the impairments in a given state of health, the question is approached iteratively, with systematic variation in the probability of death in the gamble until the point of indifference is reached, as demonstrated in the examples in Section 4.5.

It is also very helpful to provide the subject with visual aids describing the nature of the health states being evaluated, and the specific characteris-tics of the choices being presented. In the standard gamble, this is often done with pie charts depicting the probabilities of perfect health and death in the gamble. In the time trade-off, the visual aids often depict graphically the lengths of life in impaired and perfect health the subject is being asked to consider. These visual aids can range in sophistication from simple diagrams on pieces of paper given to subjects being interviewed in person or over the phone, to boards with sliding or rotating sections to represent lengths of life and probabilities, to interactive computerized utility assess-ment programs. One advantage of these computerized programs is that they insure greater standardization of the format of the utility elicitation interview. Even so, it is generally recommended that a trained interviewer be present while the subject completes the computerized interview, not only to help with the running of the program, but also to address questions

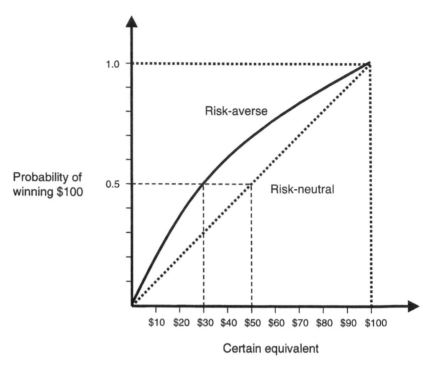

Certain equivalent

Figure 4.8   Utility curve illustrating risk aversion and risk neutrality.

that may arise. No matter what method is used, direct utility elicitation is time-consuming and resource-intensive.

4.12 Risk aversion and time preference

Imagine that you have the opportunity to play the following game. I flip a coin and you call it in the air. If you're right, I give you $1000. If you're wrong, you win nothing. Not a bad opportunity! If you play repeatedly, you will make $500 per game, on average. But I am only offering you the opportunity to play once, and there is a 50% chance you will win nothing. Now, what is the minimum amount of money you would accept rather than play this game? If you answered $500, the average value of the game, you are said to be *risk-neutral*. However, you may be willing to accept as little as $300 rather than play the game. Many individuals would opt for a smaller amount of money, offered with certainty, over a gamble with a higher value on average. These individuals are said to be *risk-averse*. In other words, they prefer a certain outcome of lower value over a gamble with a higher average value, but risk of a poor outcome.

The utilities of an individual who is risk-neutral with respect to money

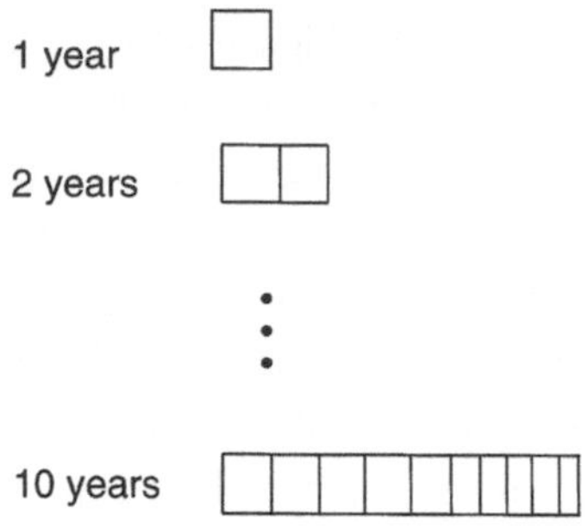

1 year

2 years

⋮

10 years

Figure 4.9   Diminishing incremental value of additional time.

would lie along the straight diagonal line in Figure 4.8. The utilities of an individual who is risk-averse would form a concave curve, above and to the left of the diagonal. An individual who prefers a gamble with a small probability of a very large payoff over a certain outcome with the same expected value is said to be *risk-seeking*. For such an individual, the utility curve would lie below the diagonal.

The same concepts can be applied to nonmonetary outcomes, including health outcomes such as years of life. Consider a gamble in which you have a 50% probability of 40 years of life and a 50% probability of 0 years of life. If you would consider a certain alternative of 20 years of life to be equivalent to this gamble, you are risk-neutral with respect to years of life. However, if you are risk-averse with respect to life-years, you will prefer a shorter, but certain, length of life over the gamble. In general, risk attitudes are inferred from expressed choices, just as values are. It is important to note that risk attitude is not necessarily a stable personality trait. An individual might be risk-seeking with respect to money (a gambler) and risk-averse with respect to years of life. The context of the attitude should be specified.

For a risk-neutral utility function, the certainty equivalent is equal to the expected value. For a risk-averse utility function, the certainty equivalent is greater than the expected value. For a risk-seeking utility function, the certainty equivalent is greater than the expected value.

The concept of risk aversion does not apply to the time trade-off, since this technique does not involve uncertainty. However, the related concept of *time preference* does. As shown in Figure 4.9, the incremental value of an additional year may not be constant.

Most people would favor an intervention that increased life expectancy from 1 year to 2, over one that increased life expectancy from 9 years to 10, for example. This has implications for the interpretation of utilities gener-

DEFINITION

Consider a gamble in which each possible outcome is expressed on some numerical scale (such as dollars or years of life). The *certainty equivalent* of a gamble is the outcome along the scale such that the decision maker is indifferent between the gamble and that certain outcome.

ated with a time trade-off. Consider Figure 4.6 once again. If future years are valued less than those in the near term, the value of u will depend on the value of t. All else being equal, the longer the life expectancy in impaired health, the higher the proportion of that life expectancy one might be willing to give up in exchange for perfect health. This follows from the fact that years of life farther in the future are valued less. Consequently, the longer the life offered in the time trade-off, the lower the utility for the impaired state of health. It is possible to adjust time-trade-off utilities for time preference, but only if you have an independent estimate of the rate of time preference (i.e., the rate at which the length of the rectangles in Figure 4.9 are diminishing; Johannesson et al., 1994).

4.13 Quality-adjusted life expectancy as a utility

We have seen that in order to be amenable to being averaged out, health-state utilities must reflect preferences under uncertainty in the sense implied by the standard gamble. We have also seen that, in order to be amenable to being used as the weights in quality-adjusted survival, they must reflect time trade-offs. In order to use averaged-out life span as a utility (i.e., life expectancy), preferences must be risk-neutral with regard to longevity. In sum, *all three* of these criteria must be met in order to be able to use quality-adjusted survival to reflect preferences in a decision analysis. This may seem an insurmountable hurdle, which may cause us to despair. However, it has been shown that if an individual's preferences satisfy only two conditions, then quality-adjusted survival can represent his or her preferences:

1 Constant proportional trade-off: the proportion of life span that an individual would give up in order to improve health from a health state to perfect health does not depend on the length of life, and

2 Risk neutrality on survival (Bleichrodt and Amiram, 1996; Wakker, 1996; Bleichrodt and Johannesson, 1997).

While the conditions for utility may not be met precisely, studies have shown them to be met approximately enough so that rankings of gambles on quality of life and survival are not unduly distorted (Johannesson et al., 1994). Finally, as we shall see in Chapters 9 and 10, an adjustment can be made for time preference by using discounting.

4.14 Other psychological issues in utility assessment

Whether or not a formal utility assessment technique is used, the focus on values emphasizes that eliciting and clarifying a patient's preferences is inherently a psychological process. We may use methods that have a foundation in a formal mathematical theory, but in another sense, the issues that arise are related to some recurrent issues in psychological scaling. The following are some of the issues that have been the focus of some discussion over the years.

1 In many cases, decision making must be made prospectively, before the patient has experience with the outcome of the treatment intervention, for example prophylactic mastectomy. How are utility assessments affected by lack of direct experience?

2 In most situations, people gradually adapt to their current reality, and what was anticipated to be a very unpleasant situation becomes at least bearable. If this is true, then a utility assessment of a yet-to-be-experienced outcome may judge it to be worse than it will subsequently prove to be. On the other hand, for a minority of patients, the new reality may turn out to be worse than they had feared. In either case, sensitivity analysis of the relevant utilities is crucial, because there is some reason to believe that either set of numbers (prospective or concurrent utilities) may be valid estimates of the patient's 'true' values.

3 All the methods of utility assessment that we have described assume that the people being assessed have preexisting preferences that are simply being uncovered by the elicitation procedure. In some situations, however, people may not have well-formed preferences, and their responses to questions may be generated 'on the fly' in response to the implicit pressure of the interview situation. In these cases, the physician or whoever is doing the utility assessment must be especially careful not to bias the responses by the manner of questioning.

4 Utility elicitation is subject to framing effects, in which the format or wording of the questions asked of subjects may influence their responses. In the standard gamble and time trade-off methods, values are inferred from choices. These choices should be stable over minor changes in the wording of the problem. This is called procedural invariance. When preferences change as a function of minor changes in the wording of the task, the assumption of procedural invariance has been violated. Systematic framing effects have been documented in a variety of situations (Kahneman and Tversky, 1984; McNeil et al., 1982; Kuhberger, 1998). Framing effects are not found in all clinical situations, for reasons that are still unclear (Christensen-Szalanski, 1984). Our understanding of the conditions evoking this effect is still imperfect. Nevertheless, when eliciting a patient's values using a preference-based method, one should take care to insure that the preferences elicited are reasonably stable across alternative, but equivalent wordings of the choice task.

5 Finally, expected-utility theory is a prescriptive theory, not a descriptive one. It describes how people ought to make decisions under uncertainty if they wish to satisfy certain axioms and principles, not necessarily how they actually make decisions in an imperfect world. It is also a 'small world' theory, since any decision model inevitably omits some factors from the decision that another decision maker may find critical. The study of how people actually make decisions, when they do not use decision analysis, forms the field of decision psychology or behavioral decision theory (Tversky and Kahneman, 1981; Kahneman and Tversky, 1984; Connolly et al., 1999; Chapman and Elstein, 2000).

4.15 Discussion: decision-making paradigms revisited

With these new tools in hand, let us return to the decision-making paradigms introduced in the beginning of the chapter. When and how should values be measured and incorporated into the decision-making process in each setting?

4.15.1 The clinical encounter with the active decision maker

The information needs of patients who wish to assume full decision-making autonomy include a thorough understanding of the nature, likelihood, and timing of the outcomes associated with each intervention under consideration. The patient may then weigh those alternatives, applying his or her own values. There is no need to supply that patient with information on other patients' utilities or values, or for formal elicitation of the patient's own values.

The only caveat is that competent patients may occasionally make decisions that seem unconventional or even unreasonable (Brock and Wartman, 1990). This may reflect unusual but deeply held beliefs or values. If so, these decisions should be accepted and honored. However, it could also reflect difficulty processing complex medical information, and/or inordinate fear of certain outcomes or medical procedures, fear that could be alleviated with further education. It is the physician's responsibility to attempt to help patients avoid making decisions that are inconsistent with their underlying goals and values. A formal analysis of the risks and benefits of alternative strategies, and perhaps an 'off-the-shelf' or back-of-the-envelope decision analysis, including utility elicitation, could help achieve this goal in two ways. First, the process of making the expected harms and benefits explicit can be useful in educating the patient about the choices (Gillick, 1988). Second, this process insures that the patient's choice reflects underlying values rather than a misunderstanding of the nature or probabilities of the various outcomes.

4.15.2 The clinical encounter with the patient wanting guidance

Most medical decisions require some value judgments. For patients who prefer a more passive role in decision making, someone's preferences must be used to weigh the outcomes associated with alternative strategies. While physicians are uniquely qualified to integrate the complex clinical data relevant to medical decision making, their values may be poor proxies for those of patients. The ideal of tailored medical decision making can only be achieved if the individual patient's preferences are somehow brought to bear on the choice among alternatives.

Occasionally, formal utility elicitation and incorporation of those utilities into a decision analysis can be the best way to achieve this goal. For example, Pauker and Pauker (1987) have used formal preference assessment to help couples decide whether to undergo a diagnostic amniocentesis (puncture to obtain fluid from a pregnant woman to diagnose abnormalities of the fetus). But often, simpler strategies are sufficient. A formal decision analysis can identify the critical utility values to which the choice of the preferred strategy is sensitive, and the thresholds of those values at which the preferred strategy changes. These results can then be used to structure qualitative, less conceptually complex questions for patients that allow the patients to express where their preferences fall relative to that threshold. For example, based on their decision analysis, Hillner and Smith (1991) concluded that whether women with newly diagnosed node-negative breast cancer should receive adjuvant chemotherapy depends on their feelings about the side-effects of chemotherapy and their concerns about recurrence of cancer. Their analysis suggested that the preferred choice for a woman at low risk of recurrence who is as frightened of chemotherapy as she is of cancer is to forgo chemotherapy (Hillner and Smith, 1991).

Some patients, such as those who are cognitively impaired or young children, may not be able to supply any information at all about their preferences. In this situation, the experiences of other patients who have faced similar choices may provide some guidance. The preferences of other patients may be inferred from the choices that they made, assuming that they were fully informed about the alternatives. Alternatively, explicit quantitative data on other patients' values for the relevant health states can form the basis for judgments about the optimal strategy for the typical patient. Such data are available in the literature for a growing number of health states, collected in cross-sectional surveys, or from participants in clinical trials.

4.15.3 Societal decision making: clinical guidelines

As discussed earlier, value judgments are embedded in most clinical guidelines. Those judgments should reflect the preferences of the population served by the guideline. But exactly who is in that population? Consider the example of a guideline about whether to use adjuvant chemotherapy in women with node-negative breast cancer. One could argue that the relevant values are those of patients facing that particular clinical decision, for example, women newly diagnosed with node-negative breast cancer. But these women are less knowledgeable about the outcomes of treatment than are women who have a history of treated node-negative disease; perhaps the preferences of that group are more informative and more relevant. But this may be too narrow a view. Since this guideline will affect women diagnosed in the future, too, one might want to solicit and incorporate the preferences of all women in the population. But men may be affected by this guideline as well, through its impact on the women in their lives, and the diversion of resources into treatment for breast cancer that might otherwise be available to fund programs targeted to men. Should their preferences be reflected in the guidelines?

The field has not yet come to consensus about these issues. There is growing interest, however, in guidelines that include preference assessment in some form as one of the steps. This is especially important for choices that are toss-ups with respect to survival outcomes, but involve important differences in quality of life.

4.15.4 Societal decision making: resource allocation

The most widespread application of quantitative utility assessment is decision making for resource allocation. Judgments about how to spend limited health-care resources should take into account the full range of the expected health benefits of alternative programs, including both length and quality of life, and should use units that allow comparisons across conditions. As a result, an international panel of experts has identified quality-adjusted survival as the preferred outcome for use in cost-effectiveness analysis (Gold et al., 1996). Calculation of quality-adjusted life years requires quantitative utility weights.

The question of whose values to use in cost-effectiveness analyses is also controversial. In this case, however, there is an emerging consensus. The Panel on Cost-Effectiveness in Health and Medicine recommended that all cost-effectiveness analyses include a 'reference case,' conducted from a societal perspective (Gold et al., 1996). To adopt a true societal perspective requires that societal preferences be used to allocate societal resources. To quantify these values, the views of a representative sample of members of the general public could be elicited using techniques introduced in this chapter, such as the standard gamble. Alternatively, as described in Section 4.8, utilities reflecting societal preferences could be derived from the results of a utility survey administered to patients in the relevant health states. We return to the role of utilities in cost-effectiveness analysis in Chapter 9.

Not all analyses require high-quality empirical utility data. If the results of the decision analysis or cost-effectiveness analysis are insensitive to the utility values, resources should not be spent on collecting them. None the less, it is important that all decision analysts understand the strengths and limitations of alternative methods of eliciting and quantifying preferences, and exercise judgment about how and when to undertake this challenging task.

4.16 Summary

Most decisions regarding alternative strategies require some value judgment about how to weigh the benefits versus the harms. The value of the outcomes may have several (competing) attributes such as length and quality of life. To compare strategies we need a scale that combines the important attributes in one metric. Quality-adjusted survival, measured in QALYs, provides such a scale. Furthermore, QALYs fulfill the criteria of a utility, that is, they can be considered a quantitative measure of the strength of a person's preference for an outcome.

Techniques for valuing outcomes include the rating scale, the standard reference gamble, the time trade-off, health indexes, willingness to pay, magnitude estimation, and the person trade-off. Other factors that may affect outcome values are risk aversion and risk-seeking attitudes and time preference.

Exercises

Exercise 4.1

Time trade-off

During the iterative process of the *time trade-off* with our osteoarthritis patient (whose natural life expectancy is 40 years in the impaired health state), it turns out that the *point of indifference* is reached when the magic curing pill is said to reduce his life expectancy to 35 years.

(a) What does this mean for the patient's utility for the current health state?

(b) Is this utility likely to be higher or lower than if it were assessed using the *standard gamble* method?

Exercise 4.2

(a) Discuss the advantages and disadvantages of using rating scale values in utility assessment.

(b) A 75-year-old patient suffered from intermittent claudication for 3 years and subsequently developed critical limb ischemia. Two years later the patient died. The utility for intermittent claudication is 0.79 and the utility for critical limb ischemia is 0.35. Calculate the QALYs for this patient.

Exercise 4.3

You are asked to participate in a study on the health-related quality of life of readers of this book. The study consists of a questionnaire with three different kinds of questions.

Read the following scenarios and give your responses to the questions.

(a) Scenario 1

Imagine that your present health state can improve if you take a magic pill. Your present health state is your average health during the past 4 weeks. If you take the magic pill you will enjoy full health, which means that your health will be comparable to that of healthy people your age. However, taking the pill carries with it a risk of immediate death. There are no other side-effects. If you do not take the pill you will go on living in your present state of health.

Questions
Would you take the magic pill if the chances of death and full health, respectively, are distributed as follows (Figure 4.10), or would you prefer to remain in your present state of health?

If your answer is yes or no, go to the next box as indicated by the arrow.
If you are indifferent, mark ?*.
You may stop when your answer is marked *.

(b) Scenario 2
(imagine that an interviewer reads this question aloud to you)
Imagine that I have a crystal ball in which I can see your future. I see that you will live another 30 years in your present state of health. That means that your health state will be as it was on average during the past 4 weeks. However, I can make you the following offer: you will enjoy full health, which means that your health will be comparable to that of healthy people your age, but your life will be shortened; you will have to give up a certain number of years.

Questions
Instead of spending 30 years in your present state of health, I am making you an offer whereby you have to give up ... years, but you will spend ... years in full health (Figure 4.11). Would you accept my offer?

If your answer is yes or no, go to the next box as indicated by the arrow.
If you are indifferent, mark ?*.
You may stop when your answer is marked *.

(c) If you had to rate your general state of health during the past 4 weeks on a scale from 0 to 100 points, where 100 is full health and 0 death, how many points would you give?

The text of the questions derives from a translation of a Dutch questionnaire and the concept of the charts used can be found in: Bosch, J.L. & Hunink, M.G.M. (1996). The relationship between descriptive and valuational quality of life measures in patients with intermittent claudication. *Med. Decis. Making*, **16**, 217–25.

(d) Which kind of measures were questions a, b, and c?

(e) Calculate your utility for questions a and b, and compare these. Compare these numbers also with your response to question c.

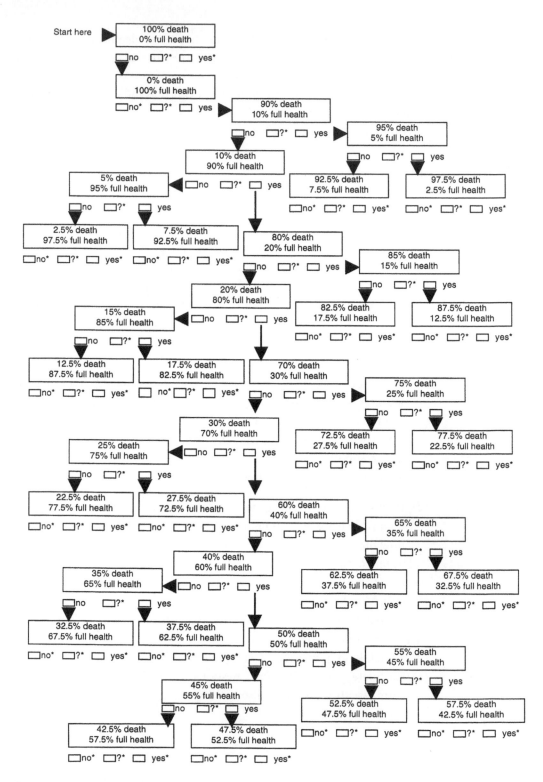

Figure 4.10   Question 1.

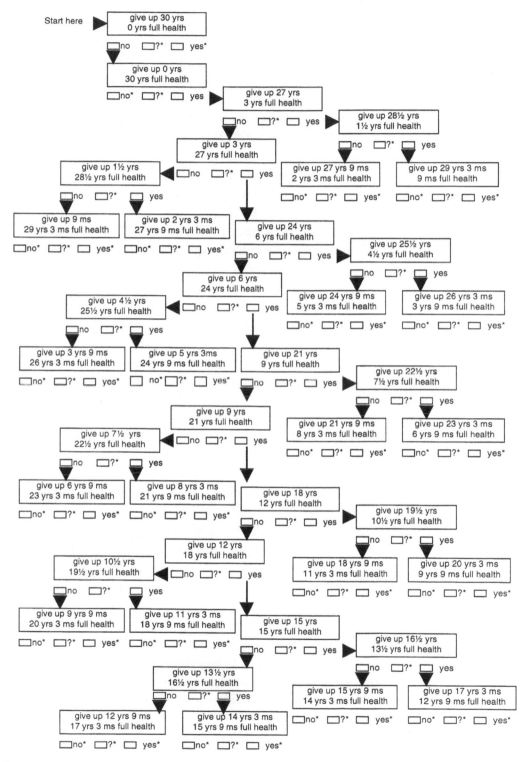

Figure 4.11   Question 2.

Exercise 4.4

In this exercise you are asked to construct your own utility curve based on your time preference. Consider the following hypothetical choice:

Looking at a glass ball we predict that you will live 20 years. Imagine that a magic pill exists that can increase your life expectancy to 40 years. However, this pill has one serious side-effect: 50% of people who take it die immediately. Do you want to take this pill?

The choice is therefore:

(A) no risk now and living 20 years for certain

(B) a very risky treatment with a chance of dying immediately of 0.50, but if treatment is successful, living 40 years

Your maximum life expectancy is 40 years and if you are indifferent between A and B, then your certainty equivalent 50 (CE50) is 20 years. That is the value of the certain period of survival of A for which A and B are perceived as equal. More specifically, that is the period of certain survival equivalent to 50% of the uncertain longer survival.

1. The first task now is to estimate x, posing the hypothetical choice:

Looking at a glass ball we predict that you will live x years. There exists a magic pill that can make you live 40 years. However, this pill has one serious side-effect: 50% of people who take it die immediately. Do you want to take this pill?

The choice is therefore:

(A) no risk now and living x years for certain

(B) a very risky treatment with a chance of dying immediately of 0.50, but if treatment is successful, living 40 years

For which value of x are you indifferent between choice A and B?

This is your CE50.

2. The next task is to estimate x for the certainty equivalent 25 (CE25).

Looking at a glass ball we predict that you will live x years. There exists a magic pill that can make you live ... (fill in your CE50) years. However, this pill has one serious side-effect: 50% of people who take it die immediately. Do you want to take this pill?

The choice is therefore:

(A) no risk now and living x years for certain

(B) a very risky treatment with a chance of dying immediately of 0.50, but if treatment is successful, living ... (fill in your CE50) years

For which value of x are you indifferent between choice A and B?

This is your CE25.

3. The last certainty equivalent that we are going to estimate is the CE12.5.

Looking at a glass ball we predict that you will live x years. There exists a magic pill that can make you live ... (fill in your CE25) years. However, this pill has one serious side-effect: 50% of people who take it die immediately. Do you want to take this pill?

The choice is therefore:

(A) no risk now and living x years for certain

(B) a very risky treatment with a chance of dying immediately of 0.50, but if treatment is successful, living ... (fill in your CE25) years

For which value of x are you indifferent between choice A and B? This is your CE12.5.

4. Construct a utility curve with the life expectancy on the x-axis and your utility (certainty equivalent 50, 25, and 12.5) on the y-axis. Are you risk-neutral, risk-averse, or risk-seeking?

Exercise 4.5

Multiattribute utility for carpal tunnel syndrome

You are conducting a cost-effectiveness analysis of treatments for carpal tunnel syndrome. You plan to assign weights to health-related quality of life defined according to two attributes: dexterity and pain. A multi-attribute utility function for these two attributes is elicited by a survey of carpal tunnel syndrome patients. The survey yielded the following responses for a typical respondent:

Rating scale (visual analog) values:

Dexterity

D1	Full use of two hands and 10 fingers	1.0
D2	Limitations in use of hands or fingers, but does not require help	0.8
D3	Limitations in use of hands or fingers, requires help with some tasks	0.4
D4	Limitations in use of hands or fingers, requires help for all tasks	0.0

Pain

P1	No pain or discomfort	1.0
P2	Moderate pain	0.6
P3	Severe pain	0.0

Standard gambles:

(i) (D1,P3) ~ {0.4 (D1,P1), 0.6 (D4,P3)}

(ii) (D4,P1) ~ {0.7(D1,P1), 0.3 (D4,P3)}

(iii) Dead ~ (D4,P3)

(~ means 'equivalent to the gamble')

(a) Show how the value-utility transformations can be used to adjust the attribute-specific utility functions for dexterity and pain. Discuss the advantages and disadvantages of using rating scale values in utility assessment.

You may want to use the following value-utility transformation formulas:

Torrance: $(1 - u) = (1 - r)^{1.6}$

Weeks: $u = 1$ (for $r > 0.85$)

$u = 1.18 \times r$ (for $r < 0.85$)

where $u =$ utility and $r =$ rating scale.

(b) Derive a set of weights that can be used in estimating quality-adjusted life expectancy consistent with these preferences. Derive weights for all 12 possible combinations of attributes. State your assumptions clearly. (See Torrance et al., 1995, 1996 for details.)

(c) Suppose instead of (iii) that

Dead ~ {0.05 (D1,P1), 0.95 (D4,P3)},

i.e., the worst health state is worse than death. What weights should now be used in calculating QALYs?

(d) Suppose now that the standard gambles yield the following, instead of (i–iii):

(i') (D1,P3) ~ {0.4 (D1,P1), 0.6 (D4,P3)}

(ii') (D3,P1) ~ {0.8 (D1,P1), 0.2 (D4,P3)}

(iii') Dead ~ (D4,P3)

What is the appropriate weight for the state (D2,P2)? Remember to state any necessary assumptions.

Exercise 4.6

Risk–risk trade-offs

A method of utility assessment that is being employed more frequently, particularly in the context of environmental risks, is the 'risk–risk trade-off' (RRTO). Like the standard gamble (SG), the RRTO involves hypothetical choices under uncertainty. Unlike the SG, in which one of the hypothetical options is the certainty of experiencing the health state of interest, the RRTO presents *both* alternatives as gambles.

For example, a Stanford University study of preferences used the following RRTO to elicit utilities for health states seen in a rare genetically transmitted disorder called Gaucher disease. Subjects were presented pictures and descriptions of a number of such states. For each state G, the following RRTO was elicited:

$$(P, H; 1 - P, G) \sim (q, H; 1 - q, D)$$

($\sim$ means 'is equivalent to')

where H denotes perfect health and D denotes death. The variable P was fixed by the interviewer, and the respondent was asked to give the value of q that results in indifference between the two risky gambles.

For one state, G^*, for which the probability P was set at 0.97, the mean response q was 0.98. (Hint: It may be helpful to draw the decision tree corresponding to the above statement.)

(a) On a scale where $u(H) = 1$ and $u(D) = 0$, what does this result imply about $u(G^*)$?

(b) In a validation question, a standard gamble involving health state G^* was administered, and the average response was 0.8. Specifically,

$$G^* \sim (0.8, H: 0.2, D)$$

Apply behavioral decision theory to explain the source of the discrepancy.

(d) Which result would you believe, and which would you use in a decision analysis of treatments for Gaucher disease? (Hint: There is no 'correct' answer!)

REFERENCES

Beck, A.T., Ward, C.H., Mendelson, M., Mock, J. & Erbaugh, J. (1961). An inventory for measuring depression. *Arch. Gen. Psych.*, **4**, 53–63.

Bell, C.M., Chapman, R.H., Stone, P.W. et al. (2001). An off-the-shelf help list: a comprehensive catalog of preference scores from published cost utility analyses. *Med. Decis. Making*, **21**, 288–94.

Bleichrodt, H. & Amiram, G. (1996). Time preference, the discounted utility model and health. *J. Health Econ.*, **15**, 49–67.

Bleichrodt, H. & Johannesson, M. (1997). The validity of QALYs: an experimental test of constant proportional trade-off and utility independence. *Med. Decis. Making*, **17**, 21–32.

Bosch, J.L. & Hunink, M.G.M. (1996). The relationship between descriptive and valuational quality-of-life measures in patients with intermittent claudication. *Med. Decis. Making*, **16**, 217–25.

Brock, D.W. & Wartman, S.A. (1990). When competent patients make irrational choices [see comments]. *N. Engl. J. Med.*, **322**, 1595–9.

Chapman, G.B. & Elstein, A.S. (2000). Cognitive processes and biases in medical decision making. In: *Decision Making in Health Care*, ed. G.B. Chapman & F.A.

Sonnenberg. New York: Cambridge University Press.

Christensen-Szalanski, J.J. (1984). Discount functions and the measurement of patients' values. Woman's decisions during childbirth. *Med. Decis. Making,* **4**, 47–58.

Connolly, T., Arkes, H.R. & Hammond, K.R. (eds) (1999). *Judgment and Decision Making: An Interdisciplinary Reader,* 2nd edn. Cambridge: Cambridge University Press.

Degner, L.F. & Sloan, J.A. (1992). Decision making during serious illness: what role do patients really want to play? *J. Clin. Epidemiol.,* **45**, 941–50.

Dolan, P. (1997). Modeling valuations for EuroQol health states. *Med. Care,* **35**, 1095–108.

Feeney, D.H., Torrance, G.W. & Furlong, W.J. (1996). Health utilities index. In: *Quality of Life and Pharmacoeconomics in Clinical Trials,* ed. B. Spilker, pp. 239–52. Philadelphia, PA: Lippincott-Raven.

Fryback, D.G., Lawrence, W.F., Martin, P.A., Klein, R. & Klein, B.E. (1997). Predicting quality of well-being scores from the SF-36: results from the Beaver Dam health outcomes study. *Med. Decis. Making,* **17**, 1–9.

Gafni, A. (1991). Willingness-to-pay as a measure of benefits. Relevant questions in the context of public decision making about health care programs. *Med. Care,* **29**, 1246–52.

Gillick, M.R. (1988). Talking with patients about risk. *J. Gen. Intern. Med.,* **3**, 166–70.

Gold, M.R., Siegel, J.E., Russell, L.B. & Weinstein, M.C. (1996). *Cost-effectiveness in Health and Medicine: Report of the Panel on Cost-Effectiveness in Health and Medicine.* New York: Oxford University Press.

Gold, M.R., Franks, P., McCoy, K.I. & Fryback, D.G. (1998). Toward consistency in cost–utility analyses: using national measures to create condition-specific values [see comments]. *Med. Care,* **36**, 778–92.

Hillner, B.E. & Smith, T.J. (1991). Efficacy and cost effectiveness of adjuvant chemotherapy in women with node-negative breast cancer. A decision-analysis model. *N. Engl. J. Med.,* **324**, 160–8.

Jansen, S.J., Stiggelbout, A.M., Wakker, P.P. et al. (1998). Patients' utilities for cancer treatments: a study of the chained procedure for the standard gamble and time tradeoff. *Med. Decis. Making,* **18**, 391–9.

Johannesson, M., Pliskin, J.S. & Weinstein, M.C. (1994). A note on QALYs, time tradeoff, and discounting. *Med. Decis. Making,* **14**, 188–93.

Kahneman, D. & Tversky, A. (1984). Choices, values and frames. *Am. Psychol.* **39**, 341–50.

Kuhberger, A. (1998). The influence of framing on risky decisions: a meta-analysis. *Org. Behav. Hum. Decis. Processes,* **75**, 23–55.

Man-Son-Hing, M., Laupacis, A., O'Connor, A.M. et al. (1999). A patient decision aid regarding antithrombotic therapy for stroke prevention in atrial fibrillation: a randomized controlled trial [see comments]. *J.A.M.A.,* **282**, 737–43.

McHorney, C.A., Ware, J.E. Jr & Raczek, A.E. (1993). The MOS 36-Item Short-Form Health Survey (SF-36): II. Psychometric and clinical tests of validity in measuring physical and mental health constructs. *Med. Care*, **31**, 247–63.

McNeil, B.J., Pauker, S.G., Sox, H.C. Jr & Tverski, A. (1982). On the elicitation of preferences for alternative therapies. *N. Engl. J. Med.*, **306**, 1259–62.

O'Brien, B. & Gafni, A. (1996). When do the 'dollars' make sense? Toward a conceptual framework for contingent valuation studies in health care. *Med. Decis. Making*, **16**, 288–99.

O'Brien, B. & Viramontes, J.L. (1994). Willingness to pay: a valid and reliable measure of health state preference? *Med. Decis. Making*, **14**, 289–97.

Patrick, D.L., Starks, H.E., Cain, K.C., Uhlmann, R.F. & Pearlman, R.A. (1994). Measuring preferences for health states worse than death. *Med. Decis. Making*, **14**, 9–18.

Pauker, S.P. & Pauker, S.G. (1987). The amniocentesis decision: ten years of decision analytic experience. *Birth Defects: Orig. Art. Ser.*, **23**, 151–69.

Raiffa, H. (1968). *Decision Analysis: Introductory Lectures on Choices under Uncertainty*, 1st edn. New York: Random House.

Richardson, J. & Nord, E. (1997). The importance of perspective in the measurement of quality-adjusted life years. *Med. Decis. Making*, **17**, 33–41.

Schrag, D., Kuntz, K.M., Garber, J.E. & Weeks, J.C. (1997). Decision analysis – effects of prophylactic mastectomy and oophorectomy on life expectancy among women with BRCA1 or BRCA2 mutations. *N. Engl. J. Med.*, **336**, 1465–71.

Stiggelbout, A.M. (2000). Assessing patients' preferences. In: *Decision Making in Health Care*, ed. G.B. Chapman & F.A. Sonnenberg, pp. 289–312. New York: Cambridge University Press.

Torrance, G.W. (1986). Measurement of health state utilities for economic appraisal; a review. *J. Health Econom.*, **5**, 1–30.

Torrance, G.W., Furlong, W., Feeny, D,H. & Boyle, M. (1995). Multi-attribute preference functions: Health Utilities Index. *PharmacoEconomics*, **7**, 503–20.

Torrance, G.W., Feeny, D.H., Furlong, W.J. et al. (1996). Multiattribute utility function for a comprehensive health status classification system. Health Utilities Index mark 2. *Med. Care*, **34**, 702–22.

Tsevat, J., Weeks, J.C., Guadagnoli, E. et al. (1994). Using health-related quality-of-life information: clinical encounters, clinical trials, and health policy. *J. Gen. Intern. Med.*, **9**, 576–82.

Tversky, A. & Kahneman, D. (1981). The framing of decisions and the psychology of choice. *Science*, **211**, 453–8.

Von Neumann, J. & Morgenstern, O. (1944). *Theory of Games and Economic Behavior*. Princeton, NJ: Princeton University Press.

Wakker, P. (1996). A criticism of healthy-years equivalents [see comments]. *Med. Decis. Making*, **16**, 207–14.

Ware, J.E. Jr & Sherbourne, C.D. (1992). The MOS 36-item short-form health survey (SF-36). I. Conceptual framework and item selection. *Med. Care*, **30**, 473–83.

5

Interpreting diagnostic information

The interpretation of new information depends on what was already known about the patient.

Harold Sox

5.1 Diagnostic information and probability revision

Physicians have at their disposal an enormous variety of diagnostic information to guide them in decision making. Diagnostic information comes from talking to the patient (symptoms, such as pain, nausea, and breathlessness), examining the patient (signs, such as abdominal tenderness, fever, and blood pressure), and from diagnostic tests (such as blood tests, X-rays, and electrocardiograms (EKGs)) and screening tests (such as Papanicolaou smears for cervical cancer or cholesterol measurements).

Physicians are not the only ones that have to interpret diagnostic information. Public policy makers in health care are equally concerned with understanding the performance of diagnostic tests. If, for example, a policy maker is considering a screening program for lung cancer, he/she will need to understand the performance of the diagnostic tests that can detect lung cancer in an early phase of the disease. In public policy making other types of 'diagnostic tests' may also be relevant. For example, a survey with a questionnaire in a population sample can be considered analogous to a diagnostic test. And performing a trial to determine the efficacy of a treatment is in fact a 'test' with the goal of getting more information about that treatment.

Obtaining information may be expensive, risky, or both. The purpose of information, however it is obtained, is to aid in deciding on the best further management. Most of this information is, however, subject to some degree of error. Both false positives and false negatives are possible, the rates of which will differ between different pieces of information. Hence we must examine how to interpret and select information to minimize the impact of such errors. Let us consider an example.

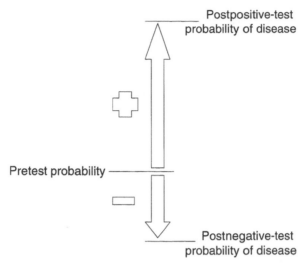

Postpositive-test
probability of disease

Pretest probability

Postnegative-test
probability of disease

Figure 5.1   Probability revision: the pretest probability is revised upward if the test is positive or downward if the test is negative.

Example	A 50-year-old man presents with fatigue, and the initial workup shows an iron-deficiency anemia. You do a fecal occult blood test (FOBT), to check whether gastrointestinal bleeding, particularly from a colorectal cancer, is present and this is found to be positive. You are aware, however, that the FOBT is not perfectly accurate in detecting cancers: some cancers are not bleeding and are missed (false negatives), and there are other causes of apparent bleeding (false positives). How do you interpret the FOBT?

This chapter will be concerned with the process of using such imperfect diagnostic information to reassess the probability that a patient has one of several possible diseases. When a test result is 'positive' we are interested in 'the probability of a disease given a positive test result' (Figure 5.1). In probability notation, this is written as $P(D+ \mid T+)$. When a test result is 'negative,' we are interested in 'the probability of a disease given a negative test result.' In probability notation, this is written as $P(D+ \mid T-)$. Sometimes the patient may have one of more than two diseases ($D_1, D_2, D_3 \ldots D_i \ldots$), and the possible test results ($R_1, R_2, R_3 \ldots R_j \ldots$) may not be easily characterized as 'positive' and 'negative.' An example might be a patient with acute abdominal pain who presents with a constellation of symptoms and signs, white blood cell counts, and other test results, and who may have appendicitis, pancreatitis, or other causes of pain. In such cases, we are interested in $P(D_i \mid R_j)$, the probability of each diagnosis given the test result(s).

DEFINITIONS

The *pretest (prior) probability of disease* is the probability of the presence of the target disease conditional on the available information prior to performing the test under consideration.

The *posttest (posterior) probability of disease* is the probability of the presence of the target disease conditional on the pretest information and the test result.

Probability revision is the process of converting the pretest probability to the posttest probability taking the test result into account.

Usually, estimates of probabilities of disease, conditional upon test results, are not readily available. Instead, one is more likely to have an assessment of the probability of a test result among patients with or without the disease. For example, there may be a study which reports $P(T+ \mid D+)$, the probability of a positive test given the presence of disease, and $P(T+ \mid D-)$, the probability of a positive test given the absence of disease. This chapter is concerned with the process of converting probabilities of this latter type (test results given disease) to probabilities of the type we usually want to help guide decision making (disease given test results). We discover quickly that this process also depends on assessing some pretest probability of the disease, $P(D+)$. The process of taking the test result into account by converting the pretest probability, $P(D+)$, to a posttest probability of disease, $P(D+ \mid T+)$ or $P(D+ \mid T-)$, is called probability revision.

The posttest probability will depend both on the pretest probability and the information obtained from the test. The aim of this chapter is to introduce both the methods of calculation and theory behind calculating the posttest probability.

We begin with a discussion on pretest probabilities, then discuss how test accuracy is measured, and subsequently examine how measures are used to calculate posttest probability. However, we emphasize here that, although it is important to understand how the calculations are done for purposes of formal decision analysis, the concepts themselves can be very helpful in the clinical setting even without explicit calculation. Charts and graphs can replace the actual calculations. This chapter will emphasize tests with two possible outcomes, and Chapter 6 will look at how and when such tests should alter clinical decisions. Chapter 7 expands upon the material in this and the next chapter, assisting the decision maker to assess more generally the value of diagnostic test information when there are more than two possible test results, and when there is more than one test available.

5.1.1 Prevalence and pretest probability

If a patient were chosen at random from a given population, the pretest probability of disease for the patient would be the disease prevalence in that population.

However, patients are not selected at random. Nor are candidates for screening selected at random. Each person who presents for a possible test has specific characteristics, including history, physical findings, and previ-

DEFINITION

Disease *prevalence* is the frequency of existing disease in the population of interest at a given point in time.

ous test results. These characteristics, along with the disease prevalence, determine the probability that an individual has any given disease at any point in time. This probability is conditional upon already available information and may be taken as the pretest probability with respect to a subsequent test. For example, the pretest probability that a patient has colorectal cancer before the FOBT level has been determined will be adjusted based on age, gender, clinical history, and family history. In that sense, the prior probability is actually a posterior probability that is conditional upon all of these factors (for example, the probability of colorectal cancer in a 50-year-old male whose mother had colorectal cancer) while it is still a prior probability with respect to the FOBT test. The prior probability here reflects the proportion of patients with similar characteristics in whom colorectal cancer would be expected.

This chapter will focus on diagnostic tests that have only two outcomes, positive $(T+)$ or negative $(T-)$, and a single disease so that we may divide the tested group into those with the disease $(D+)$ and those without the disease, the nondiseased $(D-)$.

5.1.2 The 2×2 table for the FOBT and colorectal cancer

How will you interpret positive and negative FOBTs in the example? First, we need to understand the accuracy of the test by quantifying the error rates. To obtain the error rates, you might consult the literature. You find a study of an immunochemical FOBT, the results of which are shown in Table 5.1.

The table clearly demonstrates that the FOBT is imperfect. Using the terms in Table 5.1B, there were 5 false negatives, that is, 5 patients with colorectal cancer whose FOBT was negative; there were 271 false positives, that is, people without colorectal cancer who showed a positive FOBT. We shall use Table 5.1 to define some important probabilities that describe the rates of these errors. Using these probabilities we will introduce the concept of probability revision. Specifically, we will calculate the probability that a patient has colorectal cancer (CRC) given a positive fecal occult blood test result (FOBT), or $P(\text{CRC} + \mid \text{FOBT} +)$. In the process we will also calculate several other probabilities that we will find useful for decision making. One of these is the probability that a patient has colorectal cancer given a negative FOBT, or $P(\text{CRC} + \mid \text{FOBT} -)$. Since a patient either has or does not have colorectal cancer, we can apply the summation principle to calculate the probabilities of *not* having colorectal cancer, conditional

Table 5.1. (A) Results of 7211 screens for colorectal cancer with an immunochemical test for fecal occult blood (FOBT) in 'high-risk' but asymptomatic patients. (B) Terms for the four cells of the 2 × 2 table

(A) FOBT	Disease status			(B) General	Disease status	
FOBT result	Colorectal cancer	No colorectal cancer	Totals	Test result	Disease	No disease
Positive	24	271	295	Positive	True positive TP	False positive FP
Negative	5	6911	6916	Negative	False negative FN	True negative TN
	29	7182	7211		Total disease TP + FN	Total no-disease FP + TN

(A) Data from Weller et al. (1994) with permission.

upon the test results, as 1.0 minus the corresponding probability of having cancer.

Also of interest, and a byproduct of the process of probability revision, is the probability that the FOBT will be positive, or $P(T+)$. As we will demonstrate, the probability of a positive test result is not necessarily the same as the probability that disease is present, $P(D+)$. Why might we be interested in the probability of a positive test? There may be follow-up tests and procedures induced by positive tests, which have risks and costs themselves. In the case of a positive FOBT, patients may then undergo colonoscopy (endoscopic procedure of the large intestine) to confirm the presence of cancer, a procedure that not only has a modest risk of morbidity and mortality, but also causes discomfort and anxiety (loss of quality-of-life-related utility). And from the viewpoint of a health-care payer or society, the cost of the colonoscopy would also be triggered by a positive FOBT.

5.1.3 Two important conditional probabilities: sensitivity and specificity

Consider the proportion of patients with colorectal cancer who have a positive FOBT test result. This proportion is 24/29, or about 0.83 (83%). This is the probability of a positive test result given that the disease is present; it may be expressed symbolically as $P(T+ \mid D+)$. We call this probability the *sensitivity* or *true-positive ratio* (TPR) of the test. Similarly, the proportion of patients without the disease who have a negative test result is 6911/7182 or about 0.96 (96%). This probability of a negative test result given that the disease is absent is denoted by $P(T- \mid D-)$ and is called the *specificity* or *true-negative ratio* (TNR) of the test.

Sensitivity and specificity describe how often the test is correct (in the diseased and nondiseased groups respectively); they are two independent values. The complement of the sensitivity, that is $(1.0 - TPR)$, is the proportion of patients with disease who have a negative test result, or $P(T- \mid D+)$; this is called the *false-negative ratio* (FNR) of the test. In the example the false-negative ratio is 5/29, which equals 0.17 (17%). We could have obtained FNR as $1 - TPR$, or $100\% - 83\% = 17\%$. The complement of the specificity, that is $(1.0 - TNR)$, is the proportion of patients without the disease who have a positive test result, or $P(T+ \mid D-)$; this is called the *false-positive ratio* (FPR) of the test and, for the FOBT in Table 5.1, is equal to 271/7182, which equals 0.04 (4%). We could have obtained FPR as $1 - TNR$, or $100\% - 96\% = 4\%$.

Thus, we have derived four proportions from the 2×2 table: sensitivity and specificity which are two independent values to describe how often the test is correct, and the false-negative and false-positive ratios which are two independent values to describe how often the test is in error. The formal definitions of these terms are as follows:

DEFINITIONS

Consider a test with two results, positive $(T+)$ and negative $(T-)$, used to distinguish between two disease states, $D+$ (disease present) and $D-$ (disease absent).

The *sensitivity* or *true-positive ratio (TPR)* is the proportion of patients with the target disease who have a positive test result. In probability notation this is $P(T+ \mid D+)$.

The *specificity* or *true-negative ratio (TNR)* is the proportion of patients without the target disease who have a negative test result. In probability notation this is $P(T- \mid D-)$.

The *false-positive ratio (FPR)* is the proportion of patients without the target disease who have a positive test result. In probability notation this is $P(T+ \mid D-)$.

The *false-negative ratio (FNR)* is the proportion of patients with the target disease who have a negative test result. In probability notation this is $P(T- \mid D+)$.

A sensitive test, one with a high true-positive (and low false-negative) ratio, is very good at detecting patients with the target disease (sensitive to the presence of disease). A specific test, one with a low false-positive (and high true-negative) ratio, is very good at screening out patients who do not have the disease (and hence specific to that disease). Remember that test sensitivity applies to patients with the disease; test specificity applies to patients without the disease. A test may have a high sensitivity and a low specificity, a low sensitivity and a high specificity, both a high sensitivity and a high specificity, or both a low sensitivity and a low specificity.

Observe that the true-positive ratio and the false-negative ratio sum to 1.0, or 100%, and that the true-negative ratio and false-positive ratio also sum to 1.0, or 100%. An ideal test has a true-positive ratio of 1.0 (and therefore a false-negative ratio of 0.0) and a false-positive ratio of 0.0 (and therefore a true negative ratio of 1.0). The definitions of these probabilities and others to be introduced in this chapter are summarized in Table 5.2.

5.1.4 Posttest probabilities: the postpositive-test and postnegative-test probabilities

> **DEFINITIONS**
>
> The *postpositive-test probability of disease* or *predictive value positive* is the probability that a patient with a positive test result has the target disease. In probability notation it is written as $P(D+ \mid T+)$.
>
> The *postnegative-test probability of disease* is the probability that a patient with a negative test result has the target disease. In probability notation it is written as $P(D+ \mid T-)$.

Although sensitivity and specificity are important characteristics of a test, they are not the probabilities we need to decide how to treat a patient. Sensitivity and specificity are the probabilities of test results given the presence or absence of disease. However, in health-care practice we do not know whether or not someone has the disease, but rather we find a test result is positive or negative, and from this information we wish to infer the probability of disease. Thus we usually need to know the probabilities of disease given positive or negative test results, which, as we shall see, may turn out to be very different.

For an individual selected randomly from the study population upon which the estimates of sensitivity and specificity were based (Table 5.1), the probability of disease given a positive test result, $P(D+ \mid T+)$, may be obtained from the 2×2 table. This probability is calculated as TP/(TP + FP), which is the proportion of those with positive test results (TP + FP) who also have the disease (TP). We call this the *postpositive-test probability of disease* or *predictive value positive* of the test. (Our terminology here follows Vecchio. Some authors use other terms for this proportion, and the same is true for many other concepts defined in this book. Since there are no universally recognized conventions, we have tried to adopt the most widely used nomenclature.) In our study population the postpositive-test probability of disease would be 24/295, which is approximately 0.08 or 8%. *The postnegative-test probability of disease* is the conditional probability of having the disease given a negative test result, or $P(D+ \mid T-)$. It may be calculated as FN/(FN + TN) from Table 5.1B. In the example the postnegative-test probability in the study population is 5/6916, or approximately 0.0007.

A related term is the *predictive value negative*, which is the probability

Table 5.2. Various probabilities related to diagnostic tests

Common name	Meaning	Probability notation	Equivalent probability	Estimate from 2×2 table from study sample
Sensitivity True-positive ratio (TPR)	Frequency of positive test results in those with the target disease	$P(T+ \mid D+)$	$1 - P(T- \mid D+)$	TP/(TP + FN)
False-negative ratio (FNR)	Frequency of negative test results in those with the target disease	$P(T- \mid D+)$	$1 - P(T+ \mid D+)$	FN/(TP + FN)
Specificity True-negative ratio (TNR)	Frequency of negative test results in those without the target disease	$P(T- \mid D-)$	$1 - P(T+ \mid D-)$	TN/(TN + FP)
False-positive ratio (FPR)	Frequency of positive test results in those without the target disease	$P(T+ \mid D-)$	$1 - P(T- \mid D-)$	FP/(TN + FP)
Pretest probability of disease	Frequency of target disease in the population of interest. Prevalence in population of interest	$P(D+)$	$1 - P(D-)$	Requires independent estimate
Pretest probability of nondisease	Frequency of absence of target disease in the population of interest	$P(D-)$	$1 - P(D+)$	Requires independent estimate
Postpositive-test probability of disease (predictive value positive)	Frequency of target disease in those with positive results	$P(D+ \mid T+)$	$1 - P(D- \mid T+)$	Requires knowledge of pretest probability
Postnegative-test probability of nondisease (predictive value negative)	Frequency of absence of target disease in those with negative results	$P(D- \mid T-)$	$1 - P(D+ \mid T-)$	Requires knowledge of pretest probability
Ratio of test positives	Frequency of positive test results in the population	$P(T+)$	$1 - P(T-)$	Requires knowledge of pretest probability

that a patient with a negative test does not have the target disease, that is, $P(D- \mid T-)$. In terms of the discussion at the beginning of the chapter, the predictive value positive and the predictive value negative are both examples of posttest (or posterior) probabilities.

We have seen that patients in the study population who have a positive FOBT have an 8% probability of colorectal cancer. But recall that this study population was asymptomatic. In that population 29 persons had colorectal cancer and 7182 persons did not have colorectal cancer. Would these posttest probabilities also apply to patients with iron-deficiency anemia, as in our clinical example? Would they apply to a more generally selected population, such as in mass screening? In general, the answer is no to both questions. The estimates of the posttest probabilities obtained directly from Table 5.1 apply only to the study population. Unless the proportion of patients with the disease in the study population equals the proportion of patients with the disease in the population in which the test will be applied, these posttest probabilities will not apply. In general, the test characteristics sensitivity and specificity are conditional on whether disease is present or not and are usually generalizable across settings. The posttest probabilities are not test characteristics and are not generalizable because they depend on the pretest probability of disease.

To estimate the posttest probabilities for our patients, we need an independent estimate of the probability of the disease in the population from which our patient is selected, an estimate of the pretest (or prior) probability of disease. That is, we require a procedure that will permit us to carry over our information from the study population to the target population of interest. One way to do this, as we shall now see, is to construct a hypothetical table as if the study had been done in a population with the pretest probability in which we are interested.

5.1.5 Probability revision: using the 2 × 2 table

Let us return to the clinical example of the man with iron-deficiency anemia. In the study population of Table 5.1, 24 of 295 positives had cancer, and hence the postpositive-test probability was 24/295 or about 8.1%. Because this study was in an asymptomatic population, however, this estimate would be incorrect, because it assumes that the prevalence of the disease in the population from which our patient was selected is the same as the prevalence in the study population (0.4%). For patients presenting with iron-deficiency anemia, three recent studies showed cancer

Table 5.3. The steps in probability revision for the fecal occult blood test (FOBT) for the diagnosis of colorectal cancer (CRC) for a patient with a pre-test probability of CRC of 8%

FOBT result	CRC	No CRC	Total by row
Step 1: Use prevalence to fix column totals: 8% × 10 000 = 800			
Positive			
Negative			
Total by column	*800*	*9200*	*10 000*
Step 2: Use sensitivity to fill in disease column: 83% × 800 = 664			
Positive	*664*		
Negative	*136*		
Total by column	800	9200	10 000
Step 3: Use specificity to fill in nondisease column: 96% × 9200 = 8832			
Positive	664	*368*	
Negative	136	*8832*	
Total by column	800	9200	10 000
Step 4: Compute row totals: 664 + 368 = 1032			
Positive	664	368	*1032*
Negative	136	8832	*8968*
Total by column	800	9200	10 000

in 19 of 170, 11 of 100, and 2 of 114 patients. Pooling these results suggests a rate of 32 per 384 or about 8%, which is already almost as high as that among the FOBT positives in Weller's group.

The first step is to modify the column totals of Table 5.1 so that they reflect the prevalence in the population of concern. This is shown in Step 1 of Table 5.3, where the probability of colorectal cancer is fixed at 8% of a hypothetical cohort of 10 000 similar patients. The second step is to use the known true-positive ratio, or test sensitivity, to fill in the first column of the table. Since the sensitivity is 83%, this means that 83% of the 800 colorectal cancers, or 664 members (6.64%) of the hypothetical population, have the disease *and* a positive test result.

Similarly, 17% of those with colorectal cancer have a negative test result; hence, 17% of the 800, or 136 members (1.36%) of the population have the disease *and* a negative test result.

The third step (Table 5.3) is to use the known true-negative ratio, or test specificity, to fill in the second column of the table (i.e., the joint probabilities of no colorectal cancer and each possible test result). Since the true-negative ratio is 96%, this means that 96% of 9200 or 8832 members

(88.32%) of the population have no colorectal cancer and a negative test result and that 4% of 9200 or 368 members (3.68%) of the population have no colorectal cancer and a positive test result.

Finally, we complete the 2×2 table by filling in the numbers and proportions of test positives and test negatives. Those are simply the totals across the rows. Notice that the probability of a positive test is 10.32%, even though the pretest probability of cancer is only 8%. Evidently the false positives outnumber the false negatives. This is true even though the false-positive ratio of the test (4%) is less than its false-negative ratio (17%). Do you understand how this can be? (Hint: There are many more people without the disease than with the disease.)

With the 2×2 table completed, we can compute the probability of colorectal cancer given a positive FOBT test result in this population. Of the 1032 with positive test results, 664 have colorectal cancer and the remaining 368 do not. Therefore, 664/1032, or approximately 64%, of patients with iron-deficiency anemia and a positive FOBT test results actually have colorectal cancer. Contrast this result with the 8% that was obtained by implicitly assuming a disease prevalence of 0.4% (Table 5.1) rather than a prevalence of 8%. Clearly, the prevalence makes a difference!

The process we have just worked through is called probability revision. We start with a pretest probability of colorectal cancer, which in this case is 0.08. We observe a test result, which in this example is a positive FOBT test result. We revise the probability to obtain a posttest probability of colorectal cancer given the positive test result. In this example the posttest probability is 0.64.

The method shown in Table 5.3 can also be used to compute the postnegative-test probability of colorectal cancer. In Table 5.3, Step 4, the total number of patients with a negative test result is 8968. Included among these patients with a negative test result are 136 who have colorectal cancer. Therefore, the postnegative-test probability in this population is 136/8968 or approximately 0.015. This leaves a probability of not having colorectal cancer, given a negative test result, of 1.0 minus 0.015 or 0.985 (the predictive value negative).

To summarize the results for our 50-year-old man with anemia, we have revised our pretest probability of colorectal cancer as follows:
- Without an FOBT, we would assess $P(\text{CRC}) = 0.08$.
- If the FOBT result is positive, we calculate $P(\text{CRC} \mid \text{FOBT} +) = 0.64$.
- If the FOBT result is negative, we calculate $P(\text{CRC} \mid \text{FOBT} -) = 0.015$.
- The probability of a positive FOBT is $P(\text{FOBT} +) = 0.1032$.

5.1.6 The effect of prevalence in screening

We have seen that the interpretation of a test depended on the test characteristics (sensitivity and specificity) and on the pretest probability. Let us look at another example of this phenomenon in the context of screening.

Example

Your practice has called together a committee to consider screening all adult patients using FOBTs. You are concerned about the potential for missing cancers, and also about the anxiety and unnecessary investigation caused by falsely positive tests. Since you do not know how often these may occur, and how their occurrence may vary across different patient groups, you seek more detail about the accuracy and diagnostic implications of the test.

How should your committee interpret the FOBT in this screening setting? For this task you need to estimate the prevalence of colorectal cancer in a screening population. In a recent large trial, Mandel et al. (1999) provided figures from which we can calculate the prevalence of colorectal cancer as approximately 1 per 1000, 2 per 1000, and 3.5 per 1000 for persons aged 50–59, 60–69, and 70 + respectively. How does this observation modify the analysis? Let us repeat the steps above, but for the prevalence in the 50–59 age group, that is, 1 per 1000. Take a few minutes to try this yourself by filling out a 2×2 table using the four steps above before consulting Table 5.4. To facilitate the calculations it is prudent to start out with a total group of 100 000 subjects, or if you prefer to work with probabilities, be sure to carry at least five digits after the decimal point.

Now the posttest probability after a positive test result is 83/4079 or about 2%. In terms of probabilities this is 0.00083/0.04079, or about 0.02.

This postpositive-test probability of cancer for a screened person is less than the *pretest* probability for the 50-year-old anemic patient in our first clinical example, and similar to his *postnegative*-test probability. Clearly, the posttest probability depends strongly on the pretest probability of the group we apply the test to, and will strongly influence both how the person should be managed and what he or she should be told. For example, if we investigate patients with a positive FOBT in this screened group, the patient should know that, of 100 follow-up colonoscopies, only about two will show colorectal cancer.

Figure 5.2 illustrates how the post-FOBT probability varies according to the pre-FOBT probability.

In the next section we offer an alternative approach to probability

Table 5.4. The steps in probability revision for the fecal occult blood test (FOBT) for the diagnosis of colorectal cancer (CRC) in a screening situation with a pre-test probability of CRC of 0.1%

FOBT result	CRC	No CRC	Total by row
Step 1: Use prevalence to fix column totals			
Positive			
Negative			
Total by column	100	99 900	100 000
Step 2: Use sensitivity to fill in disease column			
Positive	83		
Negative	17		
Total by column	100	99 900	100 000
Step 3: Use specificity to fill in nondisease column			
Positive	83	3996	
Negative	17	95 904	
Total by column	100	99 900	100 000
Step 4: Compute row totals			
Positive	83	3996	4079
Negative	17	95 904	95 921
Total by column	100	99 900	100 000

revision, using the mathematics of probability. This device, known as Bayes' formula, is numerically equivalent to the method that uses 2×2 tables, although it may be easier to use in some circumstances. While not essential to the remainder of this book, an understanding of the formula and the mathematical basis of probability revision will help the reader with the applications that will be discussed in the next two chapters.

5.2 Bayes' formula

5.2.1 A review of probability notation

The manipulation of a contingency table and probability notation can be combined to yield an important generalization for the revision of pretest probabilities. Let us review the notation introduced in Chapter 2.

Recall that the expression $P(E)$ indicates the probability of event or condition E; $P(E \mid F)$ denotes the probability of E contingent upon the presence of F; and $P(E, F)$ stands for the probability of the joint occurrence

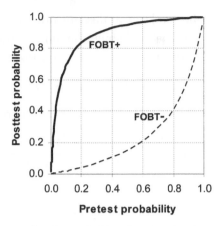

Figure 5.2 Postfecal occult blood test (FOBT) probability depending on the pre-FOBT probability and the test result, either positive (FOBT +) or negative (FOBT −).

of both E and F. The term $P(D+)$, therefore, simply means the probability of disease, or the prevalence; $P(T+ \mid D+)$ denotes the probability that an individual has a positive test result given the presence of disease, which is a relation we expressed earlier in this chapter as the test sensitivity; and $P(T+, D+)$ means the probability of both a positive test result and the presence of disease.

With this notation in mind, let us return to the example of FOBT and colorectal cancer.

5.2.2 Derivation of Bayes' formula

Recall from the laws of probability that we can write the joint probability in terms of conditional probabilities:

$$P(T+, D+) = P(D+ \mid T+) \, P(T+)$$

Dividing both sides of the equation by $P(T+)$ we get:

$$P(D+ \mid T+) = P(T+, D+)/P(T+) \tag{5.1}$$

that is, the probability of disease among patients with a positive test result equals the proportion of those with a positive result that are also diseased.

What proportion of patients have a positive test result? Positive results can occur in two ways: true positives among the diseased and false positives among the nondiseased. That is:

$$P(T+) = P(T+, D+) + P(T+, D-)$$

Each term on the right-hand side of this equation can be factored according to the laws of conditional probability, but now we will condition on the presence or absence of disease rather than on the test result:

$$P(T+) = P(T+ \mid D+)\, P(D+) + P(T+ \mid D-)\, P(D-) \tag{5.2}$$

If we substitute Equation 5.2 into Equation 5.1, we derive the following:

$$P(D+ \mid T+) = \frac{P(T+ \mid D+)\, P(D+)}{P(T+ \mid D+)\, P(D+) + P(T+ \mid D-)\, P(D-)}$$

(Bayes' formula) $\tag{5.3}$

Equation 5.3 is known as Bayes' formula for a dichotomous ($+$ or $-$) test and two disease states. In the next two chapters we will generalize this expression for multiple test outcomes and multiple diseases. We could also write Equation 5.3 using words rather than probability notation, as follows:

Postpositive-test probability =

$$\frac{\text{Sensitivity} \times \text{pretest probability}}{(\text{Sensitivity} \times \text{pretest probability} + (1 - \text{specificity}) \times (1 - \text{pretest probability}))}$$

More generally, we can write the above equation for interpreting any test result, R, as,

$$P(D+ \mid R+) = \frac{P(R \mid D+)\, P(D+)}{P(R \mid D+)\, P(D+) + P(R \mid D-)\, P(D-)}$$

(Bayes' formula) $\tag{5.4}$

The derivation is identical to the derivation in the dichotomous case.

5.2.3 Applying Bayes' formula

Applying Bayes' formula to our first example of a 50-year-old-man with iron-deficiency anemia, we can calculate his posttest probabilities of having colorectal cancer as follows:

If he has a positive FOBT:

$$P(\text{CRC}+ \mid \text{FOBT}+) = 0.83 \times 0.08/(0.83 \times 0.08 + 0.04 \times 0.92) = 0.64$$

If he has a negative FOBT:

$$P(\text{CRC}+ \mid \text{FOBT}-) = 0.17 \times 0.08/(0.17 \times 0.08 + 0.96 \times 0.92) = 0.015$$

Both of these results agree with what we obtained in the analysis using 2×2 tables. The above equations are both forms of Bayes' formula (also called

Bayes' theorem: Bayes' theorem was developed by the eighteenth-century mathematician Reverend Thomas Bayes). They incorporate two kinds of data: pretest probabilities of the presence or absence of disease, and information about the characteristics of a given test in individuals with and without disease, or a test's true-positive and false-positive ratios. This information is combined to yield a new probability of the presence of disease in the patient who is the subject of the test. It is in this sense that we refer to test results as revising or modifying our pretest probabilities of disease.

We began this analysis in response to the question: 'What is the probability of disease in an individual with a positive test result?' The result is given in Bayes' formula by the ratio of the number of individuals who have the disease and whose test results are positive to the number of all those individuals whose test results are positive.

5.3 Bayes' theorem with tree inversion

Thus far we applied Bayes' theorem using a 2×2 table and subsequently using a formula. If you look back at the arithmetic you performed while filling in the 2×2 table and the arithmetic involved in using the formula you will notice that, in fact, it was exactly the same arithmetic. There is yet another method to do the exact same exercise which may be more appealing to some. Using a chance tree we can visualize the probabilities and then invert the chance tree.

Figure 5.3 visualizes the probabilities relevant for the first case example. The upper chance tree first divides into colorectal cancer vs. no colorectal cancer with the associated pretest probability of disease. Subsequently, conditional on the presence or absence of colorectal cancer, the probabilities of a positive vs. negative FOBT result are depicted. This chance tree represents the pretest probability of disease and the test sensitivity and specificity (Figure 5.4). To calculate the posttest probabilities of disease we need to invert the chance tree so that the tree first models the test result and then the disease status conditional on the test result (Figure 5.4). We calculate the number of cases (or equivalently the probability) for each path through the tree (Figure 5.3), which is equivalent to filling in the cells of the 2×2 table. These numbers are copied to the ends of the branches of the inverted chance tree. The frequency of a positive test result is calculated by summing the true- and false-positive results and the frequency of a negative test result is calculated by summing the true- and false-negative results, which is equivalent to computing the row totals of the 2×2 table. Finally, we can calculate the posttest probabilities by dividing the path

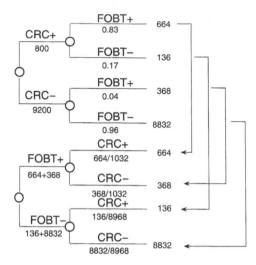

Figure 5.3   Tree inversion to perform probability revision for the fecal occult blood test (FOBT) for the diagnosis of colorectal cancer (CRC) for a patient with a pretest probability of colorectal cancer of 8%.

frequencies by the test result totals. Again, notice the analogy to what we did using the 2×2 table.

In Chapter 3 we discussed the importance of sequencing chance nodes in the correct order. Going from left to right, a decision tree should depict the sequence of events as they may occur over time. To model chronologically we would want to model the test result first and then the true disease status. As we can see here, it can sometimes be convenient to model it the other way round, that is, model disease status first followed by the test result. The advantage is that you can use the pretest probability of disease and sensitivity and specificity in your tree and let the model do the probability revision for you. Because the path probabilities are the same, the end result is the same provided that there are no intervening decisions or events that may influence the course of the disease or affect the probabilities thereafter. The next management decision should always be modeled conditional on the test result, which you observe, and not on the true disease status, which is the underlying truth but unknown to the decision maker as long as a reference test has not (yet) been performed.

5.4 The odds-likelihood-ratio form of Bayes' formula

Bayes' formula, even in the dichotomous (disease vs. nondisease) situation, is too complicated for most people to do as a mental calculation. The 2×2

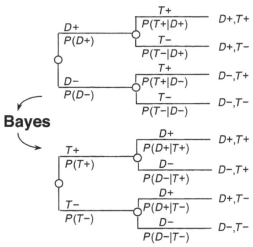

Figure 5.4 Tree inversion to perform probability revision with probability notation.

table also requires calculation aids. For a situation when a quick estimate of revised probabilities is needed, many people find the odds-likelihood-ratio version of Bayes' formula easier to use. This version of Bayes' formula is also instructive in that it highlights the relations between the pretest and posterior probabilities. It makes use of the concepts of odds and likelihood ratio, which we define at this point. It also forms the basis for a simple pocket nomogram for rapidly working out posttest probabilities. Finally, we shall find this form of Bayes' theorem invaluable when we turn to the analysis of multiple-valued or continuous-valued test results and the choice of a positivity criterion for such tests, a subject to which we turn in Chapter 7.

5.4.1 Odds

DEFINITION

Let P be the probability of an event. Define the following:

Odds favoring the event
$(O) = P/(1-P)$

Odds against the event
$(O_A) = (1-P)/P$

If the probability that an event will occur is P, then the probability that it will not occur is $1 - P$. An event that has a 20% chance of occurring has a corresponding 80% chance of not occurring. Recall from Chapter 2 that the ratio of P to $1 - P$, or $P/(1 - P)$, is called the *odds* favoring the occurrence of an event. The odds against the occurrence of an event can be expressed as $(1 - P)/P$.

If an event has a 0.20 probability of occurrence, the odds favoring are $0.2/0.8$, or 0.25, and the odds against are $0.8/0.2$, or 4 (sometimes written $4:1$ and read 'four to one'). If an event has a 50% chance of occurrence, then odds favoring and odds against are both $0.5/0.5$, or $1:1$, which are called 'even odds.' As probability varies from 0.0 to 1.0, the corresponding

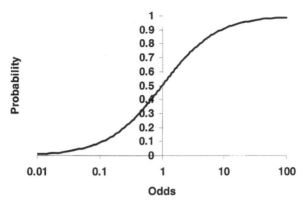

Figure 5.5   Relationship between odds and probability.

odds favoring range from 0 to infinity, and the odds against range from infinity to 0. The relationship of odds and probability may be shown graphically as in Figure 5.5, where each unit on the horizontal axis increases by a multiple of 10.

We can also reverse the calculation if we know the odds (or odds against) and want to determine the probability by using the equations:

$$P = O/(1+O)$$

and

$$P = 1/(1+O_A)$$

(In a horse race, the odds given each horse are odds against that horse winning. Thus, if a horse is given odds of $4:1$, its probability of winning is 20%, because $0.2 = 1/(1+4)$.)

5.4.2 Probability revision using odds

The posttest probability of disease is related to the pretest probability and the test characteristics, through Bayes' formula (Equation 5.4):

$$P(D+ \mid R) = \frac{P(R \mid D+) \ P(D+)}{P(R \mid D+) \ P(D+) + P(R \mid D-) \ P(D-)}$$

Now consider the analog of Bayes' formula for the nondiseased state:

$$P(D- \mid R) = \frac{P(R \mid D-) \ P(D-)}{P(R \mid D+) \ P(D+) + P(R \mid D-) \ P(D-)}$$

If we divide the first equation by the second equation, we get the simple formula:

$$\frac{P(D+ \mid R)}{P(D- \mid R)} = \frac{P(D+)}{P(D-)} \frac{P(R \mid D+)}{P(R \mid D-)} \tag{5.5}$$

This version of Bayes' formula is expressed in terms of odds rather than probabilities. Remember that the odds favoring an event with a probability of P equals $P/(1-P)$. The first ratio on the right-hand side of the equation, $P(D+)/P(D-)$, is therefore the pretest odds favoring disease. For example, if we started with a pretest probability $P(D+)$ equal to 0.1, the pretest odds would be $0.1/0.9$, or $1/9$. The ratio on the far left, $P(D+ \mid R)/P(D- \mid R)$, is the posttest odds given the test result; it is the odds corresponding to the posttest probability $P(D+ \mid R)$.

To obtain the posttest odds, we multiply the pretest odds by the ratio $P(R \mid D+)/P(R \mid D-)$. Let us interpret this ratio. The numerator, $P(R \mid D+)$, is the probability of obtaining the test result we saw, assuming that the individual has the disease. The denominator, $P(R \mid D-)$, is the probability of obtaining the same test result, but assuming that the person does not have the disease. The ratio of the two is a measure of the *relative* likelihood of observing this test result, comparing persons with the disease with persons without the disease. It is called the *likelihood ratio* for the test result R. Evidently, this ratio summarizes all the information we need to know about the test for purposes of revising the probability of disease.

For a dichotomous test, the likelihood ratio for a positive test result is denoted $LR+$. It is the true-positive ratio, $P(T+ \mid D+)$, divided by the false-positive ratio, $P(T+ \mid D-)$, or:

$$LR+ = \text{sensitivity}/(1 - \text{specificity}) = TPR/FPR$$

The likelihood ratio for a negative test result from a dichotomous test, $LR-$, is the false-negative ratio, $P(T- \mid D+)$, divided by the true-negative ratio, $P(T- \mid D-)$, or:

$$LR- = (1 - \text{sensitivity})/\text{specificity} = FNR/TNR$$

Now let's apply the odds-likelihood-ratio formula to our FOBT example. The $LR+ = 0.83/(1-0.96) = 20.8$; and the $LR- = (1-0.83)/0.96 = 0.18$. The pretest probability for the 50-year-old anemic man was 0.08, and hence the odds were $0.08/(1-0.08) = 0.087$. After a positive FOBT, the posttest odds would be $0.087 \times 20.8 = 1.8$. But this is an odds, and we have to convert it to a probability using the relation $P = O/(1+O)$. Hence the

---

DEFINITION

The *likelihood ratio* associated with a test result is the ratio of its probability of occurrence if the disease is present to its probability of occurrence if the disease is absent. In probability notation, the likelihood ratio$= P(R \mid D+)/P(R \mid D-)$.

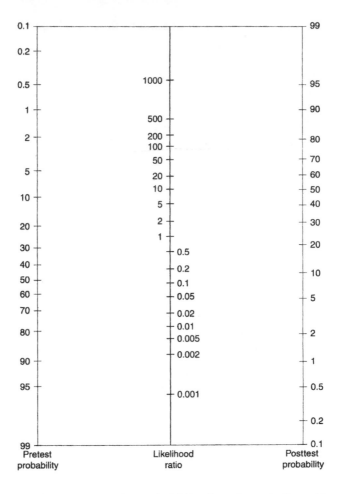

Figure 5.6   Bayes' nomogram. The probabilities have been indicated in percentages. The posttest probability is found by drawing a line from the pretest probability through the likelihood ratio of the test result to the posttest probability. Reproduced from Fagan, T.J. (1975). Nomogram for Bayes' theorem. *N. Engl. J. Med.*, **293**, 257, with permission. Copyright © (1975) Massachusetts Medical Society. All rights reserved.

posttest probability would be $1.8/(1.8+1) = 0.64$, which is the answer we had obtained previously.

The odds-likelihood-ratio version of Bayes' theorem forms the basis for a simple nomogram (Figure 5.6) that could, in practice, be carried around by clinicians in their pockets or on their mobile computers. The construction of the nomogram takes advantage of the fact that the logarithmic version of the odds-likelihood-ratio formula is additive, rather than multiplicative; that is, log(posttest odds) = log(pretest odds) + log(LR). Given the likelihood ratios and the pretest probability, the posttest probability can be read off with a ruler.

Thus we have five ways of revising probabilities: the 2×2 table, Bayes' formula, tree inversion, the odds-likelihood-ratio version of Bayes' formula, and the nomogram. All give the same answers.

5.4.3 Using the odds-likelihood-ratio formula to revise probabilities mentally

To show how easy it is to use the odds-likelihood form of Bayes' formula, one of the authors of this book (MCW) recalls the following episode:

When my wife thought she had become pregnant for the first time, about 20 years ago, she went to her gynecologist to have a pregnancy test. Although she felt she was pregnant, the test was negative. She was naturally disappointed and asked her doctor whether the test could be wrong. He told her that about 10% of pregnant women have a negative result on the first pregnancy test. I met her at the doctor's office and found her disheartened by the doctor's report.

I asked her how likely she had thought it that she was pregnant before the test, and she said, 'I was very sure.' I said, 'You mean maybe 95%?' and she answered, 'Yes, about 95%.' I assumed that the false-positive ratio was virtually nil, and calculated in my head the posttest probability using the odds-likelihood formulation. Since the pretest odds favoring pregnancy were about $20:1$ and the likelihood ratio for a negative result about $1:10$, I immediately calculated the posttest odds favoring pregnancy as $(20)(1/10)$, or 2. This was easy for me to convert in my head to a posttest probability of about $2/3$. With this conclusion, reached in a matter of seconds, I was able to reassure myself as well as my wife. Our first child is almost 20.

Even though the pretest odds used in this illustration were rounded off (from $19:1$ to $20:1$), this author got a serviceable approximation in a matter of seconds. In a patient-care setting, a pocket calculator or Bayes' nomogram can provide a more exact and secure estimate in as little time.

5.5 Finding (subjective) information about pretest probabilities

This book views diagnostic inference as a problem of revising opinion with imperfect information. Research has shown that the conclusions of unaided opinion revision, the kind physicians do every day, often differs systematically from conclusions they would reach by applying Bayes' formula or other formal aids. Our discussion has focused on posttest probabilities and the cognitive processes involved in getting to a posttest probability. But Bayesian analysis must begin with a pretest probability. Where do those come from?

In general, as discussed in Chapter 2, we recommend that epidemiological sources and relevant databases be consulted for the starting point of the reasoning process – the pretest probability. As with finding studies of test accuracy or therapeutic efficacy, this takes some facility with searching computerized databases.

Despite these efforts, published frequency data that seem truly relevant and applicable to your particular case may not be available. The data may have been published so long ago that you wonder if the figures are still correct. Or the study was done in a community quite unlike yours, and you wonder if the disease prevalence there applies to your locale. For these reasons, and others, clinicians sometimes have to rely upon subjective probabilities – personal opinions formulated as probabilities – to begin to apply Bayes' formula.

Although the mechanics of the calculation with Bayes' formula is the same whether one relies on subjective probabilities or has access to large data sets, there are important possibilities for error and bias in the assessment of subjective probabilities. First and foremost, any individual clinician, or 'probability assessor,' is unlikely to have observed a large enough number of cases to be able to provide a reliable estimate. Furthermore, psychologists have identified three heuristic principles that are commonly employed to generate subjective probability estimates: availability, representativeness, and anchoring and adjustment, which may lead to biased judgment (Tversky and Kahneman, 1974).

5.5.1 Availability: reliance on the easily recalled

Availability is employed when the probability of an event (or an underlying disease) is judged by how easy it is to recall instances or occurrences of similar events. When a clinician estimates a probability by remembering a patient very much like the one being evaluated, availability may operate. What is wrong with using this principle to estimate probability? Recall can be affected by factors other than frequency and probability. More recent events ('I just had a patient last week who . . .') are often better remembered than more distant ones. On the other hand, memory is also affected by how strange and unusual an event is: commonplace events tend to be forgotten but unusual events are usually remembered very well. We are more likely to remember what we ate at a particularly outstanding banquet years ago than what we had for dinner two weeks ago Monday. Every clinician remembers a very unusual case seen just once, and the result is that the probability of such events is likely to be overestimated. A partial remedy for this bias is to take the precaution of dividing the number of observed cases by the total number of patients one has seen, thereby making reference to the relative frequency of the observed event.

5.5.2 Representativeness: focusing on features at the neglect of prevalence

Representativeness is used when the probability of a disease for a particular patient is judged by how closely the clinical picture resembles a larger class of events, such as the 'typical picture' of that disease. Most of the time, this is a rather safe principle to use: physicians commonly diagnose a patient by how closely the clinical picture resembles a classic description. But suppose the clinical picture of a particular case resembles but does not exactly match the typical description of two alternative diseases, or resembles disease A in some respects and disease B in other respects. Let's assume, too, that A is more common than B and that the patient does not have both diseases. In such a situation clinicians may judge A and B to be equally probable, because the observed findings of the case fit both A and B equally well. In doing so, the different prevalences of the two diseases have been neglected. In other words, the representativeness heuristic is insensitive to pretest probabilities.

5.5.3 Anchoring and adjustment: underadjustment for new information

Suppose a clinician consults some epidemiological sources to obtain estimates of the local prevalence of various diseases. She decides that none of the published data really fits her community or her patients and that these numbers have to be revised, up or down. The published estimates serve as an anchor, and her subjective probabilities of the prevalence in her community are the result of adjustment. The problem is that adjustments are frequently insufficient; the starting point overly influences people. This implies that we could arrive at two different subjective probabilities for a disease, depending on whether we started out with the prevalence of 'disease' and adjusted up or if we started with the prevalence for 'no disease,' adjusted down, and then converted that subjective probability back to $P(D+)$. Clearly, we should have the same subjective $P(D+)$ regardless of where we started. The anchoring and adjustment heuristic says that frequently these numbers will not be the same.

5.5.4 Value-induced bias

In decision analysis, estimates of probability (the likelihood of an event) and utility (which reflects its value) should be made independently and kept in separate accounts, to be combined during the stage of evaluation. But, in practice, this may be hard to do. Concern about the consequences of a possible disaster makes it more salient and vivid, and these contribute to the workings of availability, so the disaster may seem more likely. Insurance companies use this principle to induce people to buy insurance for very specific, imaginable, but narrowly defined classes of events. In medicine, the probability of serious illness may be overestimated, because the penalties for missing a serious disease are much greater (a malpractice suit?) than the penalties for excessive testing to rule out unlikely possibilities. For example, a patient complains of headache and a medical student concludes the problem is brain cancer. Perhaps the probability of a malignancy is overestimated because of the adverse consequences of missing the case.

5.6 Finding and assessing the quality of studies of test accuracy

In all we have done so far, we have assumed that information on sensitivity and specificity is readily available. Rather than doing the study yourself, you will at least want to find the studies that have already been carried out. You may try searching for the combination of the diagnostic test and the disease you are interested in, e.g., ultrasound and abdominal aneurysm. However, this may lead to many studies that are not about diagnostic tests. So we will want to narrow this down to just the diagnostic studies. Sometimes these are indexed by MEDLINE (the MeSH headings – Medical Subject Headings), such as the keywords such as 'diagnosis' and 'sensitivity-and-specificity' (as a single term). Those that are not indexed by keyword will need to be found by text word searches, using, e.g., specificity, or predictive value. We will explore such searches more fully in Chapter 8. In the meantime, the best single term you might use is 'specificity' as a text word. But be warned, this will miss many good studies.

It is also important to be aware that there are many pitfalls in carrying out studies of diagnostic accuracy. It is therefore important that after having found the appropriate studies you will be able to appraise their validity, as was discussed in Chapter 2. In Chapter 8, we will look at methods for systematically identifying, appraising, selecting, and combining such studies.

5.7 Summary

In this chapter we discussed how information can be interpreted and used to aid decision making. Although we focused on diagnostic (clinical) information that is used to make treatment decisions, the same principles apply to any information that is obtained to guide a decision.

Most information is subject to some degree of error – both false-positive and false-negative results are possible. The accuracy of a test can be summarized with the sensitivity and specificity of the test (or with the true- and false-positive ratios). The sensitivity (or true-positive ratio) is the proportion of patients with the target disease who have a positive test result. The specificity (or true-negative ratio) is the proportion of patients without the target disease who have a negative test result. The false-positive ratio is the proportion of patients without the target disease who have a positive test result. The false-negative ratio is the proportion of patients with the target disease who have a negative test result. A sensitive test, one with a high true-positive (and low false-negative) ratio, is very good at detecting patients with the target disease (sensitive to the presence of disease). A specific test, one with a low false-positive (and high true-negative) ratio, is very good at screening out patients who do not have the disease (and hence specific to that disease).

Our interpretation of the test result, i.e., our estimate of the posttest probability of disease, depends in part on the pretest probability of disease and in part on the sensitivity and specificity (or true- and false-positive ratios) of the test. Probability revision is the process of converting the pretest probability of disease to the posttest probability of disease taking the test result into account. Probability revision can be performed with a 2×2 table, Bayes' formula, tree inversion, odds-likelihood-ratio form of Bayes' theorem, or with a nomogram. In essence all methods do the same thing: the estimate of the probability of disease prior to performing the test (the pretest probability of disease) is combined with the information from the test result (sensitivity and specificity, or true- and false-positive ratio, or the likelihood ratio) to derive the probability of disease after performing the test (the posttest probability of disease). The process can be used to calculate the postpositive-test probabilities of disease and no disease and the postnegative-test probabilities of disease and no disease.

The use of Bayes' formula can help to overcome various biases in estimating probabilities such as the bias due to availability, representativeness, anchoring and adjustment, and value-induced bias.

Table 5.5.

Clock-drawing errors	True disease state	
	Normal	Dementia
1 or 0	48	5
More than 1	14	53

Exercises

Exercise 5.1

Screening for dementia

The clock-face drawing test ('Draw a circle and mark in it the clock numbers 1 to 12; now draw hands indicating quarter to 11') appears to be a simple test for dementia. The data in Table 5.5 were compiled from a series of patients being assessed for dementia (*J. Am. Geriatr. Soc.*, 1992; **40**, 579–84) by both this simple test and a full history, examination, and laboratory tests (the 'reference standard').

(a) Given that a patient has dementia, what is the probability that the patient makes more than one error on clock drawing? (What is this quantity called?)

(b) Given that a patient does *not* have dementia, what is the probability that the patient does *not* make more than one error on clock drawing? (What is this quantity called?)

(c) Given that a patient makes more than one error on clock drawing, what is the probability that the patient has dementia? (What is this quantity called?)

(d) Given that a patient does *not* make more than one error on clock drawing, what is the probability that the patient does *not* have dementia? (What is this quantity called?)

(e) Calculate the posttest probabilities that result from testing a person with a pretest probability of 5% using the method of revising probabilities.

(f) Answer question (e) again, but now by using Bayes' formula (odds-likelihood-ratio form).

Exercise 5.2

Screening for breast cancer

In a breast cancer screening program, initial mammography would detect 87% of undiagnosed cancers of the breast in women aged between 40 and

49 and would falsely detect as positive about 5% of those without cancer (*J.A.M.A.*, 1996; **276**, 33–8, 39–43). About 0.1% of women screened in that age range will have cancer.

(a) Estimate in your head the probability that a woman with a positive test result (an abnormal mammogram) actually has breast cancer. (No computations; use your intuition!)

(b) Now calculate: (i) the probability that a woman has cancer if the test result is positive and (ii) the probability that a woman has cancer if the test result is negative (not using Bayes' formula).

(c) If the woman had a strong family history of breast cancer, the pretest probability might rise to 0.5%. Recalculate (b) with this value.

(d) Answer questions (b) and (c) again but now using Bayes' formula.

Exercise 5.3

Urinary screen for *Chlamydia*

Treating screen-detected asymptomatic chlamydial infection reduces the subsequent risk of pelvic inflammatory disease (*N. Engl. J. Med.*, 1996; **334**, 1362–6). The prevalence of *Chlamydia trachomatis* among young adults in your clinic is 7%. The ligase chain reaction assay of urine is a simple test for detecting *Chlamydia* and has a sensitivity of 94% and a specificity of 99.9% (*Lancet*, 1995; **345**, 213–16).

(a) Use the likelihood ratio version of Bayes' formula to calculate the probability that a young adult with a positive test result (LCR+) has *Chlamydia.*

(b) Use the likelihood ratio version of Bayes' formula to calculate the probability that a young adult with a negative test result (LCR−) has *Chlamydia.*

(c) Repeat (a) and (b) using the Bayes' nomogram. Is the result the same?

(d) Now use the nomogram to repeat the calculations but assuming the prevalence in your clinic was 1% and then 0.1%.

Exercise 5.4

Fecal occult blood test (FOBT) and colorectal cancer (CRC)

Look back at the first example in Chapter 5. FOBT has a sensitivity of 83% and a specificity of 96% for colorectal cancer. Let's say that colonoscopy is performed if the postpositive FOBT probability of colorectal cancer is at least 1%. If it is less than 1%, FOBT is repeated after some months.

Above what prevalence of colorectal cancer will a positive FOBT lead to the decision to perform a colonoscopy?

Exercise 5.5

Think about the analogy between a diagnostic test performed with the purpose of obtaining more clinical information and a clinical trial performed with the purpose of obtaining more information about a treatment. How do the sensitivity and specificity (or true- and false-positive ratios) relate to the significance and power of the trial?

Exercise 5.6

If a likelihood ratio is 1, then the corresponding test result is uninformative – the pretest and posttest probabilities are the same. Given that the likelihood ratio for a positive test result is the sensitivity/(1 – specificity), for what sensitivities and specificities is the test result uninformative? Similarly, given that the likelihood ratio for a negative test result is the (1 – sensitivity)/specificity, for what sensitivities and specificities is the test result uninformative? Can you formulate a general rule for a test to be informative or uninformative?

REFERENCES

Mandel, J.S., Church, T.R., Ederer, F. & Bond, J.H. (1999). Colorectal cancer mortality: effectiveness of biennial screening for fecal occult blood. *J. Natl Cancer Inst.,* **3**, 434–7.

Tversky, A. & Kahneman, D. (1974). Judgment under uncertainty: heuristics and biases. *Science,* **185**, 1124–34.

Weller, D., Thomas, D., Hiller, J., Woodward, A. & Edwards, J. (1994). Screening for colorectal cancer using an immunochemical test for faecal occult blood: results of the first 2 years of a South Australian programme. *Aust. N. Z. J. Surg.,* **64**, 464–9.

6

Deciding when to test

Before ordering a test ask: What will you do if the test is positive? What will you do if the test is negative? If the answers are the same, then *don't do the test.*

Poster in an Emergency Department

6.1 Introduction

In the previous chapter we looked at how to interpret diagnostic information such as symptoms, signs, and diagnostic tests. Now we need to consider when such information is helpful in decision making. Even if they reduce uncertainty, tests are not always helpful. If used inappropriately to guide a decision, a test may mislead more than it leads. In general, performing a test to gain additional information is worthwhile only if two conditions hold: (1) at least one decision would change given some test result, and (2) the risk to the patient associated with the test is less than the expected benefit that would be gained from the subsequent change in decision. These conditions are most likely to be fulfilled when we are confronted with intermediate probabilities of the target disease, that is, when we are in a diagnostic 'gray zone.' Tests are least likely to be helpful either when we are so certain a patient has the target disease that the (false) negative result of an imperfect test would not dissuade us from treating, or, conversely, when we are so certain that the patient does not have the target disease that a positive result of an imperfect test would not persuade us to treat. These concepts are illustrated in Figure 6.1, which divides the probability of a disease into three ranges:

(a) do not treat (for the target disease) and do not test, because even a positive test would not persuade us to treat;

(b) test, because the test will help with treatment decisions or with follow-up; and

(c) treat and do not test, because even a negative test would not dissuade us from treating.

In the following section we use a simple example to demonstrate how one can decide when a test will be useful by calculating two threshold probabilities that separate the three zones: the no treat–test threshold and the

157

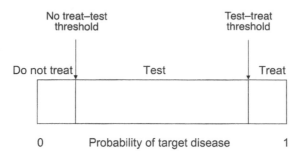

Figure 6.1   Division of the probability of a disease into three ranges: (a) do not treat (for the target disease) and do not test, because even a positive test would not persuade us to treat, (b) test, because the test will help with treatment decisions; and (c) treat and do not test, because even a negative test would not dissuade us from treating.

test–treat threshold (Pauker and Kassirer, 1980).

Let us begin by revisiting the issue of when treatment is warranted despite an uncertain diagnosis. We then look at how and when the results of a diagnostic test should alter the treatment chosen and hence avoid inappropriate treatment.

Example   Thrombolytic therapy in suspected myocardial infarction

A 45-year-old man presents to the Accident & Emergency department with 3 h of severe central chest pain. Patients presenting with central chest pain may have one of several conditions requiring different treatments, the most serious common condition being acute myocardial infarction (a 'heart attack'). Acute myocardial infarction is caused by a clot in one of the coronary arteries which supply the heart muscle with blood. Dissolving the clot with thrombolytic agents (such as streptokinase or recombinant tissue plasminogen activator) has been demonstrated to reduce mortality, provided that the thrombolytic therapy is given sufficiently early. If the patient has another cause of chest pain, which may be clinically indistinguishable from acute myocardial infarction, thrombolytic therapy will do no good at all and may even occasionally induce major bleeding. If we are uncertain about whether a patient has a myocardial infarction, should we treat early (and risk bleeding), or wait for several hours until serial electrocardiograms (EKGs) and blood tests will give a definite diagnosis (but thrombolytic therapy will be less effective)?

To keep the analysis relatively simple, let us assume that if we choose to delay treatment and move from the 0–6-h window to the 7–12-h window, we will then know for certain (based on repeated EKGs and blood tests) whether or not the patient has a myocardial infarction. Hence waiting will

Table 6.1. Clinical balance sheet for alternative management strategies for a patient with suspected myocardial infarction

	Outcome	Wait	Immediate thrombolytic	Urgent testing
AMI	Deaths prevented (includes fatal bleeding[a])	20 per 1000	30 per 1000	Intermediate
	Other adverse reactions	Nil	Acute hypotension (10%)	Intermediate
	Cost	$250	$250	$250 + test cost
No AMI	Bleeding	Nil	4 per 1000	Intermediate
	Other adverse reactions	Nil	Acute hypotension (10%)	Intermediate
	Cost	Nil	$250	Test cost

AMI, acute myocardial infarction.
[a]Due to thrombolytic therapy.

let us treat only those patients who truly have myocardial infarction, and avoid treating those without. However, the delay also means the benefits of thrombolytic treatment are diminished. Let us now tabulate the options in a clinical balance sheet (Table 6.1). To be able to do this, we will need some further information.

> Example (*cont.*) A 45-year-old man with a myocardial infarction who is not treated with thrombolytic agents has an estimated short-term mortality risk of 11%. A combined analysis of the major randomized trials (Fibrinolytic Therapy Trialists' Collaborative Group, 1994) showed that giving thrombolytics between 0 and 6 h after the start of chest pain prevents 30 deaths per 1000 patients; between 7 and 12 h it prevents only 20 deaths per 1000 patients treated. Thus, with delayed thrombolysis the mortality risk is reduced to 9%, and with immediate thrombolysis it is reduced to 8%. These estimated risks include the risk of complications from thrombolytic therapy, including gastrointestinal and intracerebral bleeding.

It is clear that no strategy is dominant: any option we choose will have some advantages and disadvantages when compared to the others. The choice between the two options of 'wait' and 'immediate thrombolytic' is complex, and it will help to calculate the expected value of each option. One way to do this is to draw the decision tree, which will help us structure the sequence of events and probabilities over time. This is shown in Figure 6.2.

As we have done previously, to find the expected value we work backwards from the right-hand side of the tree successively averaging at each chance node. Thus overall the expected survival for the immediate

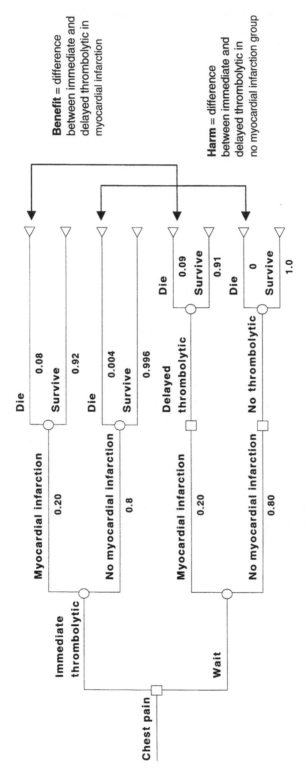

Benefit = difference between immediate and delayed thrombolytic in myocardial infarction

Harm = difference between immediate and delayed thrombolytic in no myocardial infarction group

Chest pain

Immediate thrombolytic

Myocardial infarction 0.20
Die 0.08
Survive 0.92

No myocardial infarction 0.8
Die 0.004
Survive 0.996

Wait

Delayed thrombolytic
Myocardial infarction 0.20
Die 0.09
Survive 0.91

No thrombolytic
No myocardial infarction 0.80
Die 0
Survive 1.0

Figure 6.2   Decision tree comparing two strategies for suspected myocardial infarction. The benefit and harm of immediate thrombolytic therapy, conditional on presence or absence of myocardial infarction, are indicated.

thrombolytic arm is 981 per 1000 patients treated (as usual, we prefer final results expressed in a frequency format); and for the 'wait' option the survival is 982 patients per 1000 patients treated. So waiting is marginally better than treating in terms of survival – one extra survivor per 1000 patients not treated immediately. Checking our clinical balance sheet (Table 6.1), it is also better in terms of minor adverse effects and costs, so it is clearly the preferred of these two options (though we still need to analyze the 'urgent test' option, which we shall come to shortly).

6.2 The treatment threshold revisited

The aim of diagnostic testing is to improve treatment decisions by reducing diagnostic uncertainty. Hence, understanding the treatment decision is important in devising a diagnostic strategy. The treatment threshold is the pivot around which diagnostic testing turns. Diagnostic testing may be viewed as an attempt to place a patient clearly on one side or the other of the treatment threshold. Once testing can no longer change the choice of treatment, it is unhelpful. We must choose despite any residual uncertainty. Conversely, testing is most helpful when we are near the treatment threshold, since tests can still change the choice of treatment. Hence we begin the analysis by reviewing the treatment threshold.

To find the treatment threshold we must compare the benefits and harms of immediate vs. delayed treatment – a common medical problem. As illustrated in Figure 6.2, the benefit of early thrombolytic therapy is the greater mortality reduction with earlier treatment. For patients with definite myocardial infarction, immediate thrombolytic therapy results in a 0.09 (9%) probability of mortality with delayed treatment but 0.08 (8%) mortality with immediate treatment. Thus, there is a survival benefit of 0.01, or 10 lives saved per 1000 patients with myocardial infarction treated compared with waiting (Figure 6.2). What about the harms to those without myocardial infarction? There were four additional intracranial bleeds per 1000 patients treated, resulting in two fatal, one major stroke, and one minor stroke; in addition, there were seven other major but nonfatal bleeds. We could evaluate all these outcomes on a scale from healthy survival to dead using the utility assessment methods from Chapter 4, but let us assume that the combined events are considered equivalent to four deaths per 1000 patients. Thus, for patients without myocardial infarction, the harm of immediate thrombolytic therapy is four deaths per 1000 patients treated compared with waiting, or a reduction in survival equivalent to 0.004 (Figure 6.3).

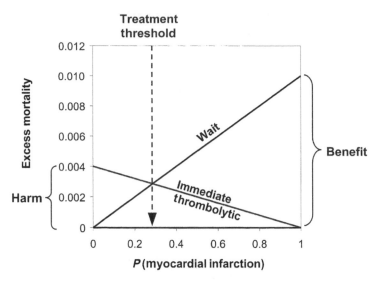

Figure 6.3 The excess mortality of immediate thrombolytic therapy compared to delayed treatment as a function of the probability of myocardial infarction. The benefit and harm of immediate thrombolytic therapy compared to waiting have been indicated. Waiting has the lowest excess mortality (disutility) for low probabilities of myocardial infarction whereas immediate thrombolytic therapy has the lowest disutility for high probabilities of myocardial infarction. The excess mortality of immediate thrombolytic therapy and waiting are equal at the treatment threshold (dashed line).

Recall in Chapter 3 we derived the general equation for the treatment threshold as:

$$\text{Threshold} = \text{harm}/(\text{harm} + \text{benefit}) \tag{6.1}$$

Using this for immediate vs. delayed thrombolytic gives us a treatment threshold for the probability of myocardial infarction of:

$$P(\text{MI}) = \text{harm}/(\text{harm} + \text{benefit}) = 0.004/(0.01 + 0.004) = 0.29 \tag{6.2}$$

Hence, assuming that we can do no further tests, we would prefer to wait if the chance of a myocardial infarction were less than 29%; and we would prefer immediate treatment if it were greater than 29%. The aim of testing will be to shift our probability assessment under or over this threshold.

6.3 Test thresholds: defining the 'gray zone'

In general, a test will only be helpful if a positive result can shift from a tentative treatment of 'wait' to 'treat' or a negative result can shift us from

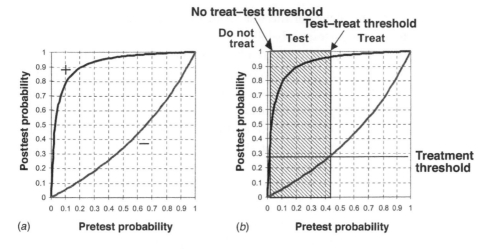

(a) Pretest probability   (b) Pretest probability

Figure 6.4   (*a*) Graph of the relationship between pretest and posttest probabilities for the positive and negative troponin test result, and (*b*) including the treatment threshold and the consequent zone where testing can change the decision.

'treat' to 'wait.' That is, the test must be able to shift the probability across the test threshold. If a test cannot cause one or the other change in the treatment plan, then its result can have no value, because the action is the same no matter what it says.

There will be a range of probabilities around the treatment threshold for which the diagnostic test is capable of changing the choice of treatment. The boundaries defining this 'gray zone' of uncertainty are known as the *test thresholds*.

Now let us return to the question of whether to perform further testing on our patient.

Example (*cont.*)	One test to reduce the uncertainty is the cardiac troponin serum level (a biochemical assay indicative of myocardial infarction). This test has a high specificity of 98%, but at 3 h after onset of chest pain has a sensitivity of only 50% (Antman et al., 1995). Hence it has a good ability to 'rule in,' but not to 'rule out' myocardial infarction.

When will the serum troponin be useful? Let us first calculate the posttest probabilities for all possible pretest probabilities. This was done using the methods explained in Chapter 5 and is shown in Figure 6.4*a*.

When should the results change the treatment decision? In Figure 6.4*b* the treatment threshold (29%) has been marked on the posttest probability axis, and the zones where testing can change the decision have been

DEFINITION

The *test–treat threshold* is the probability at which we are indifferent between testing and immediate treatment. It is the probability for which the expected utility of testing and treating is equal.

indicated. The ability of the test result to change the treatment choice depends on the pretest probability. For example, at a pretest probability of 15%, a negative troponin test result would lower the probability of disease slightly, indicating that the decision not to treat remains best, whereas a positive troponin test result would increase the probability substantially (to over 80%), suggesting immediate treatment. At a pretest probability of 70%, however, both a negative and positive troponin test result would leave us above the treatment threshold, and hence the test does not contribute to the decision.

At some pretest probability of myocardial infarction the troponin test switches from being helpful to being unhelpful in deciding which treatment is optimal. This occurs where the curve of negative troponin results crosses the treatment threshold, which is at a pretest probability of 44%. At all probabilities higher than the pretest probability of 44%, both the postpositive-test and postnegative-test probabilities are above the treatment threshold, implying that we would choose to treat no matter what the test result. This is the *test–treat threshold*.

By a similar process we can find a lower threshold below which the best treatment is 'wait,' irrespective of whether the test is positive or negative. The lower threshold is where the positive result curve crosses the treatment threshold, which is at a pretest probability of about 2%. At all probabilities lower than this threshold, both the postpositive-test and postnegative-test probabilities are below the treatment threshold, implying that we would choose to wait no matter what the test result. This is the *no treat–test threshold*.

Figure 6.4*b* shows both of these test thresholds. Within the shaded 'gray zone,' the test is capable of changing the treatment decision, whereas outside this zone it actually does not. That is, if you tested and believed the result (that is, you base your treatment decision on the result), then you would do worse than not testing at all. This is an important point, so we shall repeat it. Inappropriate tests may do more harm than good because of the subsequent inappropriate treatment decisions. At low probabilities the risk is believing false positives, whereas at high probabilities the risk is believing false negatives. Of course, if the pretest probability is outside the 'gray zone,' and the test has already been performed, a wise decision maker would be better off ignoring the result than be lulled into acting on it (medical–legal considerations notwithstanding)!

A general solution to finding any threshold is to draw the decision tree and then perform an appropriate threshold or sensitivity analysis. This is preferably done using decision analytical software. Here we will illustrate

DEFINITION

The *no treat–test threshold* is the probability at which we are indifferent between testing and not treating. It is the probability for which the expected utility of testing and not treating is equal.

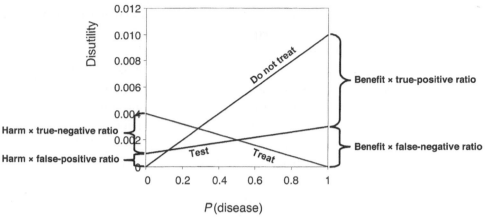

Figure 6.5 Disutility vs. probability of disease showing how a single test influences the treat vs. do not treat decision. For low probabilities of the disease, do not treat has the lowest disutility. For high probabilities of the disease, treat has the lowest disutility. In between there is a gray zone in which testing has the lowest disutility. (Not drawn to scale, for illustrative purposes.)

an equivalent graphical approach that provides several insights about the effects of individual components of the problem. Let us first modify the benefit vs. harm graph (Figure 6.3) by adding an additional line to represent the test. Figure 6.5 presents the disutility of the do not treat, test, and treat options for the range of probabilities of disease. Notice that the option with the lowest disutility is optimal: do not treat for low probabilities of disease, treat for high probabilities of diease, and test for intermediate probabilities (the gray zone). At this stage we have not yet introduced any 'toll' from the test itself.

As before, the harm from treating those without the target disease is represented by the height of the 'treat' line on the left-hand vertical axis (where $P(D) = 0$). The benefit from treating those with the target disease is represented by the height of the 'do not treat' line on the right-hand vertical axis (where $P(D) = 1$).

Now consider what happens with testing at the extreme probabilities of 0 and 1. When the pretest probability of disease is 0, no one has the target disease, and all patients with false-positive results would undergo the harm of treatment (0.004). Hence the expected harm from performing the test instead of not treating is harm × false-positive ratio ($0.004 \cdot 0.02 = 0.00008$, or eight per 100 000). This is the point at which the 'test' line intersects the y-axis in Figure 6.5 (if the graph had been drawn to scale). However, by doing the test, the patients with true-negative test results are spared the harm of treatment. Hence, the expected harm avoided by performing the test instead of treating equals harm × true-negative ratio $(0.004 \cdot 0.98 = 0.00392)$. This is shown in Figure 6.5 as the vertical distance between the 'test' line and the 'treat' line along the y-axis. Similarly, when the pretest probability of disease is 1, then everyone has the target disease. In that case, all patients with false-negative test results would miss out on the benefit of treatment. Hence the expected loss of utility from doing the test instead of treating is benefit × false-negative ratio $(0.01 \cdot 0.50 = 0.005)$. This is shown in Figure 6.5 as the height of the 'test' line on the right-hand side of the graph where $P(\text{disease}) = 1.0$. Also, by doing the test, patients with true-positive test results are given the benefit of treatment. Hence, the expected benefit gained by performing the test instead of not treating equals benefit × true-positive ratio. This is shown in Figure 6.5 as the vertical distance between the 'test' line and the 'do not treat' line on the right-hand side of the graph where $P(\text{disease}) = 1.0$.

The test thresholds may now be read directly from the graph, if the graph has been drawn to scale. However, we can obtain a more exact and general result using a geometric method. To find the no treat–test threshold (the left-hand test threshold), focus on the triangles made by the 'test' and 'do not treat' lines together with the vertical axes. At the no treat–test threshold, the ratio of the pretest probability of disease, $P(D)$, to its complement, $1 - P(D)$, is the same as the ratio of the vertical axis bases of these triangles. If you have trouble seeing this, look back at Chapter 3 where we explained the geometric proof.

Therefore, we derive:

$$\frac{P(D)}{1 - P(D)} = \frac{\text{Harm} \times \text{false-positive ratio}}{\text{Benefit} \times \text{true-positive ratio}} \tag{6.3}$$

And hence, adding the numerator to the denominator on both sides to convert from odds to probability (i.e., from $x/y = w/z$ follows $x/(x+y) = w/(w+z)$), the threshold is:

$$\text{No treat–test threshold} = \frac{\text{Harm} \times \text{false-positive ratio}}{\text{Harm} \times \text{false positive ratio} + \text{benefit} \times \text{true-positive ratio}} \tag{6.4}$$

Similarly, focusing on the triangles made by the 'test' and the 'treat' lines together with the vertical axes, the test–treat threshold can be derived as:

$$\text{Test–treat threshold} = \frac{\text{Harm} \times \text{true-negative ratio}}{\text{Harm} \times \text{true-negative ratio} + \text{benefit} \times \text{false-negative ratio}} \tag{6.5}$$

These formulae are for tests without a toll, and would enable us to find the exact test thresholds (Figure 6.5).

Using the benefit, harm, and test accuracy results for the troponin test, we can calculate the no treat–test threshold using the above formulae as about 2%, and the test–treat threshold as about 44%. Note that the thresholds cannot be read directly from Figure 6.5 because the graph representing the test has not been drawn to scale for illustrative purposes. The actual calculations can easily be performed in a spreadsheet program.

Alternatively, we could have drawn a full decision tree which includes the option of the troponin test. This is shown in Figure 6.6. Using a decision tree is the most general and comprehensive method to analyze the value of testing strategies and to calculate testing thresholds. With a decision tree it is fairly straightforward to add additional concerns such as failure to complete the test, or morbidity and mortality from an invasive test. The latter issues can be added to the disutility graph, but this is not always straightforward. Let us examine such 'tolls' now. Again we will illustrate this with the disutility graph because it provides helpful insights.

6.4   Thresholds for tests with a 'toll'

How would the test thresholds change if the test had some risk, adverse effect, or other 'toll'? The most straightforward examples of 'tolls' from tests are (a) direct health consequences such as direct harms or risks from the invasive nature of the test, e.g., mortality risk (usually small), permanent complications such as stroke, acute adverse events such as infections, or discomfort. We shall show how these types of consequences can be incorporated into the utilities and reflected in the analysis of the test thresholds. A more subtle type of effect of a test would be (b) to delay treatment while awaiting test results. Delay may aggravate the disease and require another treatment, or the test result may become useless if the treatment decision is time-sensitive. For example, a delay in the diagnosis of acute appendicitis increases the risk of perforation of the appendix. Tests may also impose (c) psychological harm, such as anxiety while waiting for results. For example, women with false-positive mammograms may wait several days or weeks before getting definitive negative results and during this time they may experience considerable anxiety. A final negative consequence of tests is (d) the economic costs of the test. Here we will use the term 'toll' to include only the first three of these: the economic costs will be considered separately (Chapter 9).

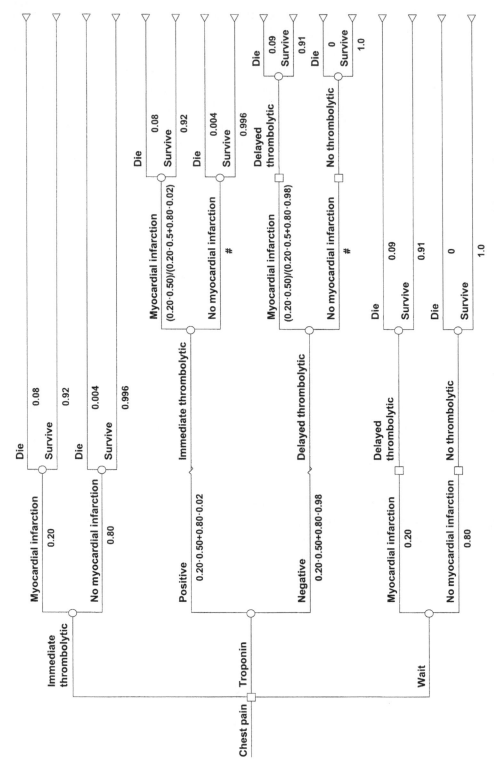

Figure 6.6   Decision tree for suspected myocardial infarction including the option of an initial troponin test.

Example (*cont.*)	In the example thus far, we assumed that the troponin test was available immediately and did not have a risk or cost associated with it. For a first estimate of the usefulness of the test, that is reasonable. But what if the test were unavailable where the patient was seen – for example, in a rural location? This delay would reduce the benefit of early treatment. Such 'harms' of testing narrow the range in which the test is useful; the test thresholds move in towards the treatment threshold.

Let us suppose there is a 'toll' for testing in those with disease of $toll_{D+}$, and for testing in those without the disease of $toll_{D-}$. In Figure 6.7 these two tolls are added to the heights of the intersection of the 'test' line with the left and right axes respectively. Using the same geometric approach as previously we may derive the test threshold with tolls as follows:

No treat–test threshold =
$$\frac{Harm \times \text{false-positive ratio} + toll_{D-}}{Harm \times \text{false-positive ratio} + benefit \times \text{true-positive ratio} + toll_{D-} - toll_{D+}} \quad (6.6)$$

Test–treat threshold =
$$\frac{Harm \times \text{true-negative ratio} - toll_{D-}}{Harm \times \text{true-negative ratio} + benefit \times \text{false-negative ratio} + toll_{D+} - toll_{D-}} \quad (6.7)$$

These formulae are simpler if the 'tolls' are equal for testing in the diseases and nondiseased group, as the 'toll' term drops out of the denominator. However, the tolls are often unequal, particularly if delaying treatment to wait for the test leads to a loss of benefit. However, there are other circumstances in which the tolls differ, e.g., when doing a lumbar puncture for suspected meningitis there is a risk of 'coning' in those with meningitis that does not occur in those without meningitis; similarly, endoscopic and angiographic procedures are often more difficult and hence more hazardous in those with the target disease.

Again, these thresholds may be calculated using either a decision tree with a threshold or sensitivity analysis or via these formulae, using for example a spreadsheet. Whichever method is used, it is valuable to obtain the sensitivity graph over the pretest probability range (Figure 6.7), because this gives a visual representation of where and how the test is useful.

6.5 The expected value of clinical information

The test thresholds define when a test is useful, but *how useful* is the test in different parts of this range? Particularly near the test thresholds, the

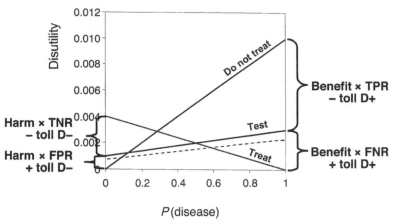

Figure 6.7   Disutility graph showing how a single test influences the treat vs. do not treat decision when the test includes a 'toll' (solid line) compared to a toll-free test (dashed line). $D+$, in the presence of disease; $D-$, in the absence of disease; TNR, true-negative ratio; FPR, false-positive ratio; TPR, true-positive ratio; FNR, false-negative ratio. (Not drawn to scale, for illustrative purposes.)

incremental gain from testing may be relatively small. The graphs in the previous section enable us to quantify precisely the value of the test.

6.5.1 Expected value of perfect information

DEFINITION

The *expected value of perfect information* (EVPI) is the difference between the averaged-out outcome value with a test and the averaged-out outcome value without any test when the test reveals the true disease state with certainty and is assumed to have no toll.

Imagine if we had a perfect and toll-free test. This would enable us to treat all patients with the target disease, and none without. There would be no errors, delays, side-effects, or costs! While such tests do not exist, they do give us an upper limit to the potential benefit from any test. The gain from such an imaginary perfect test is the expected value of perfect information (EVPI).

The EVPI can be read from Figure 6.8 as the distance between the horizontal axis and the 'do not treat' line for probabilities less than the treatment threshold, and the 'treat' line for probabilities greater than the treatment threshold. The EVPI reaches a maximum at the treatment threshold where we are most uncertain whether to treat or not. As we move away from the treatment threshold, the EVPI diminishes, and it is zero at pretest probabilities of 0 or 1.

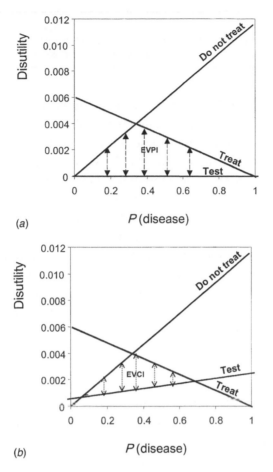

(a)

(b)

Figure 6.8   (a) Disutility graph showing the expected value of perfect information (EVPI) (obtained with a toll-free test that provides perfect information). (b) Disutility graph showing the expected value of clinical information (EVCI) (obtained with a diagnostic test that provides imperfect information). If the test line takes into account the toll of the test, (b) represents the net EVCI. Note that the EVPI and EVCI reach their maximum value at the treatment threshold probability of disease.

6.5.2 Expected value of clinical information

Very few tests in clinical medicine are perfect. For example, our troponin test had both false-positive and false-negative results. An imperfect test can remove only some of our uncertainty, and hence testing gains only a portion of the EVPI. This lesser value is known as the expected value of (imperfect) clinical information.

> **DEFINITION**
>
> The *expected value of clinical information* (EVCI) obtained from a test is the difference between the averaged-out outcome value with the test and the averaged-out outcome value without the test, assuming that the test has no toll.

> **DEFINITION**
>
> The *net expected value of clinical information* (net EVCI), obtained from a test, is the difference between the averaged-out outcome value with the test and the averaged-out outcome value without the test when the risks of the test itself (the toll) are taken into consideration.

The EVCI can be read from Figure 6.8 as the distance between the 'test' line and the 'do not treat' line for probabilities less than the treatment threshold, and between the 'test' line and the 'treat' line for probabilities greater than the treatment threshold. As with the EVPI, the EVCI reaches a maximum at the treatment threshold where we are most uncertain whether to treat or not. As we move away from the treatment threshold, the EVCI diminishes, and is zero at each of the test thresholds. It is negative outside the test thresholds, reminding us that using and selecting treatment based on a test outside the test threshold leads to more harm than good.

Finally, we need to take into account the toll of the test. Again this can be read from our disutility graph if we have plotted the 'test' line, taking into account the toll or it can be calculated as the difference between two strategies in the decision tree.

What about the economic costs of the test? We could take a ratio of the net EVCI to the financial cost of the test and obtain an approximate cost-effectiveness ratio. However, this ignores any downstream costs of the test. For example, if there are further treatment or investigation costs for the false-positive results, this needs to be incorporated in the economic analysis of the test. Without doing this, all we can say is that the cost-effectiveness ratio can only be favorable when the net EVCI is positive and is likely to be best near the treatment threshold. We will deal with this more thoroughly in Chapter 9.

6.6 Number-needed-to-test

If the scale for the expected value is in natural units, such as events or deaths averted, then we can also express the EVCI as its inverse – the number-needed-to-test. This is simply an alternative expression of the same information. For example, for troponin testing in patients with chest pain, the maximum EVCI is at the treatment threshold ($P(MI) = 29\%$), where the gain is 1.3 deaths averted per 1000 patients tested. Inverting this gives a number-needed-to-test of 769, that is, we need to undertake 769 troponin tests on patients with chest pain of uncertain cause to prevent one death.

The EVCI (and hence the number-needed-to-test) will vary with the pretest probability. As we move away from the threshold, the EVCI decreases (and hence the number-needed-to-test increases). The EVCI becomes 0 at both the test thresholds, in which case the number-needed-to-test becomes infinite.

6.7 Summary

Whether or not you explicitly calculate the test thresholds, the important concept in this chapter is that diagnosis is focused around the treatment threshold, and that there is a 'gray zone' around the treatment threshold where testing is worthwhile. There are several different ways of calculating the test thresholds.

Method 1. Use the pretest posttest graph and the treatment threshold.

Method 2. Draw the decision tree, then do a threshold or sensitivity analysis on the probability of disease to find the two thresholds. This is the most general method.

Method 3. Use the disutility graph, which is useful for visualizing the effects of changes in the parameters. This can add a 'toll' to allow for test morbidity and mortality conditional on whether the patient has the disease or not.

Method 4. Use an extended version of the threshold formula. This can give exact values for the thresholds and be readily incorporated in spreadsheet programs.

Whichever method is used, the central concern is to recognize the existence of the gray zone where testing is desirable.

Exercises

Exercise 6.1

Treating a hypothetical disease decreases mortality by 4%. However, if a healthy person is treated, his or her mortality risk increases by 2%. An invasive perfectly accurate (reference) test carries a mortality risk of 1%.

(a) Compute the treatment threshold and test thresholds using the formulas in this chapter.

(b) Construct a decision tree to model the trade-offs using mortality as outcome value. Calculate the thresholds algebraically or using decision analysis software.

(c) Draw the disutility graph (using mortality as outcome value) to understand how the risks influence the thresholds.

(d) Construct a decision tree to model the trade-offs using survival as outcome value. Calculate the thresholds algebraically or using decision analysis software.

(e) Draw the utility graph (using survival as outcome value) to understand how the utility influences the thresholds.

(f) An alternative noninvasive test has no risk but has a sensitivity of 90% and specificity of 80%. Compute the test–treat and test–no treat thresholds.

Exercise 6.2

Primary prevention of cardiovascular death by aspirin

Assume that aspirin will lower the mortality due to myocardial infarction and ischemic stroke from 10/1000 to 3/1000 in patients at risk but that it will increase the mortality due to major bleeding from 1/1000 to 2/1000 in all people you treat.

There is a possibility of selecting patients at high risk for myocardial infarction or ischemic stroke by measuring the ankle–brachial systolic blood pressure ratio.

(a) Within what range of probabilities (risk for cardiovascular death) would you use the ankle–brachial pressure index if you found that the sensitivity is 60% and the specificity is 70%?

(b) Within what range of probabilities would you use this ankle–brachial pressure index if you found that the sensitivity and the specificity of this test are both 50%?

Exercise 6.3

In the example given in this chapter, the outcome measure excess mortality was used to analyze the consequences of treating a possible acute myocardial infarction. However, the life expectancy of survivors differs for those with and without myocardial infarction and this was not taken into account in the analysis. Suppose that a patient with nonspecific chest pain has, on average, a life expectancy of 26 years and that patients with a myocardial infarction have an average life expectancy of 16 years (this number includes the increase in mortality from treatment plus the ongoing risks from cardiovascular disease).

(a) Determine the treatment threshold using life expectancy as outcome measure.

(b) Calculate the test thresholds for troponin using life expectancies.

(c) What happened to the test thresholds compared to the analysis using excess mortality? Did you expect this?

Exercise 6.4

You are a doctor on an ocean cruise liner a few hundred miles off the Hawaiian islands. A 50-year-old woman comes in one morning with a calf swelling suggestive of deep venous thrombosis (DVT: a clot of the deep veins of the calf). If she has a DVT, the main concern is that the thrombosis may extend into the thigh veins where some may break off (embolize) and travel to the lungs (pulmonary embolism), which can be fatal. You can't tell for sure whether or not a DVT exists, but you assess the chance at about 25%. You have two treatment options: (a) observe for symptoms suggestive of pulmonary embolism (such as chest pain and shortness of breath) before starting treatment, or (b) immediate treatment consisting of anticoagulation, using medication which slows down blood clotting: heparin, which works immediately, then warfarin, a tablet that takes several days to work. Anticoagulation will stop most thromboses but risks serious bleeding. If a DVT is present, without anticoagulation the chance that it will extend to the thigh is 25%, and if so the chance it will embolize is 50%, of which 10% would be fatal. Anticoagulation with heparin followed by warfarin would prevent 80% of these fatalities. However, about 5% of patients treated with anticoagulation would have a major bleeding episode, of which 5% would be fatal (data from *Arch. Intern. Med.*, 1992; **152**, 165–75).

(a) What are (quantitatively) the benefits and harms of anticoagulation in those with and without DVT? You may find it helpful to draw a probability tree to visualize the possible events.

(b) What is the treatment threshold?

(c) Ultrasound of the leg has a sensitivity of 97% and a specificity of 98%. Calculate the test thresholds.

Reference: Quintavalla, R., Larini, P., Miselli, A. et al. (1992). Duplex ultrasound diagnosis of symptomatic proximal deep vein thrombosis of lower limbs. *Eur. J. Radiol.*, **15**, 32–6.

Exercise 6.5

Giardia is a protozoan – a single-celled animal – that can infect the gut and cause both acute and chronic infections. The symptoms of chronic infection are a sense of fullness, nausea, and sometime diarrhoea. Several drugs can be used to treat the infection, the best being a single dose of tinidazole, though this causes a couple of days of nausea and dizziness in about 20% of patients.

(a) If chronic *Giardia* symptoms last on average for 3 months, and if these symptoms are equivalent in severity to the 2 days of adverse effects from tinidazole, then what is the treatment threshold?

(b) The usual test for *Giardia* is to look for the organism in fecal samples. A single sample will detect only about 50% of infected cases; but when the organism is seen, identification is 100% specific. What are the test thresholds (the test–no treat threshold and the test–treat threshold) for a single test?

(c) Because the test has a low sensitivity, we could consider repeating the test. Assuming that the two test results are conditionally independent, what is the sensitivity of the combined two tests if you consider the combined test positive if either one of the two test results is positive and negative otherwise? What are now the test–no treat and the test–treat thresholds?

REFERENCES

Antman, E.M., Grudzien, C. & Sacks, D.B. (1995). Evaluation of a rapid bedside assay for detection of serum cardiac troponin T. *J.A.M.A.*, **273**, 1279–82.

Fibrinolytic Therapy Trialists' (FTT) Collaborative Group (1994). Indications for fibrinolytic therapy in suspected acute myocardial infarction: collaborative overview of early mortality and major morbidity results from all randomised trials of more than 1000 patients. *Lancet*, **343**, 311–22.

Pauker, S.G. & Kassirer, J.P. (1980). The threshold approach to clinical decision making. *N. Engl. J. Med.*, **302**, 1109–17.

7

Multiple test results

Even though the diagnostic radiologist examines black-and-white images, the information that is derived from the images is hardly ever black-and-white.

(M.G. Myriam Hunink)

7.1 Introduction

In the previous chapters we focused on dichotomous test results, e.g., fecal occult blood is either present or absent. Test results can conveniently be dichotomized, and thinking in terms of dichotomous test results is generally helpful. Distinguishing patients with and without the target disease is useful for the purpose of subsequent decision making because most medical actions are dichotomous. In reality, however, most test results have more than two possible outcomes. Test results can be categorical, ordinal, or continuous. For example, categories of a diagnostic imaging test may be defined by key findings on the images. These categories may be ordered (intuitively) according to the observer's confidence in the diagnosis based on the findings. As an example, abnormalities seen on mammography are commonly reported as definitely malignant, probably malignant, possibly malignant, probably benign, or definitely benign. As we shall see later in this chapter, it makes sense to order the categories (explicitly) according to increasing likelihood ratio (LR). Some test results are inherently ordinal, e.g., the five categories of a Papanicolaou smear (test for cervical cancer) are ordinal. Results of biochemical tests are usually given on a continuous scale, which may be reduced to an ordinal scale by grouping the test results. Thus, a test result on a continuous scale can be considered a result on an ordinal scale with an infinite number of very narrow categories. Scores from prediction rules are on an ordinal scale if there are a finite number of possible scores, and on a continuous scale if there are an infinite number of scores. When test results are categorical, ordinal, or continuous, we have to consider many test results R_i, where i can be any value from 2 (the case we have considered in Chapters 5 and 6, $T+$ and $T-$) up to any number of categories. Interpretation of a test result on an ordinal scale can be considered a generalization of the situation of dichotomous test results.

177

In this chapter, we first generalize the ideas discussed in the context of dichotomous test results and apply them to interpreting diagnostic test information from tests with multiple results. We then discuss the trade-off between true-positive and false-positive ratios, summary indices for comparing diagnostic tests, and the choice of an optimal positivity criterion for making a diagnosis and proceeding to a treatment decision. Subsequently, we extend the ideas to combining multiple results from multiple tests. Finally, we address some other issues that are important in evaluating and interpreting diagnostic tests with multiple results. The discussion will focus on the clinical example introduced in Chapter 3, but now in an earlier phase of the workup.

Example	A 30-year-old, 7-month-pregnant woman presents at your clinic with right-sided chest pain that gradually increased overnight. She is breathing faster than usual (tachypneic) with 20 breaths/min and has a mildly increased pulse rate (88 beats/min). An electrocardiogram shows no signs of right heart strain (ventricular overload). Because she is pregnant, you want to avoid performing a chest X-ray. You suspect that she has a blood clot in her lungs (pulmonary embolism or PE) and consider performing a special diagnostic test of her lungs – a ventilation/perfusion scan (V/Q scan). The V/Q scan is generally reported in four categories: normal, low, intermediate, or high probability. We start by addressing the following question: if we decide to perform the test, how do we combine the pretest probability with the information from one of these four categories?

7.2 Posttest probabilities using multicategory test results

In Chapter 5 we encountered the odds-likelihood ratio version of Bayes' formula. We also saw that Bayes' formula can be generalized from the case of a dichotomous test $(T+, T-)$ to any type of test result (R). This yielded the following generalized formulation of Bayes' formula, in odds-likelihood ratio format:

$$\frac{P(D+|R)}{P(D-|R)} = \frac{P(D+)}{P(D-)} \frac{P(R \mid D+)}{P(R \mid D-)} \tag{7.1}$$

This formula, which relates the posterior odds of disease to the prior odds of disease, holds whether R is a result from a two-category or multicategory test. For a dichotomous test result, we replace R with either $R+$ or $R-$. For a test with multicategory results $i = 1 \ldots i$, R becomes R_i. For a continuous test, we simply let R be a representative result from among the (possibly infinite) set of possible results $\{\mathbf{R}\}$.

The above expression can also be written as:

$$\text{Posttest odds} = \text{pretest odds} \times \text{likelihood ratio of result } R \quad (7.2)$$

Expressed in plain English, this means that the information after doing the test (posttest odds) equals the information before doing the test (pretest odds) combined with the information obtained from the test (LR). We will apply this generalized formulation of Bayes' formula to our clinical example of the V/Q scan.

7.2.1 Pretest probability

To determine the potential value of performing a V/Q scan in this setting, you need to consider the pretest probability of PE and the LRs of the four possible test results. To estimate the pretest probability of PE we would ideally like to have information from a setting-specific database that contains information about patients with similar clinical characteristics, i.e., her age, sex, pregnancy, type of chest pain, and prior history. Rarely do we have such a database available.

The next best would be to search for this information in the literature. For example, we could look for a clinical algorithm, a clinical prediction rule, or a neural network estimate of the probability of PE based on the history and signs and symptoms (Patil et al., 1993; Susec et al., 1997; Miniati et al., 1999). Our choice of reference depends on which described patient population is the most representative of the patient in front of us, and which study we think provides the best available evidence for the problem (Chapter 8). For example, the study by Susec et al. (1997) describes 170 ambulatory patients, of whom 65% were women. Our patient would fall into the intermediate risk group of this study, which would imply that she has a pretest probability of PE of $14/107 = 13\%$. The study by Miniati et al. (1999) describes 500 patients, of whom 51% were women. In this cohort the investigators found that patients with sudden onset dyspnea, chest pain, and fainting (singly or in combination) had a probability of PE of 53%. Without electrocardiographic abnormalities (which applies to our patient) and radiographic abnormalities (which is unknown for our patient) the probability of PE was 16%. Finally, in the Prospective Investigation of Pulmonary Embolism Diagnosis (PIOPED) study (Worsley and Alavi, 1995), among 627 patients without immobilization, surgery, trauma to the legs, or central venous instrumentation, 21%

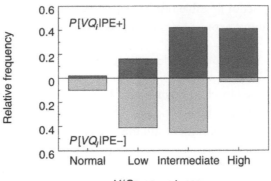

V/Q scan category

Figure 7.1   Histogram of the Prospective Investigation of Pulmonary Embolism Diagnosis (PIOPED) data. Data from PIOPED investigators (1990).

had PE. So, even though we do not have a perfect clinical prediction rule available, we have estimates for the probability of PE of 13%, 16%, and 21%, which combined give an average of 19% when each probability is weighted for sample size. So we use 0.19 as the prior probability of PE, $P(D+)$.

7.2.2 Likelihood ratios of the test categories

To decide whether a V/Q scan could provide useful information we need to know how good this test is in distinguishing patients with PE from patients without embolism. The diagnostic performance of the V/Q scan was evaluated in the PIOPED study (PIOPED investigators, 1990) and the results are presented in Figure 7.1.

The heights of the bars above the x-axis (Figure 7.1) represent the frequency distribution of V/Q scan results among patients who *have PE*. These four proportions sum to 100%. The depths of the bars below the x-axis represent the frequency distribution of V/Q scan results among patients who *do not have PE*. These four proportions also sum to 100%.

It is evident from the figure that the 'intermediate probability' category is the most frequent among patients with and without PE. It is also evident, however, that the *ratio* of the frequency among patients with PE to the frequency among patients without PE steadily increases as we move from the 'normal' to 'high probability' categories. This relative frequency, the ratio of the heights of the bars, is the LR for each of the four test results. Using the tabulated information (Table 7.1) we can calculate the LRs for each of the V/Q scan categories. For example, the frequency of a high-

Table 7.1. Data from the Prospective Investigation of Pulmonary Embolism Diagnosis (PIOPED) study using pulmonary angiography as reference standard

V/Q scan category	Pulmonary embolism		
	Present	Absent	Likelihood ratio
High probability	102	14	$(102/251)/(14/480) = 14$
Intermediate probability	105	217	$(105/251)/(217/480) = 0.9$
Low probability	39	199	$(39/251)/(199/480) = 0.4$
Normal	5	50	$(5/251)/(50/480) = 0.2$
Total	251	480	

V/Q, ventilation–perfusion.

High probability: At least two large or two moderate and one large or four moderate segmental perfusion defects without corresponding ventilation or chest X-ray abnormalities.

Intermediate probability: Difficult to categorize as low or high.

Low probability: Nonsegmental perfusion defects; single moderate perfusion defect with normal chest X-ray; large or moderate segmental perfusion defects with matching ventilation defects either equal or larger in size; or small segmental perfusion defects.

Normal: No perfusion defects.

Data from PIOPED investigators (1990).

probability result equals 102/251 among patients with PE, and only 14/480 among patients without PE. Hence, the LR equals $(102/251)/(14/480) = 14$. Similarly, for the intermediate category the LR equals 0.9, for the low probability 0.4, and for the normal category 0.2.

If you recall the lessons from Chapter 5, you might be asking whether these LRs would apply to a population in which the prior probability of PE is different from that in the PIOPED study. That would be a good question, but the answer is generally that they would apply. Like the sensitivity and specificity of a test, it is generally reasonable to assume that the distribution of test results conditional upon disease status does *not* depend on the prevalence of disease. In fact, because of the conditionality, the true- and false-positive ratios and the LRs do not depend on the prevalence of disease. Sometimes, however, the observed prevalence may be indicative of other variables which influence the distribution of test results. For example, the observed prevalence of liver metastases will depend on the detectability and thus the size of the metastases. The distribution of test results conditional on disease status may then appear to depend on prevalence but in fact it depends on the size of the metastases in the examined

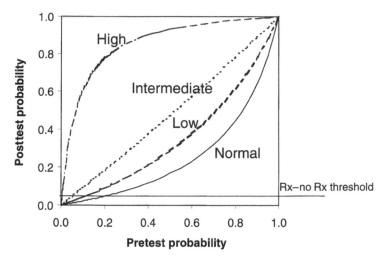

Figure 7.2 The posttest probability of disease as a function of the pretest probability of disease for the four possible categories of the ventilation–perfusion scan, using the likelihood ratios from Table 7.1. The treat–no treat (Rx–no Rx) threshold is indicated.

patient population. Thus, factors such as the distribution of disease severity may influence both the observed prevalence and test characteristics. Such situations are best handled with multivariate prediction rules, discussed later in this chapter.

7.2.3 Posttest probability

Using the LRs corresponding to each specific category, we can calculate the posttest probability of disease conditional on the pretest probability of PE and the test result. Thus, given a pretest probability of 19% and a high-probability V/Q scan result, the posttest probability equals 77%. This is obtained from Equation 7.1, as follows. First we convert the pretest probability of 0.19 to a pretest odds of $0.19/0.81 = 0.2346$. We multiply this prior odds by the LR for the high probability result (LR = 14) to obtain the posttest odds of $14 \cdot 0.2346 = 3.28$. Finally, we convert this odds back to a probability and obtain the posttest probability $3.28/(1+3.28) = 0.77$. We can repeat this exercise for varying pretest probabilities and different LRs.

Figure 7.2 presents the relationship between the posttest probability of disease and the pretest probability of disease for the four different V/Q scan categories. As expected, the graph for the intermediate category is close to the diagonal. Why do we expect this? Notice that if the LR for a test result is exactly equal to 1.0 (i.e., it is equally frequent among diseased and non-diseased patients), then the posterior odds equals the prior odds. The test result contributes no information in that case, and the relationship in Figure 7.2 would be a diagonal line. For the intermediate category in Figure 7.2, the curve is just slightly lower than the diagonal, because the LR is just slightly less than 1.0. Hence the posttest probability is little different from the pretest probability. The graph for the high probability result lies to the upper left because of the high LR (14), and the graphs for the low and normal probability results lie to the lower right because of their low LRs. For very low pretest probabilities, the posttest probability is also low, irrespective of the test result. Similarly, for very high pretest probabilities, the posttest probability is also high, irrespective of the test result.

Performing a test is, in general, most useful in the gray zone where one is uncertain of the presence or absence of disease. For example, if the pretest probability of disease is somewhere between, say, 20% and 80%, we might be most ambivalent about what intervention, if any, to take next. In such situations the test can have a large impact on the estimated probability of disease. For our patient, with an estimated pretest probability of 19%, the posttest probability ranges from 4% if the V/Q scan is normal to 77% if the V/Q scan shows high probability.

As we saw in Chapter 6 for a dichotomous test, however, the usefulness of a test in a specific setting is determined by the effect it has on the decision to treat or not. Even if a test result induces a big change in the probability of disease, it is not going to change a decision unless the posttest and pretest probabilities are on opposite sides of some decision threshold. In our patient, the decision is whether or not to anticoagulate. Suppose that we have estimated, using the methods of Chapter 3, that the threshold probability of disease for treating the patient is 5%. Then by superimposing the treat–no treat threshold probability of disease on the y-axis of the graph (Figure 7.2), we can determine how this threshold cuts the pretest probability into different regions:

- Pretest probability less than 0.004: don't perform the V/Q scan, don't anticoagulate.
- Pretest probability between 0.004 and 0.05: perform the V/Q scan and anticoagulate if the result is high probability.
- Pretest probability between 0.05 and 0.11: perform the V/Q scan and anticoagulate if the result is high or intermediate probability.
- Pretest probability between 0.11 and 0.20: perform the V/Q scan and anticoagulate if the result is high, intermediate, or low probability.

- Pretest probability more than 0.20: anticoagulate, don't perform the V/Q scan.

Thus, in this particular setting, the V/Q scan is valuable for pretest probabilities between 0.004 and 0.20, and it has no decisional value if the pretest probability is outside this range. Inside this range, its expected value of clinical information (EVCI) for the V/Q scan is greater than zero; outside this range, it has no value in decision making. (In order to calculate the EVCI of the V/Q scan, we would need more information about the benefits and harms of anticoagulation in a patient who truly has or does not have a PE.)

7.3 Trade-offs between true-positive and false-positive ratios

Tests with continuous or ordinal multiple results typically have two features: (1) a measurable *test variable*, i.e., a measurable property on a categorical, ordinal, or continuous scale that relates to a particular disease, and (2) a *positivity criterion*, which is a particular value of the measured variable that distinguishes patients with the target disease from those without the target disease. If we are interested in hypertension, for example, one possible variable would be the average diastolic blood pressure at three successive readings, and we might choose as our positivity criterion a diastolic blood pressure of 90 mmHg. In the diagnosis of tuberculosis, the variable might be the size (in mm) of the indurated papule induced by injection of a small quantity of antigen into the skin, and the positivity criterion might be a particular size, e.g., 10 mm.

Biologic variables often show a substantial spread in values for populations with and without the target disease. Furthermore, the values in the two groups usually overlap. This overlap makes it impossible to define a positivity criterion that distinguishes perfectly all those with a disease from all those without it. Most clinical tests share this imperfection, but it does not render them useless. Our task is to discover the positivity criterion that makes the best possible separation of those in the population who have the target disease from those who do not have it. Although in reality we commonly have to deal with a variety of diseases and varying degrees of severity of disease, it is useful to dichotomize a continuous test variable into 'positive' and 'negative' regions. This is because most medical action is dichotomous: we decide to operate or not to operate, to initiate treatment or not to initiate it. Even if more than two actions are possible, the problem can generally be redefined as a two-stage process consisting of two dichotomous actions. As we shall see later in this chapter, the choice of an optimal positivity criterion depends on the context in which the test is to be used to reach a clinical decision.

For example, we need to decide whether to anticoagulate (administer heparin to) our 30-year-old pregnant patient with suspected PE based on the V/Q scan result. In this situation we want to avoid performing a pulmonary angiogram. Which patients in this situation would you anticoagulate? Only those with a high-probability V/Q scan? Or would you also anticoagulate those with an intermediate V/Q scan result? In other words, where would we draw our threshold for the choice between anticoagulating vs. not anticoagulating the patient? First, we need to know how changing the threshold influences the test characteristics, i.e., the true-positive and false-positive ratios.

7.3.1 Graphical representation of the trade-off: ROC curves

Consider the PIOPED data presented in Table 7.1 and as a histogram in Figure 7.1. If we choose to set the threshold between the high and intermediate categories, for example, we will incorrectly withhold treatment from 149 patients with PE (Figure 7.3A).

If we relax the positivity criterion (i.e., move it down in the table or to the left in the histogram; Figure 7.3B; Table 7.2), we will increase the fraction of patients with PE who are correctly identified as such (true-positive results). Alas, at the same time we will also increase the number of subjects without PE who are incorrectly labeled as having the disease (false-positive results). If we tighten the positivity criterion (move the threshold up in the table or to the right in the histogram), the proportion of patients without PE whose test results are positive will decrease (false-positive results). But, we will also decrease the proportion of patients with PE whose positive test results correctly identify the disease (true-positives). Moving the positivity criterion thus entails a trade-off between true-positive and false-positive ratios (Table 7.2). A receiver operating characteristic (ROC) curve demonstrates these trade-offs graphically (Figure 7.4).

An ROC curve thereby evaluates overall test performance independently of the ultimately chosen decision criterion. The points (0,0) and (1,1) are inherent to all ROC curves. The point (0,0) represents the most stringent possible positivity criterion: no patients in any of the test categories are labeled as having the target disease. The point (1,1) represents the most relaxed positivity criterion: all patients are labeled as having the target

DEFINITION

A *receiver operating characteristic (ROC) curve* is a plot of pairs of possible combinations of true-positive and false-positive ratios achievable with a test as the positivity criterion is varied.

Table 7.2. Data from the Prospective Investigation of Pulmonary Embolism Diagnosis (PIOPED) study (1990): calculating cumulative true-positive and false-positive ratios

	Pulmonary embolism		Cumulative proportions	
V/Q scan categories that are considered positive	Present	Absent	True-positive	False-positive
None	0	0	0	0
High	102	14	0.41	0.03
High/intermediate	102 + 105	14 + 217	0.82	0.48
High/intermediate/low	102 + 105 + 39	14 + 217 + 199	0.98	0.90
All	102 + 105 + 39 + 5	14 + 217 + 199 + 50	1.00	1.00
Total	251	480		

V/Q, ventilation–perfusion.

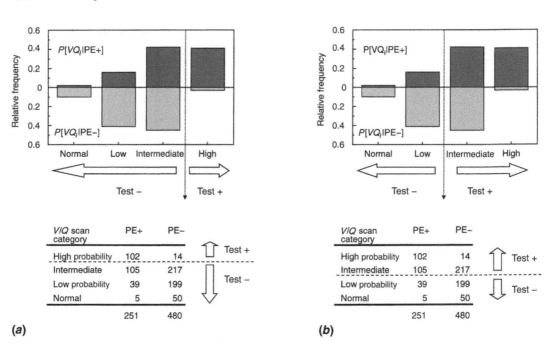

(a)   (b)

Figure 7.3   Varying the positivity criteria of the ventilation–perfusion (V/Q) scan. Data from PIOPED investigators (1990).

disease. Points on the curve closer to the lower left corner (Figure 7.4) represent situations in which strict criteria are used to make the diagnosis. In that part of the curve there will be few false-positive test results (low false-positive ratio) but at the expense of missing the diagnosis in a considerable number of patients (low true-positive ratio). Points on the

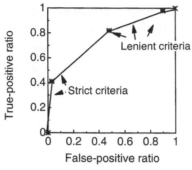

Figure 7.4   Receiver operating characteristic (ROC) curve for the ventilation–perfusion (V/Q) scan data.

curve closer to the upper right-hand corner represent situations in which lenient criteria are used to make the diagnosis. In that part of the curve many patients are identified as having the target disease (high true-positive ratio), but many nondiseased subjects are also labeled as having the target disease (high false-positive ratio).

If the diagnostic test has results with numerical values, such as with biochemical tests, the positivity criterion will be a particular value, above which (or below which, depending on the test) a test will be called positive or negative. With diagnostic imaging this approach is usually not possible, because no numerical value indicating the presence or absence of disease is produced. However, specific characteristics on the image, such as an ill-defined nodule and microcalcifications on a mammogram, can be used to categorize the results. Alternatively, the reader of the image can (and in the clinical routine usually does) express his or her confidence in the diagnosis based on various criteria.

ROC analysis (in the past also known as relative operating characteristic analysis) was developed by signal detection theorists who needed to distinguish signal from noise, for example in analyzing radar data. The technique is also used in psychology, polygraph lie detection, and weather forecasting. Since the 1970s the technique has been applied to diagnostic tests in medicine.

7.3.2 Likelihood ratios and the ROC curve

In using the term 'likelihood ratio' one needs to distinguish the result-specific LR from the cumulative LR of a dichotomized test result. For the V/Q scan, Table 7.1 shows the result-specific LRs for each of the four

DEFINITION

The *result-specific likelihood ratio* for a particular test result is the ratio of the probability of observing that result conditional on the presence of the target disease, to the probability of observing that result conditional on the absence of the target disease. When the results are grouped into categories, we refer to this quantity as the *category-specific likelihood ratio.*

possible results. However, once a positivity criterion has been selected (such as intermediate or higher), a cumulative LR can be defined for the group of 'positive' results (intermediate and high) and for the group of 'negative' results (low or normal). These can be derived from Table 7.2 as 0.82/0.48, which equals 1.7.

The result-specific likelihood ratio is generally implied when using the term 'likelihood ratio.' It is the most useful ratio because it contains the most information. In probability notation, the result-specific (or category-specific) likelihood ratio (LR_i) of the test result R_i is:

$$LR_i = \frac{P(R_i \mid D+)}{P(R_i \mid D-)} \tag{7.3}$$

where $P(R_i \mid D+)$ is the probability of the test result R_i given presence of the target disease, and $P(R_i \mid D-)$ is the probability of the test result R_i given absence of the target disease. Note that for dichotomous test results the above equation is equivalent to the ratio introduced in Chapter 5.

Notice that we can generate the operating points on the ROC curve by starting at the origin (0,0), and then, beginning with the category-specific probabilities of the high-probability V/Q scan result, adding one-by-one the category-specific probabilities (Table 7.3) to the cumulative true-positive and false-positive ratios. Going from one (strict) operating point to the next (less strict) point, we add the category-specific probability given no disease to the cumulative false-positive ratio (the x-axis in ROC space), and we simultaneously add the category-specific probability given disease to the cumulative true-positive ratio (the y-axis in ROC space). Thus, the slope of the line joining two operating points of the ROC curve is equivalent to the ratio of the category-specific probabilities given disease and given no disease, which, as we defined above, equals the category-specific LR. Using strict positivity criteria in the left-lower corner, the slope of the ROC curve (and the corresponding category-specific LR) is high. Walking up the ROC curve the slope of the curve, and the category-specific LR, decrease (Figure 7.5a). For continuous data the categories are infinitesimally small and the LR equals the tangent of the curve (Figure 7.5b).

7.3.3 Likelihood ratios and uninterpretable test results

The fact that the slope of the ROC curve, and the category-specific LR, decrease as we go from strict to lenient criteria can be helpful in determining the value of uninterpretable test results. If uninterpretability is unre-

Table 7.3. Data from the Prospective Investigation of Pulmonary Embolism Diagnosis (PIOPED) study (1990): calculating the category-specific true- and false-positive ratios and the corresponding likelihood ratios

	Pulmonary embolism		Category-specific probabilities		Category-specific LR
			Probability given disease	Probability given no disease	$P(VQ_I \mid PE+)/$
V/Q scan category	Present	Absent	$P(VQ_I \mid PE+)$	$P(VQ_I \mid PE-)$	$P(VQ_I \mid PE-)$
High probability	102	14	0.41	0.03	14
Intermediate probability	105	217	0.42	0.45	0.9
Low probability	39	199	0.16	0.41	0.4
Normal	5	50	0.02	0.10	0.2
Total	251	480			

VQ, ventilation–perfusion scan; PE, pulmonary embolism; LR, likelihood ratio.

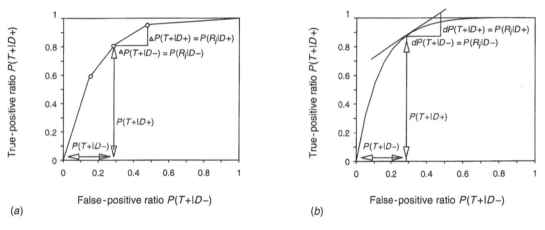

Figure 7.5   Likelihood ratios and the receiver operating characteristic curve (*a*) for categorical data and (*b*) for continuous data.

lated to the presence or absence of the target disease, we would expect to find an equivalent proportion of uninterpretable test results among those with and without the disease, i.e., the LR would equal one, and the uninterpretable test result would convey no meaningful information. The intermediate V/Q scan category, for example, is commonly referred to as the equivocal or indeterminate category because the LR is very close to one (Table 7.3). If, on the other hand, uninterpretable test results are seen relatively more often in patients without the target disease than in those with the disease, then an uninterpretable result would contain information

Table 7.4 Ultrasound for appendiceal disease

Ultrasound result (US_i)	AppDis +	AppDis −	$P(US_i/$ AppDis +)	$P(US_i/$ AppDis −)	LR
Positive	39	0	0.75	0.00	Infinity
Dubious	3	3	0.06	0.10	0.60
Appendix not visualized	10	28	0.19	0.90	0.21

AppDis, appendiceal disease; US, ultrasound; US_i, specific ultrasound findings as indicated by row: positive, dubious, or appendix not visualized; LR, likelihood ratio.

(low LR) and would reduce the probability of disease. This was the case in a study evaluating the use of ultrasound in the diagnosis of appendicitis (Table 7.4; Puylaert et al., 1987), in which a low LR was found for appendices not visualized with ultrasound. Pathophysiologically, the findings can be explained in that a normal appendix is not swollen and thus about 2–5 mm in diameter, which can be very difficult to identify among the bowel loops using ultrasound.

7.4 Summary indices for comparing diagnostic test performance

Should we use spiral computer tomography (CT) or a V/Q scan for the diagnosis of PE? Clinicians, local purchasers, and policy makers often need to decide which is the better diagnostic technique to use or have available. One of the important components of this decision should be the relative accuracy of the methods. In summarizing and comparing diagnostic test performance, we need useful indices that measure the information content of a test result or the test as a whole. To ensure generalizability, such indices should (ideally) be independent of the setting in which the study was performed, in other words independent of the disease prevalence and the costs and benefits associated with true- and false-positive and true- and false-negative test results. In Chapter 5 we discussed the LR and odds ratio in the context of dichotomous test results. In this chapter we have used LRs in the context of multicategory test results. Here we discuss the area under the ROC curve. The relationship with odds ratios will be discussed in the context of prediction rules at the end of this chapter.

7.4.1 The area under the ROC curve

ROC curves that go up steeply from (0,0) and reach near (0,1) describe a test that is nearly perfect in discriminating subjects with and without the

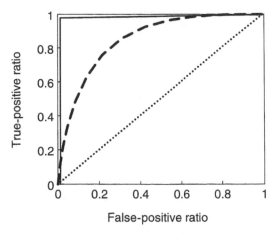

False-positive ratio

Figure 7.6 Receiver operating characteristic (ROC) curves of perfect (continuous line), good (dashed line), and useless (dotted line) tests, illustrating how the area under the ROC curve is an overall measure of the diagnostic performance of a test.

target disease. Curves close to the diagonal have little or no discriminatory power (Figure 7.6), the LR being near 1.0 for every point on the curve. Most tests have an ROC curve somewhere between these two extremes. Thus, the area under the ROC curve is a summary measure of test performance. An area of 1 represents a perfect test, whereas an area of 0.5 indicates a test with no discriminatory power. Note that the area under the curve is a measure of test performance independent of the chosen operating point on the curve and thus independent of the probability of disease and the benefits and harms associated with test outcomes. The area under the ROC curve also has an intrinsic meaning: it equals the probability that a randomly chosen pair of normal and abnormal images will be correctly categorized.

7.4.2 Nonparametric estimates of the area under the ROC curve*

The most convenient way of calculating the area under the ROC curve is by connecting the calculated points and adding the areas of the trapezoids underneath each part of the curve (Figure 7.7) This is a nonparametric method, that is, no assumptions are made regarding the underlying probability distributions of test results. The method is equivalent to the Mann–Whitney–Wilcoxon U statistic from nonparametric statistics. The U

* This is advanced material and can be skipped without loss of continuity.

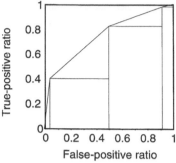

True-positive ratio / False-positive ratio

Figure 7.7　Calculating the area under the empirical, nonparametric receiver operating characteristic (ROC) curve of the ventilation–perfusion (V/Q) scan results from the Prospective Investigation of Pulmonary Embolism Diagnosis (PIOPED) study (1990). The area calculated nonparametrically is 0.79.

statistic is normally used to test whether the value of a quantitative variable is generally larger in one population compared to another population. Its value in this context is that, in addition to providing a formula for calculating the area, we can also easily determine its standard error according to the Hanley–McNeil algorithm or using a bootstrap algorithm (Hanley and McNeil, 1983; Efron and Tibshirani, 1993). The nonparametric method is adequate, provided that enough data points are present and the points are spread along the curve. The area under the ROC curve is slightly underestimated with this method compared to a parametric estimate, but if comparing tests is the major issue, the underestimation of the area is of little concern.

7.4.3 Parametric estimates of the area under the ROC curve*

Parametric methods are based on the assumption that the test results conform to some well-defined underlying probability distribution (Figure 7.8). The most commonly used parametric method is the one introduced by Dorfman and Alf (1968), which assumes that the underlying distributions of the test results are Gaussian, or normal. Although the distributions of test results are often not Gaussian, it has been shown that the binormal ROC model gives accurate results for many non-Gaussian distributions (Hanley, 1988). Other underlying distributions include chi-squared, log-normal, and the negative exponential (Hanley, 1988).

* This is advanced material and can be skipped without loss of continuity.

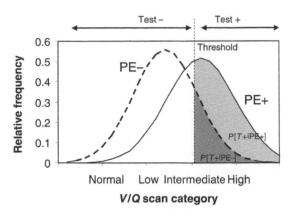

Figure 7.8   The binormal distribution of the results of the ventilation–perfusion (V/Q) scan among patients with and without pulmonary embolism (PE) in the Prospective Investigation of Pulmonary Embolism Diagnosis (PIOPED) study (1990). An arbitrary threshold has been indicated. Areas under the distributions to the right of the threshold represent the true- and false-positive ratios associated with that threshold. Compare this with the histogram (Figure 7.1). The parametric receiver operating characteristic curve has an area under the curve of 0.83.

When using the binormal ROC model the basic procedure is to convert the true- and false-positive ratios to their corresponding normal deviate values. The ROC curve plotted on binormal deviate axes is a straight line (Swets, 1979). A maximum likelihood estimation algorithm is subsequently used to calculate the slope and intercept of the line (Dorfman and Alf, 1968). Finally, the predicted values are transformed back to ROC space.

7.4.4 Comparing the areas under two or more ROC curves*

A plot of the competing ROCs is helpful to visualize the range of values and relative accuracy of the two tests. In particular, it should be noted whether or not the two curves cross, suggesting that each may be better but in different areas. To compare the overall performance we need a statistical method. In comparing the area under two ROC curves a two-sided paired t-test is used. If the test results were derived from the same set of patients, one should take into account the correlation between test results (Hanley and McNeil, 1983). The z-statistic is calculated using the formula:

---

* This is advanced material and can be skipped without loss of continuity.

$$z = \frac{A_1 - A_2}{\sqrt{SE_1{}^2 + SE_2{}^2 - 2rSE_1SE_2}} \tag{7.4}$$

where A_1 and A_2 are the areas under the ROC curves of the two tests, SE_1 and SE_2 are the standard errors of the areas, and r is the correlation coefficient between the areas under two ROC curves derived from the same cases (Hanley and McNeil, 1983). To determine the parameter r we need to calculate the Kendall tau (for categorical scales) or Pearson product moment correlation (for continuous scales) between the two test results for nondiseased (r_N) and diseased (r_D) patients. The parameter r is based on the average area of the two ROC curves and the average of r_N and r_D and can be found in published tables or with software packages.

7.5 Choosing a positivity criterion

Not all positivity criteria of the test variable, and thus the associated operating points on an ROC curve, result in equivalent outcomes. In using diagnostic tests with multiple results, we need to identify the optimal positivity criterion, i.e., the best threshold value or cutoff point of the test variable. This optimal positivity criterion represents the combination of true- and false-positive ratios that yield the greatest expected utility when applied to a particular decision problem. Utility, as we have seen, can be defined in terms of survival, life expectancy, quality-adjusted life expectancy, or any other metric suitable for the problem at hand. The choice of an optimal positivity criterion is equivalent to choosing a point on the ROC curve – an optimal 'operating point' on the curve.

As we shall demonstrate using decision analysis, the optimal operating point depends upon the pretest probability of disease, the expected net benefit of correctly diagnosing the disease (true positives), and the expected net harms associated with false-positive results (Phelps and Mushlin, 1988). These factors are combined in an expression that equals the slope of the ROC curve, and thus the LR of the test result, at the optimal operating point. We will show that the optimal operating point will shift to a less stringent positivity criterion (i.e., higher sensitivity and lower specificity, lower LR, and less steep slope) if the probability of disease is higher, the net benefit of diagnosing the disease is larger, or the net harm associated with false-positive results is smaller.

For example, consider the case example of the 30-year-old pregnant woman with which we started our discussion. There is a fairly low pretest probability of PE of 19%. Treatment with anticoagulants has risks not only

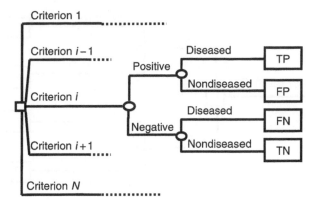

Figure 7.9   A generic decision model to determine the optimal positivity criterion of a test variable. TP, true positive; FP, false positive; FN, false negative; TN, true negative.

for the mother but also potentially for the fetus. These circumstances make it desirable to set a relatively stringent cutoff point, which is to the left on the ROC curve (Figure 7.4) in an effort to minimize the number of false-positive test results. On the other hand, if PE is likely – as would be the case in a bedridden patient following surgery for cancer – or if PE has serious consequences if left untreated (which is the case in the example), then we would prefer to shift our positivity criterion to a more lenient criterion. In that situation we would want to shift the operating point more to the upper right on the ROC curve, in order to increase test sensitivity in spite of the increased number of false-positive results.

Balancing the risks and benefits to determine the optimal positivity criterion can be done explicitly using decision models (Figure 7.9) in which every possible positivity criterion is considered a choice option. Here we shall instead use an analytical approach based on a decision tree (Figure 7.10) to derive a general equation for calculating the optimal positivity criterion. This approach is especially useful when a test has a large number of categories or for continuous data. We will, however, apply it to our example with the V/Q scan that has only four categories. As an exercise we ask the reader to determine the optimal positivity criterion by explicitly modeling all the possible thresholds and comparing the results.

Figure 7.10 presents a generic decision tree for the decision to treat versus not treat conditional on test result R_i. Thus, $D+$ and $D-$ in our case example indicate presence and absence of PE, R_i indicates the V/Q scan result, EU means expected utility, and 'u' is used to indicate the net health benefit or utility associated with an outcome: uFP for false positives, uFN for false negatives, uTP for true positives, and uTN for true negatives.

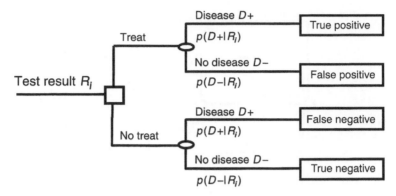

Figure 7.10   Decision tree to derive a general equation for calculating the optimal positivity criterion. The decision is to treat or not treat conditional on test result R_i.

Averaging out the decision tree we get:

$$EU(treat) = P(D+|R_i) \cdot uTP + P(D-|R_i) \cdot uFP$$
$$EU(no\ treat) = P(D+|R_i) \cdot uFN + P(D-|R_i) \cdot uTN \tag{7.5}$$

To optimize the expected outcome we would use the decision rule: Treat if:

$$EU(treat) > EU(no\ treat) \tag{7.6}$$

Thus, substituting the above expressions, treat if:

$$P(D+|R_i) \cdot uTP + P(D-|R_i) \cdot uFP > P(D+|R_i) \cdot uFN + P(D-|R_i) \cdot uTN \tag{7.7}$$

This can be rearranged algebraically as follows:

$$P(D+|R_i) \cdot (uTP - uFN) > P(D-|R_i) \cdot (uTN - uFP) \tag{7.8}$$

and this simplifies to the following comparison of ratios:
Treat if:

$$\frac{P(D+|R_i)}{P(D-|R_i)} > \frac{(uTN - uFP)}{(uTP - uFN)} \tag{7.9}$$

We recognize the left side of this inequality as the posttest odds given the test result R_i. The posttest odds can be rewritten as the product of the pretest odds and the LR of R_i. Thus, the criterion becomes:
Treat if:

$$\frac{P(D+)}{P(D-)} \cdot \frac{P(R_i|D+)}{P(R_i|D-)} > \frac{(uTN - uFP)}{(uTP - uFN)} \tag{7.10}$$

Dividing by the pretest odds ratio on both sides yields the decision rule:
Treat if:

$$\frac{P(R_i|D+)}{P(R_i|D-)} > \frac{P(D-)}{P(D+)} \cdot \frac{(u\text{TN} - u\text{FP})}{(u\text{TP} - u\text{FN})} \qquad (7.11)$$

which can also be written as:

$$LR_i > \frac{1}{\text{Pretest odds}} \cdot \frac{\text{Net loss due to a false-positive}}{\text{Net loss due to a false-negative}} \qquad (7.12)$$

Thus, we have identified the parameters that need to be considered in our choice of a threshold value of the test variable. These are the LR for each of the test results, the pretest probability (or pretest odds) of disease, the net harm associated with incorrectly labeling someone 'diseased' who isn't (a false-positive compared with a true-negative outcome), and the net benefit associated with making a correct diagnosis (a false-negative compared with a true-positive outcome).

Here we have considered utility in a very generic sense. We can optimize the criterion for whatever outcome we choose. For example, this may be life expectancy, quality-adjusted life years, monetary costs, or a measure that combines effectiveness and costs. An example of the last factor is net health benefit, which is the health gain expected from a strategy minus the health gain the decision maker would demand in order to justify the cost incurred (effectiveness – cost/G, where G is the threshold cost-effectiveness ratio; Stinnett and Mullahy, 1998). (See Chapter 11 for more details.)

Now let us again consider our patient with suspected PE. PE is a serious condition with a case fatality rate of 25% if left untreated. Treatment with anticoagulation reduces the risk of mortality to 1%. However, the risk of mortality due to anticoagulation in patients without PE equals 0.8% (van Erkel and Pattynama, 1998). For our patient we want to use the V/Q scan to choose whether or not to anticoagulate, thereby avoiding a pulmonary angiogram. Thus, if the V/Q scan is positive we would anticoagulate the patient and if it is negative we would neither anticoagulate nor perform any further tests. Using the quoted data, the excess mortality risk (or loss in survival probability) in undiagnosed and untreated patients is 0.24 compared to those diagnosed and treated. The corresponding excess mortality risk in subjects incorrectly diagnosed and treated for PE is 0.008 compared to subjects identified as not having PE and not treated. Assuming the patient has a pretest probability of 0.19 and using the derived equation, we would maximize the survival chances of this patient by anticoagulating her if the test result has a LR of more than $(0.81/0.19) \cdot (0.008/0.24) = 0.14$. This implies that we should anticoagulate her irrespective of the V/Q scan result, because even a normal result has a higher LR than 0.14.

We have not explicitly taken into account the outcome of the fetus but instead assumed that maximizing the woman's chances of survival by anticoagulating her with heparin would also maximize the fetus's chances of survival.

Other examples where a similar analysis would be useful in determining the optimal positivity criterion include:

- Determining the optimal cutoff value of the peak systolic velocity as measured by ultrasound for the decision to proceed to angiography and possibly carotid endarterectomy for suspected carotid artery stenosis in patients with a transient ischemic attack or stroke.
- Determining the optimal cutoff value of the ankle–brachial index (the ratio of the systolic blood pressure measured at the ankle and the arm) for the decision to refer a patient with intermittent claudication for angiography and possibly revascularization.
- Determining the optimal threshold of signs and symptoms for the decision to operate for suspected appendicitis.
- Determining the optimal combination of a clinical prediction rule and the V/Q scan category for the decision to anticoagulate in patients with suspected PE.

The last examples take the analysis one step further in that they not only consider the optimal threshold of the results from one particular test but combine the results from various tests, which we consider in the next section.

7.6 Combining results from multiple tests

In many decision-making situations, it is possible to obtain more than a single test. In using the tests to make treatment decisions, the results from multiple tests are combined. Decisions must be made about which tests to perform, in what sequence to perform them with each test decision contingent on the results of previous tests, and how to treat based on the composite information from all the chosen tests. Here we focus on the task of estimating the posttest probabilities of the disease of interest, in the presence of multiple test data. The choice of sequential testing strategies is best handled with decision trees, although the probabilities required in the trees will be obtained using the methods described here.

Each test may yield dichotomous results, or results in multiple categories, or results along a continuum. Consider, for example, the two categorical tests that were evaluated in the PIOPED study, the clinical assessment (CLIN) and the V/Q scan category (VQ), for the diagnosis of PE. The generalized form of Bayes' formula still applies, but now instead of a single result R we have the combination of results from multiple (in this example, two) tests. In our example, each combination of the two tests may be denoted as $R = (\text{CLIN, VQ})$. Combining the results from these two tests yields the following formulation of Bayes' formula:

$$\frac{P(\text{PE}+ \mid \text{ CLIN, VQ})}{P(\text{PE}- \mid \text{ CLIN, VQ})} = \frac{P(\text{PE}+)}{P(\text{PE}-)} \cdot \frac{P(\text{CLIN, VQ} \mid \text{PE}+)}{P(\text{CLIN, VQ} \mid \text{PE}-)} \qquad (7.13)$$

7.6.1 Conditional dependence and independence of multiple tests

Combining the results of the clinical assessment and V/Q scan requires information of the test characteristics $P(\text{CLIN, VQ} \mid \text{PE}+)$ and $P(\text{CLIN, VQ} \mid \text{PE}-)$ for each possible combination of the test results, i.e., the joint distribution of the test results conditional on disease status.

Often it is not possible to find data on the joint distribution of two or more tests conditional upon the disease we are interested in. If we have the test characteristics per test separately, it would be helpful to be able to derive the joint distributions conditional on disease status from the individual test distributions.

Suppose that the two tests were *independent*, conditionally upon the presence or absence of disease. Recall that two events E and F are independent if their joint probability equals the product of their individual probabilities: $P(E, F) = P(E) \cdot P(F)$. But in the setting of testing, the relevant probabilities of test results are conditional upon disease status, $D+$ or $D-$. Independence conditional upon a common third event, such as the presence of a disease, is called *conditional independence*.

DEFINITION

Two tests, T and U, are said to be *conditionally independent, given disease status D* if, for all possible pairs of results (T, U):

$$P(T, U \mid D) = P(T \mid D) \cdot P(U \mid D) \qquad (7.14)$$

Note that the qualifier 'given disease status D' is part of the definition of conditional independence. It is possible that two tests are conditionally independent given disease status $D+$, but conditionally *dependent* given $D-$, or vice versa.

Also take heed that two tests which are conditionally independent given $D+$ and $D-$ are not usually *unconditionally* independent. If both tests are associated with the presence or absence of disease D, then they will generally be dependent, through the association with D. In other words, if tests T and U are both good tests for D, a highly positive result on T will tend to be associated with a positive result on U, because D is more likely to be present. As the following example illustrates, this can happen even if the tests are conditionally independent.

If we are able to assume conditional independence of the test results given disease status, then the posttest odds of disease for the combination of CLIN and VQ becomes:

$$\frac{P(\text{PE}+\mid \text{CLIN, VQ})}{P(\text{PE}-\mid \text{CLIN, VQ})} = \frac{P(\text{PE}+)}{P(\text{PE}-)} \cdot \frac{P(\text{CLIN}\mid \text{PE}+)}{P(\text{CLIN}\mid \text{PE}-)} \cdot \frac{P(\text{VQ}\mid \text{PE}+)}{P(\text{VQ}\mid \text{PE}-)} \quad (7.15)$$

Posttest odds = pretest odds $\cdot$ $\text{LR}_{\text{CLIN}} \cdot \text{LR}_{\text{VQ}}$

Note that this equation assumes conditional independence of the test results in the presence of disease and conditional independence of the test results in the absence of disease. If conditional independence holds in both disease statuses, then the LRs for the combined results equal the products of the LRs for the individual results.

The data presented by the PIOPED investigators give us the opportunity to test the conditional independence assumption for the clinical assessment category and the V/Q scan category for the diagnosis of PE. Table 7.5 presents the LRs calculated from the actual observed data on the combination results and the LRs calculated from the individual test results when combined assuming conditional independence, this time using the test results with angiography or follow-up as the reference test. The results demonstrate that the two sets of LRs are very similar, indicating that conditional independence is a reasonable assumption in this particular setting. Notice, however, that the LRs from the observed data are (with one exception) always closer to 1.0 than the LRs calculated from the marginal probabilities of each test assuming conditional independence. This implies that, although the assumption of conditional independence is reasonable, it is not fully correct and that in reality the actual combination categories contain slightly less information than we would expect based on the conditional independence assumption.

Note that the combination test categories are by definition categorical and not ordinal. There is no inherent ordering of combinations of test results if ordered by their category names as done in Table 7.5. To order the

Table 7.5. Observed data of the tests clinical assessment, the ventilation–perfusion scan, and the combination of the two in the Prospective Investigation of Pulmonary Embolism Diagnosis study (PIOPED Investigators, 1990). The likelihood ratios for the combination test have been calculated from the actual observed data of the combined results and from the likelihood ratios of the individual test results combined assuming conditional independence

CLIN category	V/Q scan category	PE +	PE −	$P(R_i/PE+)$	$P(R_i/PE-)$	LR_{OBS}	$LR_{CLIN} \cdot LR_{VQ}$
High		61	29	0.242	0.046	5.30	
Intermediate		170	399	0.675	0.628	1.07	
Low		21	207	0.083	0.326	0.26	
	High	103	15	0.409	0.024	17.30	
	Intermediate	104	241	0.413	0.380	1.09	
	Low	40	256	0.159	0.403	0.39	
	Normal	5	123	0.020	0.194	0.10	
High	High	28	1	0.111	0.002	70.56	91.71
High	Intermediate	27	14	0.107	0.022	4.86	5.76
High	Low	6	9	0.024	0.014	1.68	2.09
High	Normal	0	5	0.000	0.008	0.00	0.54
Intermediate	High	70	10	0.278	0.016	17.64	18.58
Intermediate	Intermediate	66	170	0.262	0.268	0.98	1.17
Intermediate	Low	30	161	0.119	0.254	0.47	0.42
Intermediate	Normal	4	58	0.016	0.091	0.17	0.11
Low	High	5	4	0.020	0.006	3.15	4.42
Low	Intermediate	11	57	0.044	0.090	0.49	0.28
Low	Low	4	86	0.016	0.135	0.12	0.10
Low	Normal	1	60	0.004	0.094	0.04	0.03
Total		252	635				

CLIN, clinical assessment; V/Q, ventilation–perfusion scan; PE, pulmonary embolism; R_i category-specific test result, with i the category number; LR_{OBS}, likelihood ratio based on the observed results of the combined tests clinical assessment and V/Q scan; $LR_{CLIN} \cdot LR_{VQ}$ product of the likelihood ratios of the clinical assessment category and V/Q scan category, i.e., assuming conditional independence.

combinations of test results correctly we have to refer to their composite LRs. If we order the combination categories according to decreasing LR, i.e., by the diagnostic information of the combination result, we can then construct a ROC curve for the combination test. In our example of the combination of the clinical assessment and V/Q scan, we could use either of the last two columns of Table 7.5 for this purpose. Which column we would use would depend on whether we had more confidence in the estimates based on the joint data, despite small sample sizes in each combination, or in the assumption of conditional independence.

7.6.2 Multivariable Bayes' and multivariable prediction rules*

If instead of one test we have multiple tests, Bayes' formula applies in a generalized formulation. In the multivariable case, the test result R becomes a set of variables $X = (X_1, X_2, X_3, X_4 \ldots X_i \ldots)$ with each X_i being either a dichotomous or multicategory variable and i indicating the category number. The set of variables X may be a combination of clinical variables, diagnostic test variables, and even response variables to previous treatment. The variables (or covariates) are combined with regression coefficients (using logistic regression analysis) to derive a score, which may be considered the diagnostic test variable of the combination test. For example, for the PIOPED data (Miettinen et al., 1998):

$$
\begin{aligned}
\text{Score} = \beta_0 + \beta_1 \cdot \text{age} + \beta_2 \cdot \text{sex} + \beta_3 \cdot \text{symptoms} + \ldots \\
+ \beta_i \cdot \text{\# mismatched defects} + \beta_{i+1} \cdot \text{\# matched defects}
\end{aligned}
\tag{7.16}
$$

Logistic regression analysis in this context has favorable properties and has been used to derive prediction rules for various combination tests (Hunink et al., 1990; Moons et al., 1997, Krijnen et al., 1998; Miettinen et al., 1998). The probability of disease given the set of variables (or vector) X can be expressed as:

$$
P(D+\,|\,X) = \frac{1}{(1 + e^{-\text{score}})}
\tag{7.17}
$$

The posttest odds of disease given the set of variables X can be expressed as:

$$
\frac{P(D+\,|\,X)}{1 - P(D+\,|\,X)} = e^{\text{score}} = e^{\beta_0 + \beta_1 \cdot X_1 + \beta_2 \cdot X_2 + \beta_3 \cdot X_3 + \ldots}
\tag{7.18}
$$

Substituting $e^{\beta_0} = P(D+)/(1 - P(D+))$ the above expression can also be written as:

$$
\frac{P(D+\,|\,X)}{1 - P(D+\,|\,X)} = \frac{P(D+)}{1 - P(D+)} \cdot e^{\beta_1 \cdot X_1 + \beta_2 \cdot X_2 + \beta_3 \cdot X_3 + \ldots}
\tag{7.19}
$$

in which case $P(D+)$ is the pretest probability of disease in the reference group. The above expression emphasizes that prediction rules based on

---

* This is advanced material and can be skipped without loss of continuity.

combination tests are an extension from the univariable formulation of Bayes' formula to a multivariable formulation, i.e.:

Posttest odds = pretest odds $\cdot$ LR$_X$
where LR$_X$ is the likelihood ratio of the set of variables X

$$(7.20)$$

Note that LR$_X$ is the LR of the set of variables (vector) X with X expressed in comparison to the reference group. Because of the multiplicative nature of the logistic regression model, LR$_X$ is the product of the individual LR$_i$s of each variable:

$$\mathrm{LR}_X = e^{\beta_1 \cdot X_1 + \beta_2 \cdot X_2 + \beta_3 \cdot X_3 + \ldots} = \prod_i (\mathrm{LR}_i)^{X_i} \qquad (7.21)$$

If the test variables are conditionally independent, then the LR$_X$ can be derived from studies evaluating each test individually and multiplying the LRs. To account for conditional dependence requires data from a group of patients among whom all the test variables are known. Such a dataset allows for derivation of the LRs adjusted for the effect of other variables. Interaction terms between variables can also be included in the formulation to account for effect modification. Because the odds ratio (OR) for each group equals the LR in the group with the variable present ($X_i = 1$) divided by the LR in the reference group ($X_i = 0$), and because for each variable i the LR in the reference group equals 1, it follows that in this context the OR$_i$ equals the LR$_i$.

7.6.3 ROC curves and the optimal positivity criterion of combination tests: multivariable prediction rules*

Analogous to shifting the cutoff criterion along the scale of a test variable, we can also shift the cutoff along the scale of the combined categories of multiple tests. We can use, for example, the predicted probability of disease (or event) or the score function from a multivariable prediction rule which may include signs, symptoms, laboratory tests, radiological tests, and response to treatment. The 'test' is now a combination test and the 'test variable' is the predicted probability or score function from the regression model. True-positive and false-positive ratios are calculated by determining the probability of the score being larger than a particular (shifting)

* This is advanced material and can be skipped without loss of continuity.

value, x, conditional on true disease status, i.e., $P((\text{score} > x)|D+)$ and $P((\text{score} > x)|D-)$.

Analogous to the calculation of the optimal positivity criterion of a test variable, we can also calculate the optimal positivity criterion for a combination test or for a multivariable prediction rule. For example, combining the clinical assessment categories and the V/Q scan categories from the PIOPED study led to 12 combination categories (Table 7.5). Similar to the calculation we performed to determine the optimal positivity criterion of the V/Q scan result we can determine the optimal positivity criterion of the reordered combination categories. This is left as an exercise for the reader.

7.7 Other issues

7.7.1 Analyzing multiple diseases and multiple disease states

Current methods for diagnostic test evaluation and interpretation, such as prediction rules and ROC analysis, typically focus on discriminating the 'diseased' from the 'nondiseased' population. In reality, multiple diseases generally need to be distinguished. For example, infections, metabolic diseases, malignancy, benign disease, or no disease are diagnoses that need to be distinguished. Furthermore, varying degrees of severity of disease need to be distinguished. Significant carotid artery disease was previously defined as a stenosis of 70% or more, whereas distinguishing a 0–49%, 50–69%, 70–99% stenosis and an occlusion is more consistent with the results of recent trials of carotid endarterectomy. Finally, different locations of the disease need to be distinguished. For example, diagnosing a stenosis in the tibial artery if the real problem is in the iliac artery can have very serious consequences.

Bayes' formula can be extended to multiple diseases ($D_1, D_2, D_3, D_4 \ldots D_i \ldots D_n$) as follows:

$$P(D_i|R) = \frac{P(R|D_i) \cdot P(D_i)}{P(R|D_1) \cdot P(D_1) + \ldots + P(R|D_i) \cdot P(D_i) + \ldots + P(R|D_n) \cdot P(D_n)} \quad (7.22)$$

The problem of differential diagnosis in the presence of multiple tests and multicategory tests is complicated. Extensive decision models are needed in order to optimize the use of multiple tests in differential diagnosis and no simple algorithms such as we have seen for single tests exist. Although some suggestions have been made in the literature on how to handle multiple disease states, these methods have not come into common use, probably because of their complexity (Steinbach and Richter, 1987; Chakraborty and

Winter, 1990; Harrell et al., 1998; Dreiseitl et al., 2000). The most promising of these involves an application of multinomial diagnostic prediction rules and a multinomial type of ROC analysis. The challenge for the future is to apply these advanced statistical techniques in such a manner that the method and results are understandable for the doctor who will apply the conclusions (Harrell et al., 1998).

7.7.2 Focusing the development of new diagnostic technologies

The challenge of evaluating diagnostic techniques is to do so in a timely fashion. Ideally, one is 'ahead of the game,' i.e., as a new technology emerges target values are estimated that a 'new' technology would have to meet to be cost-effective compared to the 'old' technology. One such method exists: challenge ROC regions (Phelps and Mushlin, 1988; Hunink et al., 1999). Challenge ROC curves represent the threshold pairs of true-positive and false-positive ratios that a new test would have to attain to be cost-effective compared to an established test considering all possible operating points on the ROC curve of the established test. All pairs of true-positive and false-positive ratios to the upper left of the challenge ROC curve represent performance parameters for which a new test would be cost-effective compared to the established test. Clearly this method can be used to explore new diagnostic technology and focus its development (Phelps and Mushlin, 1988; Hunink et al., 1999). The limitations of the method lie in the fact that it focuses on replacing one test with another and focuses on discriminating between two disease states instead of multiple states.

7.8 Summary

In this chapter we discussed the generalized form of Bayes' formula in the context of tests with multicategory results. The generalized form of Bayes' formula is:

Posttest odds = pretest odds × likelihood ratio of result R

or, in plain English, the information after doing the test (posttest odds) equals the information before doing the test (pretest odds) combined with the information obtained from the test (LR). We saw that for very low pretest probabilities, the posttest probability is also low, irrespective of the test result. Similarly, for very high pretest probabilities, the posttest probability is also high, irrespective of the test result. Performing a test is, in general, most useful in the gray zone where one is uncertain of the presence or absence of disease.

An ROC curve is a plot of pairs of possible combinations of true-positive and false-positive ratios achievable with a test as the positivity criterion is varied. An ROC curve thereby evaluates overall test performance independently of the ultimately chosen decision criterion. The area under the ROC curve is a summary measure of test performance.

Not all positivity criteria of the test variable, and thus the associated operating points on an ROC curve, result in equivalent outcomes. In using diagnostic tests with multiple results, we need to identify the optimal positivity criterion, i.e., the best threshold value or cutoff point of the test variable. This optimal positivity criterion represents the combination of true- and false-positive ratios that yield the highest expected utility when applied to a particular decision problem. The optimal positivity criterion (operating point on the ROC curve) depends upon the pretest probability of disease, the expected net benefit of correctly diagnosing the disease (true positive compared with false negative results), and the expected net harms associated with false-positive (compared with true-negative) results. The optimal operating point shifts to a less stringent positivity criterion (i.e., higher sensitivity and lower specificity, lower LR) if the probability of disease is higher, the net benefit of diagnosing the disease is larger, or the net harm associated with false-positive results is smaller.

Finally, we showed that prediction rules based on combination tests are an extension from the univariable formulation of Bayes' formula to a multivariable formulation.

Exercises

Exercise 7.1

Optimizing the positivity criterion for the diagnosis of PE

PE is a serious condition that is fatal in 25% of cases if left untreated. With anticoagulation, the risk of mortality is reduced to 1%. However, the risk of mortality if anticoagulation is given to patients without PE is 0.8%. The reference test for determining the presence or absence of PE is pulmonary angiography. This test, however, has a mortality risk of 0.5%.

Various combinations of noninvasive diagnostic tests, including clinical parameters (clinical prediction rule), can be used to make the diagnosis of PE. The PIOPED study (PIOPED investigators, 1990) presented data on the results of using a clinical prediction rule (CLIN), a ventilation–perfusion scan (VQ), and a combination of the two tabulated by the presence or absence of PE as diagnosed by pulmonary angiography or follow-up (Table 7.5).

(a) Construct a ROC curve for the prediction of PE using the clinical prediction rule. Construct a ROC curve for the prediction of PE using the VQ scan. Which of the two ROC curves has the largest area under the curve?

(b) Construct a ROC curve and determine the optimal positivity criterion of the combination test for the choice between immediate treatment with anticoagulation and performing pulmonary angiography optimizing life expectancy. Consider a patient who is similar to someone in the PIOPED study and who has a life expectancy of 10 years if he/she survives this initial event with the associated procedures and treatment. We recommend you use a spreadsheet program to perform the calculations, for example, Excel.

(c) Construct a ROC curve for the prediction of PE using the combination test consisting of the clinical prediction rule and the VQ scan, as can be calculated from the two tests separately, but now assuming conditional independence. Calculate the area under the curve. Do you expect the area under the curve to be higher or lower than the area under the curve of the ROC based on the observed data?

Exercise 7.2

EBCT for coronary artery disease

Coronary artery disease is generally evaluated with stress testing commonly combined with a noninvasive imaging study. These tests are used in the decision to perform a coronary angiogram in patients with chest pain with the purpose of revascularization as well as identifying subjects at high risk of having a cardiac event. More recently, determining the amount of coronary artery calcification with electron beam (ultrafast) computed tomography (EBCT) is increasing in popularity. Several reports on the diagnostic performance are available for EBCT. The reported sensitivity is generally high but specificity is somewhat limited and the results demonstrate variation with differing 'cut-off' or 'threshold' values used for calling a test result positive.

A paper was published in the *Journal of the American College of Cardiology* about the costs and effectiveness of EBCT for the diagnosis of coronary

Table 7.6. Data on EBCT for the diagnosis of coronary artery disease

Calcium score	Sensitivity	Specificity
0	0.95	0.46
37	0.90	0.77
80	0.84	0.84
168	0.71	0.90

Data from Rumberger, J.A., Behrenbeck, T., Breen, J.F. & Sheedy, P.F. (1999). Coronary calcification by electron beam computed tomography and obstructive coronary artery disease: a model for costs and effectiveness of diagnosis as compared with conventional cardiac testing methods. *J. Am. Coll. Cardiol.*, **33**, 453–62

artery disease. The article attempted to find the optimal threshold value for the calcium score. The following data were used (Table 7.6).

(a) Construct a ROC curve associated with the EBCT for the diagnosis of coronary artery disease from the data provided in Table 7.6. In addition, calculate the LR associated with the different categories of EBCT.

(b) Review the formula to calculate the optimal operating point on a ROC curve. What additional information do you need to determine the optimal operating point on the ROC curve that you constructed?

(c) The authors of the original article based their cost-effectiveness analysis on the total direct costs of testing and calculated the threshold score that minimized the cost per patient correctly identified as having coronary artery disease. They concluded that a threshold of 168 should be used. What do you think of the described optimization process?

(d) Apart from using the formula presented in this chapter, what approach can you use to determine the optimal threshold?

(e) Consider the ROC curve that you have constructed. If you would find an optimal LR threshold of 5, what value of the calcium score would correspond with this?

(f) Another paper on the subject of diagnostic testing strategies for coronary artery disease presented data on the costs and quality-adjusted life years associated with various outcomes (Table 7.7) (Kuntz et al., 1999). Consider a prior probability of coronary artery disease of 0.1 and calculate the optimal LR threshold if you only consider first, the costs, and second, the quality-adjusted life years.

(g) Now combine the costs and quality-adjusted life years in one outcome measure, namely net health benefits = effectiveness − cost/G, where G

Table 7.7.

Test outcome	Cost ($)	Quality-adjusted life years
False-negative	30 706	10.670
False-positive	28 409	14.887
True-negative	23 669	14.890
True-positive	50 937	11.115

Source: Kuntz et al. (1999).

Table 7.8.

Big Blue Test result	Nondiseased	Diseased
0–1	4	24
2–6	8	19
7–12	7	10
13–15	17	8
16–20	29	6

is the societal willingness to pay and assume this is $100 000. Calculate the optimal threshold.

Exercise 7.3

Positivity criterion for hepatitis C++

Hepatitis C++ is a hypothetical disease that affects the liver of computer programmers. Without treatment, the 1-year mortality for diseased patients is 25%. Treatment reduces 1-year mortality by 40%. Of persons without disease but who are mistakenly treated, 3% will die within 1 year. Untreated persons without disease have a 99.8% chance of surviving 1 year. Of all computer programmers, one in eight has the disease. The Big Blue Test has just been developed for the diagnosis of hepatitis C++ and the following data have been collected (Table 7.8).

(a) Estimate the points along the ROC curve for the Big Blue Test and provide a plot.

(b) Estimate the area under the ROC curve. What is the interpretation of this value?

(c) Assuming your objective is to minimize 1-year mortality, what is the optimal positivity criterion for the Big Blue Test?

Hepatitis C++ is actually characterized by two stages: A and B. Without treatment, the 1-year survival for diseased patients is 80% and 65% for

Table 7.9.

Big Blue Test result	Nondiseased	Diseased	
		Stage A	Stage B
0–1	4	8	16
2–6	8	9	10
7–12	7	5	5
13–15	17	6	2
16–20	29	5	1

stages A and B, respectively. Treatment still reduces 1-year mortality by 40%, regardless of stage. One out of every three persons with hepatitis C++ has stage B. Table 7.9 shows the Big Blue Test data broken down by stage.

(d) Assuming your objective is still to minimize 1-year mortality, what is the optimal positivity criterion for the test given this new information?

(e) Although one in three persons with hepatitis C++ has stage B in the community, about 50% of the diseased patients in the study were stage B. Using the positivity criterion determined in part (d), calculate an adjusted sensitivity that accounts for this spectrum bias.

Exercise 7.4

Diagnosis of Markovian tumors

Twenty percent of patients who present with headache have an underlying (hypothetical) Markovian tumor. Life expectancy with and without a Markovian tumor (without surgery) is 25 and 30 years, respectively. If diagnosed early, effective surgery is available for patients with a tumor that increases life expectancy by 2.5 years. Persons without a tumor who inappropriately undergo surgery because of a false-positive test result face a 5% risk of death from the operation (and no benefit).

Two diagnostic tests exist to identify Markovian tumors: the Data test and the Matrix scan. Results for both tests are based on a five-point rating scale (1–5). The following data were collected in a selected group of patients with headache (Table 7.10):

(a) Estimate the points along the ROC curves for the Data test and the Matrix scan and provide a plot.

(b) What is the area under each of the curves? Describe how you would

Table 7.10.

Rating	Data test		Matrix scan	
	Tumor	No tumor	Tumor	No tumor
1	1	62	11	70
2	8	26	12	46
3	21	23	11	13
4	16	14	16	5
5	19	10	15	1

compare the overall diagnostic performance of the Data test versus the Matrix scan.

(c) What positivity criterion would you recommend for each test? What test would you use for persons presenting with headache?

(d) Consider all possible prior probabilities of tumor (0 to 1). Would you ever opt to use the Data test at a positivity criterion of 4 + (i.e., call a rating score of 4 or 5 positive and everything else negative) over the Matrix test at any positivity criteria? If so, at what prior probability of tumor (give an example of one probability)? Would you ever opt to use the Matrix test at a positivity criterion of 4 + over the Data test at any positivity criteria? If so, at what prior probability of tumor (give an example of one probability)?

(e) Within the range of prior probabilities where you would test, at what prior probability of tumor is the life expectancy for the Data test equal to that for the Matrix scan?

REFERENCES

Chakraborty, D.P. & Winter, L.H.L. (1990). Free-response methodology: alternate analysis and a new observer–performance experiment. *Radiology*, **174**, 873–81.

Dorfman, D.D. & Alf, E. Jr. (1968). Maximum likelihood estimation of parameters of signal detection theory – a direct solution. *Psychometrika*, 117–124.

Dreiseitl, S., Ohno-Machado, L. & Binder, M. (2000). Comparing three-class diagnostic tests by three-way ROC analysis. *Med. Decis. Making*, **20**, 323–31.

Efron, B. & Tibshirani, R.J. (1993). *An Introduction to the Bootstrap*. New York: Chapman & Hall.

Hanley, J.A. (1988). The robustness of the 'binormal' assumptions used in fitting ROC curves. *Med. Decis. Making*, **8**, 197–203.

Hanley, J.A. & McNeil, B.J. (1983). A method of comparing the areas under receiver operating characteristic curves derived from the same cases. *Radiology*, **148**, 839–43.

Harrell, F.E. Jr, Margolis, P.A., Gove, S. et al. (1998). Development of a clinical prediction model for an ordinal outcome: the World Health Organization multicentre study of clinical signs and etiological agents of pneumonia, sepsis and meningitis in young infants. WHO/ARI young infant multicentre study group. *Stat. Med.*, **17**, 909–44.

Hunink, M.G.M., Richardson, D., Doubilet, P.M. & Begg, C.B. (1990). Testing for fetal pulmonary maturity: an ROC analysis involving covariates, verification bias and combination testing. *Med. Decis. Making*, **10**, 201–11.

Hunink, M.G.M., Kuntz, K.M., Fleischmann, K.E. & Brady, T.J. (1999). Noninvasive imaging for the diagnosis of coronary artery disease: focusing the development of new diagnostic technology. *Ann. Intern. Med.*,**131**, 673–80.

Krijnen, P., van Jaarsveld, B.C., Steyerberg, E.W. et al. (1998). A clinical prediction rule for renal artery stenosis. *Ann. Intern. Med.*, **129**, 705–11.

Kuntz, K.M., Fleischmann, K.E., Hunink, M.G. & Douglas, P.S. (1999). Cost-effectiveness of diagnostic strategies for patients with chest pain. *Ann. Intern. Med.*, **130**, 709–18.

Miettinen, O.S., Henschke, C.I. & Yankelevitz, D.F. (1998). Evaluation of diagnostic imaging tests: diagnostic probability estimation. *J. Clin. Epidemiol.*, **51**, 1293–8.

Miniati, M., Prediletto, R., Formichi, B. et al. (1999). Accuracy of clinical assessment in the diagnosis of pulmonary embolism. *Am. J. Respir. Crit. Care Med.*, **159**, 864–71.

Moons, K.G., van Es, G.A., Deckers, J.W., Habbema, J.D. & Grobbee, D.E. (1997). Limitations of sensitivity, specificity, LR, and Bayes' theorem in assessing diagnostic probabilities: a clinical example [see comments]. *Epidemiology*, **8**, 12–17.

Patil, S., Henry, J.W., Rubenfire, M. & Stein, P.D. (1993). Neural network in the clinical diagnosis of acute pulmonary embolism. *Chest*, **104**, 1685–9.

Phelps, C.E. & Mushlin, A.I. (1988). Focusing technology assessment using medical decision theory. *Med. Decis. Making*, **8**, 279–89.

PIOPED investigators (1990). The diagnosis of pulmonary embolism. *J.A.M.A.*, **264**, 2623–5.

Puylaert, J.B., Rutgers, P.H., Lalisang, R.I. et al. (1987). A prospective study of ultrasonography in the diagnosis of appendicitis. *N. Engl. J. Med.*, **317**, 666–9.

Rumberger, J.A., Behrenbeck, T., Breen, J.F. & Sheedy, P.F. (1999). Coronary calcification by electron beam computed tomography and obstructive coronary artery disease: a model for costs and effectiveness of diagnosis as compared with conventional cardiac testing methods. *J. Am. Coll. Cardiol.*, **33**, 453–62.

Steinbach, W.R. & Richter, K. (1987). Multiple classification and receiver operating characteristic (ROC) analysis. *Med. Decis. Making*, **7**, 234–7.

Stinnett, A.A. & Mullahy, J. (1998). Net health benefits: a new framework for the analysis of uncertainty in cost-effectiveness analysis. *Med. Decis. Making*, **18**, S68–80.

Susec, O. Jr, Boudrow, D. & Kline, J.A. (1997). The clinical features of acute pulmonary embolism in ambulatory patients. *Acad. Emerg. Med.*, **4**, 891–7.

Swets, J.A. (1979). ROC analysis applied to the evaluation of medical imaging techniques. *Invest. Radiol.*, **14**, 109–21.

van Erkel, A.R. & Pattynama, P.M. (1998). Cost-effective diagnostic algorithms in pulmonary embolism: an updated analysis. *Acad. Radiol.*, **5**, S321–7.

Worsley, D.F. & Alavi, A. (1995). Comprehensive analysis of the results of the PIOPED study. Prospective investigation of pulmonary embolism diagnosis study. *J. Nucl. Med.*, **36**, 2380–7.

8

Finding and summarizing the evidence

It is surely a great criticism of our profession that we have not organised a critical summary, by specialty or subspecialty, adapted periodically, of all relevant randomized controlled trials.

Archie Cochrane

8.1 Introduction

Good decision analyses depend on both the veracity of the decision model and on the validity of the individual data elements. These elements may include probabilities (such as the pretest probabilities, the sensitivity and specificity of diagnostic tests, the probability of an adverse event, and so on), estimates of effectiveness of interventions (such as the relative risk reduction), and the valuation of outcomes (such as quality of life, utilities, and costs). Often we lack the information needed for a confident assessment of these elements. Decision analysis, by structuring a decision problem, makes these gaps in knowledge apparent. Sensitivity analysis on these 'soft' numbers will also give us insight into which of these knowledge gaps is most likely to affect our decisions. These same gaps exist in less systematic decision making as well, but there is no convenient way to determine how our decisions should be affected. In this chapter we shall cover the basic methods for finding the best estimate for each of the different elements that may be included in a formal decision analysis or in less systematic decision making.

Sometimes, but not as often as we'd like, the estimates we are looking for can be inferred from a study that someone else has done or from a series of cases that someone has reported in the literature or recorded in a data bank. This is generally considered the most satisfactory way of assessing a probability, because it involves the use of quantitative evidence. Often we will have a choice of data sources, so it is useful to have some 'rules' to guide the choice of possible estimates. A helpful concept used by many groups is the 'hierarchy of evidence' which explicitly ranks the available evidence; 'perfect' data will rarely be available, but we need to know how to choose the best from the available imperfect data. This choice will also need to be tempered by the practicalities and purpose of each decision analysis. The hierarchy we suggest is:

1 *Systematic review of primary studies.* A systematic review aims to identify all relevant primary research, undertake standardized appraisal of study quality, and synthesize the studies of acceptable quality. This is a considerable undertaking, so, if a systematic review is already available, then you will usually want to use it. If not, then you might consider doing a systematic review yourself for the most critical element(s) in the decision analysis.

   Meta-analyses are a special type of systematic review that entails quantitative rules for combining evidence from different sources. The term is used broadly to encompass methods ranging from simple pooling of observations across studies to methods that consider both within-study and between-study variability (including hierarchical models). Meta-analyses can be grounded either in frequentist theory, which restricts inference to the observed data, or in Bayesian methods that incorporate prior beliefs.

2 *'Best' single study.* A simpler alternative to a systematic review is to search for all relevant studies, but choose the largest study that meets some minimum quality criteria. For example, to estimate the effectiveness of an intervention you might choose the largest randomized controlled trial (RCT).

3 *Subjective estimates.* An estimate should not necessarily be adopted from a study or data set just because it is available. A modified assessment for an individual patient or population, based in part on your own experiences, knowledge of the patient or population, and the judgments of experts, may be required to adjust a particular estimate. Sometimes no data will be available for the estimate, and you must instead choose the most plausible value.

Finding the best data can be hard work, and sometimes impossible (firmly establishing that no data exist is often a time-consuming task). Sometimes the estimation may be straightforward. For example, suppose that you want to know the probability that a particular surgical procedure will result in perioperative death. A report in the literature states that of a series of 1000 patients who underwent the operation, 23 died in surgery. Thus, an obvious estimate of $P[\text{death}]$ is 23/1000, or 0.023. The larger the sample, the more confident we can be that the observed frequency in the sample is a good estimate of the actual probability in the general population. Based on this sample, and assuming that the patient outcomes were independent with a common mortality probability, $P[\text{death}]$, a 95% confidence interval for $P[\text{death}]$ is: 0.015 to 0.034.

Sometimes the estimation will be less straightforward: even when the data are found they may not be in the format required for the model, and may need to be adjusted, either by modeling or subjectively. For example, life expectancy is steadily increasing, and estimates based on historical or even current data will tend to underestimate the likely true value.

There are several caveats in translating the results from a single study or systematic review into an estimate for use in your particular decision problem.

First, the treatments (or diagnostic procedures) may not be entirely comparable to yours. Different personnel, equipment, facilities, or variations in the actual procedure may result in different probabilities. For example, while a study may be based on the experiences with a new surgical procedure, the performance of surgeons may have improved considerably since that time.

Second, the study population may be different in some important respects from your population or patient. Those patients in the study population may have been older or younger, or in better or worse health. They may have volunteered or have been specially selected for the treatment in question. The potential effects of this difference may best be examined by sensitivity analysis. This will enhance the ability of the analyses to be applied and adapted to a variety of situations, populations, and individuals. We will return to this in Section 8.5.

8.2 Finding the 'best' studies

The best study type will depend on the type of estimate required. We may classify most of the decision elements into the following different types of questions, which then guides our search for data:

1 *Intervention effectiveness.* What are the effects of an intervention on patients? The intervention may be a therapeutic maneuver such as a pharmaceutical, surgery, a dietary supplement, a dietary change, psychotherapy, etc. Some other interventions are less obvious, such as early detection (screening), patient educational materials, or legislation. The key characteristic is that there is some manipulation of the person or his or her environment. To study the effects of interventions requires a comparable control group without the intervention, and thus an RCT is generally the ideal design.

2 *Proportion or frequency.* How common is a particular feature or disease in a specified group? For example, what is the prevalence of osteo-

porotic fractures at various ages, or the frequency of a particular gene such as BrCa1 for breast cancer? The appropriate study design here is to perform a standardized measurement in a representative sample of people. If instead of a single frequency, we become interested in the causes of variation of that proportion or frequency, then this becomes a question of risk factors or prediction.

3 *Diagnostic performance.* How accurate is a sign, symptom, diagnostic test, or screening test in predicting the true diagnostic status of a patient? This essentially involves a comparison between the test of interest and some 'gold' or reference standard. The most commonly used measures of the diagnostic performance are the sensitivity and specificity. If the test is categorical or continuous, then we will require data on the frequency distribution of results conditional on disease status or, equivalently data for constructing an ROC curve. Note that if we move from an interest in diagnostic performance to an interest in the effects on patient outcomes, then the question becomes one of intervention – we are interested in whether the test predicts the effects of treatment on patients. Diagnostic performance is an intermediate outcome rather than the final outcome of workup and treatment. The analyst has a choice whether to model the causal chain from diagnostic accuracy to intervention to outcome, or whether to rely on direct evidence of the effect of testing on outcome.

4 *Risk or prognostic factor.* Is a particular factor, such as patient characteristic, laboratory measurement, family history, etc, associated with the occurrence of disease or adverse outcomes? This question begins with establishing a clear association between the factor and the disease. This will involve issues beyond the degree of association, such as dose–response relationships and biological plausibility. Often data on the association between risk factors and disease status is available in the form of a statistically estimated risk function relating one or more risk factors to the incidence or prevalence of disease, or to an efficacy parameter such as risk reduction. Commonly encountered statistical models of this type include logistic regression models, proportional hazard (Cox regression) models, and neural network models.

5 *Patient preferences and costs.* In all of the previous questions, additional outcomes of interest will commonly be patient preferences and costs. For example, we may be interested in not only an intervention on patient outcomes, but also in the costs of the intervention and any potential downstream cost savings caused by improved patient outcomes.

The first four (1–4) of these are probabilities. Appraising studies reporting these probabilities was covered in Chapter 2. If you find several

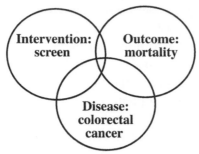

Figure 8.1   Three components of a question that might be considered in designing a search strategy.

potential studies then the appraisal should guide you to the best single study. If there are several studies which appear of equal quality, then you will need to either choose the largest or, preferably, synthesize the results using meta-analytic methods.

8.2.1 Electronic searching

The first step in the process of estimating the inputs for decision analysis is to identify sources of data. Most searching will be done electronically using words or phrases relevant to our question. A useful tactic is to break down the particular question into components: the population, the intervention (or test or risk factor), the disease, and the outcome. The search terms should include identifying potential synonyms for each component. In addition, an appropriate 'methodological filter' may help confine the retrieved set to the most valid primary research studies based on their study design. For example, if you are interested in whether fecal occult blood test screening reduces mortality from colorectal cancer (an intervention), then we may wish to confine the retrieved studies to the controlled trials evaluating screening.

It is useful to break the study question into its components, and then combine these using the special terms AND and OR. For example, in the Venn diagram of Figure 8.1, 'mortality AND screen*' represents the overlap between these two terms, i.e., only those articles that use both terms. 'screen AND colorectal cancer AND mortality', the small area where all three circles overlap, will require articles that have all three terms. Complex combinations are possible, e.g., '(mortality AND screen) OR (mortality AND colorectal cancer) OR (screen AND colorectal cancer)' captures all the overlap areas between any of the circles.

Table 8.1. Using the components of a question to guide the literature search

Component of question	Example of search term	Synonyms and related terms
Population/setting	Adult, human	
Intervention, test, or risk factor	Screen	Fecal occult blood test, early detection
Disease	Colorectal cancer	Bowel cancer, colorectal neoplasm
Outcome^a	Mortality	Death, survival
Study design^a	Controlled clinical trial	

^{a}Both outcome and study design are options needed only when the search results are unmanageable.

Though the overlap of all three parts will generally have the best concentration of relevant articles, the other areas may still contain many relevant articles. Hence, if the disease AND intervention ('colorectal cancer AND screen') combination (union of the two corresponding circles in the figure) is manageable, it is best to work with this and not restrict the search any further, e.g. using outcomes ('mortality').

When the general structure of the question is developed it is then worth looking for synonyms for each of those components. This process is illustrated in Table 8.1.

Thus a search strategy might be: '(screen* OR fecal occult blood test OR early detection) AND (colorectal cancer OR bowel cancer OR colorectal neoplasm) AND (mortality OR death OR survival)'. (The term 'screen*' is shorthand for words beginning with screen, e.g., screen, screened, screening, etc.)

In looking for synonyms one should consider both text words and key words in the database. The MEDLINE keyword system, known as the Medical Subject Headings (MeSH), is worth understanding: the tree structure of MeSH is a useful way of covering a broad set of synonyms very quickly. For example the 'explode' feature allows you to capture an entire sub-tree of MeSH terms within a single word. Thus for the colorectal cancer term in the above search, the appropriate MeSH term might be:

Colonic neoplasm (exp)

With the 'explode' the search incorporates the whole MeSH tree below colonic neoplasm, viz.,

Colorectal Neoplasms
  Colonic Polyps

Adenomatous Polyposis Coli
Colorectal Neoplasms
Colorectal Neoplasms, Hereditary Nonpolyposis
Sigmoid Neoplasms

While the MeSH system is useful, it should supplement rather than usurp the use of textwords lest incompletely coded articles are missed.

8.2.2 Methodological filters

A search may be made more specific by including terms indicative of the best appropriate study design, and hence filter out inappropriate studies (Haynes et al., 1994). For example, if you are interested in studies of an intervention's effectiveness then you may initially try to confine the studies to randomized controlled trials (RCTs). These filters might use specific methodological terms or compound terms.

What are 'methodological' terms?
MEDLINE terms not only cover specific content but also a number of useful terms on study methodology. For example, if we are considering questions of therapy, many randomized trials are tagged in MEDLINE by the specific methodological term randomized-controlled-trials to be found under publication type (pt) or as controlled-clinical trials. Be aware, however, that many studies do not have the appropriate methodological tag.

8.2.3 Electronic databases

Which databases should I use?
Which databases to use depends on the content area and the type of question being asked. For example there are general medical databases (e.g., MEDLINE), databases for nursing and allied health studies (e.g., CINHAL) and for psychological studies (e.g., Psyclit). If it is a question of intervention, then the Controlled Trials Registry within the Cochrane Library is a particularly useful resource, as it contains over a quarter of a million references for randomized trials identified by a systematic search of databases and hand-searching of selected journals.

8.3 Systematic reviews and meta-analyses

The purpose of a systematic review is to evaluate and interpret all available research evidence relevant to a particular question. A systematic review contrasts with a traditional review by its concerted attempt to identify all relevant primary research, by its standardized appraisal of study quality, and its systematic (and sometimes quantitative) synthesis of the studies of acceptable quality.

The two major advantages of systematic reviews and meta-analyses are the increase in power and the improved ability to study the consistency of results. Many studies have insufficient power to detect modest but important effects. Combining all the studies that have attempted to answer the same question considerably improves the statistical power. Furthermore, similar effects across a wide variety of settings and designs provide evidence of robustness and transferability; if the studies are inconsistent, then the sources of variation can be examined. Thus while some people see the mixing of 'apples and oranges' as a problem of systematic reviews, we see it as a distinct advantage because of its ability to enhance generalizability and transferability.

Without due care, the improved power could also be a disadvantage: it allows not only the detection of small effects, but also of small biases. All studies have flaws, ranging from the small to the fatal. Assessment of individual studies for such biases is crucial, as the added power of the systematic review will allow even small biases to result in an 'apparent' effect. For example Schulz has shown that studies evaluating treatment effects using unblinded outcome assessment gave on average a 17% greater risk reduction than those using blinded outcome assessment (Schulz et al., 1995).

A systematic review will generally require considerably more effort than a traditional review. The process is similar to primary scientific research: the careful and systematic collection, measurement, and synthesis of data (the 'data' being papers). As such, a protocol outlining the question and methods is advisable prior to starting the review; indeed this is required for all Cochrane systematic reviews (Mulrow and Oxman, 1997). The term 'systematic review' is preferred to meta-analysis because it suggests this careful review process. While it may provide a summary estimate, this is neither necessary nor sufficient to make a review 'systematic'.

It is useful to think of the process of doing a systematic review in a number of discrete steps:

1 *Listing the questions.* The process of decision analysis breaks a problem

down into many components, many of which will require relevant data. It is helpful to set up a table of the data items, their definitions, and the potential data sources.

2 *Finding studies.* The aim of a systematic review is to answer a question based on all the best available evidence, published and unpublished. Being comprehensive and systematic is important in this critical, and perhaps most difficult phase of a systematic review. Finding some studies is usually easy. Finding all relevant studies is almost impossible. However, there are a number of methods and resources that can make the process easier and more productive.

3 *Appraisal and selection of studies.* The relevant studies identified will usually vary greatly in their quality. This phase entails undertaking a critical appraisal of each of the identified potentially relevant studies, and then selecting those of appropriate quality. To avoid a selection, which is biased by preconceived ideas, it is important to use a systematic and standardized approach to the appraisal of studies.

4 *Summary and synthesis.* Next the relevant data from each of the studies needs to be extracted, summarized, and synthesized. The initial focus should be on describing the study's design, conduct, and results in a clear and simple manner – usually in a summary table. Following this, some summary plots will be helpful, particularly if there are a large number of studies. Finally, it may be appropriate to provide a quantitative synthesis. However, as indicated above, this is neither a sufficient nor necessary part of a systematic review.

5 *Generalizability and hetereogeneity.* Following the summary and synthesis of the studies we will need to ask about the overall validity, strength, and applicability of any results and conclusions. Is there a large difference in settings, methods, and results across studies? How and to whom are the results of the synthesis applicable? How will the effects vary in different populations and individuals?

It is vital to understand the type of question, and to specify the components of the question clearly before starting. This will define the process in the next three phases of: finding, appraising, and synthesizing the studies.

8.3.1 Finding relevant primary studies

Finding all relevant studies that have addressed a single question is not easy. MEDLINE indexes only about 15–20% of biomedical journals, and even the MEDLINE journals represent several hundreds of thousands of journal articles per year. Beyond sifting through this mass of literature, there are the problems of duplicate publications and with accessing the 'gray literature,' such as conference proceedings, reports, theses, and unpublished studies. A systematic approach to this literature is essential if we are to identify all of the best evidence available that addresses the question. There are various issues to take into account when searching the literature:

8.3.1.1 Has a systematic review been performed?

Published reviews may answer the question or at least provide a starting point for identifying the studies. Finding such reviews takes little effort. By qualifying your search of the electronic databases with 'review' you can limit the number of studies retrieved. For interventions a check should also be made of the Cochrane Library for a completed Cochrane Review, a Cochrane protocol (for reviews underway), or a non-Cochrane review.

8.3.1.2 Finding published original studies

It is usually easy to find a few relevant articles by a straightforward literature search, but the process becomes progressively more difficult as we try to identify additional articles. Eventually, you may sift through hundreds of articles in order to identify one further relevant study. There are no magic formulae to make this process easy, but there are a few standard tactics, which, together with the assistance of a librarian experienced with the biomedical literature, can make your efforts more rewarding.

In addition to the general methods of electronic searching described above, there are some additional methods that should be considered in a thorough search for all relevant studies.

Snowballing.
The process of identifying papers is an iterative one. We recommend starting with an electronic search strategy as described. However, this will inevitably miss useful terms, and the process will need to be repeated. The results of the initial search are used to retrieve relevant papers, which can then be used in two ways to identify missed papers:

(a) the bibliographies of relevant papers are checked for articles missed by the initial search,

(b) a citation search, using the *Science Citation Index* will identify papers that have cited the identified relevant studies, some of which may be subsequent primary research.

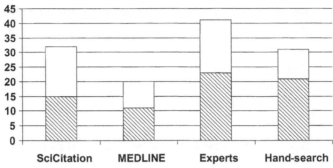

Figure 8.2   Papers identified by different search methods in a systematic review of near-patient diagnostic tests. Shaded area, unique; no shading, nonunique.

These 'missed' papers are invaluable – they provide clues on how the search may be broadened to capture further papers, e.g., by studying the keywords that have been used. The whole procedure may then be repeated. This iterative process is sometimes referred to as 'snowballing'.

Hand-searching.
If the relevant articles appear in a limited range of journals or conference proceedings, it may be feasible and desirable to search these by hand. This is obviously more important for unindexed or very recent journals, but may also pick up relevant studies not easily identified from title or abstracts. Fortunately, the Cochrane Collaboration systematically hand-searches a number of journals to identify controlled trials, and compiles them into a Master List; this should be checked before undertaking your own hand-search. However, for other question and study types there has been no such systematic search.

Is it worth writing to experts?
Experience varies on this question. However, an analysis of a recent review of the value of near-patient diagnostic tests (diagnostic tests which can be done entirely within the clinic, e.g., dipstick urine tests) showed that this may be quite useful (McManus et al., 1998). Of 75 papers eventually identified nearly one-third were uniquely identified by writing to experts. The data are shown in Figure 8.2, which also illustrates the general point that it is worth using multiple sources. However, near-patient diagnostic tests is an area of emerging technology, and a larger proportion than usual of papers are likely to be unpublished, published in less common sources, or presented at conferences.

Table 8.2. Comparison of published versus registered studies of multiagent vs. single-agent chemotherapy for ovarian cancer

	Published studies	Registered studies
Number of studies	16	13
Survival ratio	1.16	1.05
95% confidence interval	1.06–1.27	0.98–1.12
P value	0.02	0.25

Data from Simes (1987).

8.3.1.3 Publication bias

What is publication bias?

If 'positive' studies are more likely to be published than 'negative' or 'inconclusive' studies, then any review (traditional or systematic) of the published literature must be biased towards a 'positive' result. This is the essence of publication bias – the positive correlation between the results of the study and our ability to find that study. For example, a follow-up of 737 studies approved by the Institutional Review Board at Johns Hopkins University found that the odds ratio for the likelihood of publication of positive compared with negative studies was 2.5 (Dickersin et al., 1992). Interestingly, most nonpublication was because authors failed to submit, rather than that journals rejected 'negative' studies.

Does this affect the results of the reviews?

Systematic exclusion of unpublished trials from a systematic review will introduce bias if the unpublished studies differ from the published, e.g., because of the statistical significance or the direction of results. In a review (Simes, 1987) of multiagent versus single-agent chemotherapy for ovarian cancer, the authors found statistically and clinically different results between sixteen published studies and thirteen registered studies – see Table 8.2. Since the registered trials were registered at inception rather than completion, their selection for inclusion in the review is not influenced by the outcome of the study – therefore they constitute an incomplete *but unbiased* set of studies.

8.3.1.4 Duplicate publication

The converse of an unpublished study is a study that is published several times. This is often, but not always, obvious. For example, in a review of ondansetron's effect on postoperative emesis, Tramer and colleagues found 17% of trials had duplicate reports (Tramer et al., 1997). Nine trials of oral ondansetron were published as 16 reports, and 19 trials of intravenous ondansetron were published as 25 reports. One multicenter trial had published four separate reports with different first authors. But perhaps most surprisingly, four pairs of identical trials had been published that had nonoverlapping authorships! Unfortunately, there is no simple routine means of detecting such duplicates except by some careful detective work. Occasionally writing to the authors will be necessary. Clearly if duplicate publications represent several updates of the data, then the most recent should be used.

8.3.2 Appraising and selecting studies

Providing an explicit and standardized appraisal of the studies identified is often useful for two reasons. First a systematic review should try to base its conclusions on the highest quality evidence available. To do this requires a procedure to select from the large pool of studies identified so that only the relevant and acceptable quality studies are included. Second, it is important to convey to the reader the quality of the studies included as this tells us about the strength of the evidence for any recommendation made.

Is it important to perform a structured appraisal?
Unfortunately, if unstructured appraisals are made, we tend to look more critically at the studies whose conclusions we dislike. For example, 28 reviewers were asked to assess a single (fabricated) 'study' but were randomly allocated to receive either the 'positive' or 'negative' version (Mahoney, 1977). The identical Methods sections of this fabricated study were rated significantly worse by the reviewers of the 'negative' study compared with the 'positive' study! Hence, it is essential to appraise all papers equally. If warranted in a particular situation, this can be accomplished by using a standardized checklist.

How many reviewers are required?
Using more than one reviewer is rather like getting a second opinion on a medical diagnosis. When feasible and depending on the importance of the data element being sought, at least two reviewers should be used. Each of these reviewers should independently read and score each of the potentially included studies. They should then meet to resolve any discrepancies between the evaluation of the paper by open discussion. This discussion is a

useful educational procedure in itself, which probably increases the consistency and accuracy of the appraisals of the paper.

How should the appraisal be used?

The principal use of the appraisal is to decide which studies merit inclusion in the main analysis. For example, with a question of treatment, we may confine ourselves to RCTs. But even deciding whether a study is randomized or not from the report can be difficult, which emphasizes the need to appraise papers carefully.

Beyond the inclusion versus exclusion decision, there are two other ways that the appraisal can be used:

1 *Group or sort by study design and/or methodological criteria.* It is useful to consider an exploratory analysis on study design and methodological criteria. Reports may be categorized by study design (e.g., randomized, cohort, case-control) or sorted by quality features and then plotted in rank order, with or without providing summary estimators for each of the groups of studies. One then needs to determine whether this makes a difference to the results. A sensitivity analysis on quality has been suggested (Detsky et al., 1992): a cumulative meta-analysis is done looking at the best single study, the best single two studies combined, the best three studies combined, etc. However, the sorted study design/methodological plot is the most informative initial analysis.

2 *Meta-regression on design/methodological criteria.* An alternative procedure is to look at whether individual items make a difference to the effects seen in the studies. For example do the blinded studies give different results to the unblinded studies? Do the studies with good randomization procedures give different results to those with doubtful randomization procedures? It is possible to extend this further by looking at all the study design and methodological criteria simultaneously in a so-called meta-regression. However, because there will usually be a limited number of studies such techniques are probably not justified in most meta-analyses.

8.3.3 Summarizing and synthesizing the studies

How should the results of the identified studies be synthesized?

First, it is helpful simply to produce tabular and graphical summaries of the results of each of the individual studies, even if there is no attempt to combine their results. Second, if the studies are considered sufficiently homogeneous in terms of the question and methods, and this is supported by a lack of evidence of statistical heterogeneity, then it may also be appropriate to combine their results to provide a summary estimate. The method for combining studies will vary depending upon the type of questions asked and the outcome measures used.

8.3.3.1 Graphical presentation of results

The most common and useful presentation of the results of the individual studies will be the plotting of a point estimate together with some measure of uncertainty for each. Measures of uncertainty include confidence limits and posterior probability distributions. This can be done whether we are talking about the relative risk reduction or a specific measure such as reduction in blood pressure. Studies can be sorted, e.g. by publication year, by study design, or from those with the broadest to those with the narrowest range of uncertainty – and if there is a summary estimator, this should be nearest the studies with the narrowest range of uncertainty. In addition, because studies with wide uncertainty draw greater visual attention, it is useful to specifically indicate visually the contribution of the study by the size of the 'dot' at the summary estimator; specifically, the area of the dot could be made proportional to the inverse of the variance of the study's estimator. These principles are illustrated in Figure 8.3 which shows the results of the systematic review of colorectal cancer (Towler et al., 1998, 2000).

8.3.3.2 Summary estimates

Summary estimates may include the relative risk reduction, the mean difference, the proportion, or the summary receiver operating characteristic (ROC) curve (Table 8.3). Except in rare circumstances, it is not advisable to simply pool the results of the individual studies as if they were one common large study. This can be demonstrated to lead to significant biases because of confounding by the distribution of the study factor and the outcome factor. Instead the appropriate method is to obtain an estimate of the effect for each individual study, along with the measure of the random error (variance or standard error). The individual studies can then be combined by taking a weighted average of the individual estimates from each study, with the weighting being based on the inverse of the variance of each study's estimator. For example, Figure 8.3 shows, for colorectal cancer screening, the combined estimate (the center of diamonds on the line marked 'total') and its 95% confidence interval (the ends of the diamonds).

Biennial

Study	Screening n/N	Control n/N	RR (95%CI fixed)	Weight %	RR (95%CI fixed)
Funen	205 / 30967	249 / 30966		25.3	0.82[0.68,0.99]
Göteborg	121 / 34144	138 / 34164		14.0	0.88[0.69,1.12]
Minnesota	148 / 15587	177 / 15394		18.1	0.83[0.66,1.03]
Nottingham	360 / 76466	420 / 76384		42.6	0.86[0.74,0.99]
Total (95% CI)	834 / 157164	984 / 156908		100.0	0.85[0.77,0.93]

Chi-square 0.24 (df=3) P: 0.97 Z=−3.58 P: 0.8

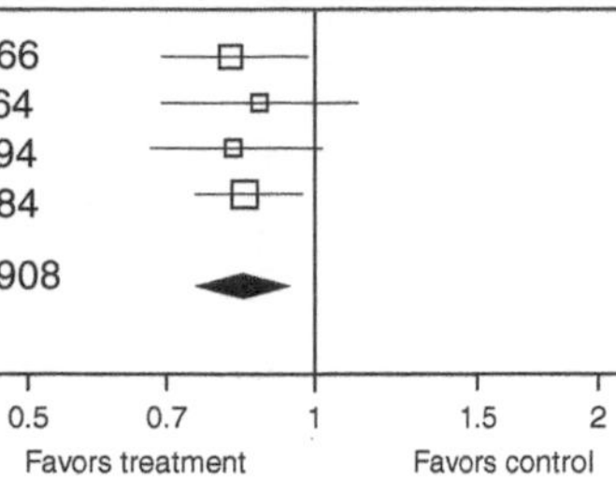

0.5 0.7 1 1.5 2
Favors treatment   Favors control

Annual

Study	Screening n/N	Control n/N	RR (95%CI fixed)	Weight %	RR (95%CI fixed)
Minnesota	121 / 15570	177 / 15394		84.2	0.68[0.54,0.85]
New York	36 / 12974	28 / 8782		15.8	0.87[0.53,1.43]
Total (95% CI)	157 / 28544	205 / 24176		100.0	0.71[0.57,0.87]

Chi-square 0.83 (df=1) P: 0.36 Z=−3.27 P: 0.4

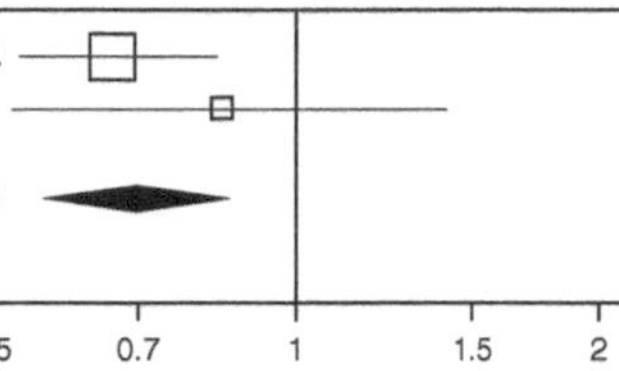

0.5 0.7 1 1.5 2

Figure 8.3   Relative risk (RR) of mortality from colorectal cancer in screened vs. unscreened randomized trials annual and biennial fetal occult blood test screening. CI, confidence interval. From Towler et al. (1998, 2000) with permission.

Although this principle is straightforward, there are a number of statistical issues, which make it far from straightforward. For example, the measures of effect have to be on a scale that provides an approximate normal distribution to the random error (for example using the log odds ratio rather than just the odds ratio), and allowance must be made for zeros in the cells of 2×2 tables or outliers in continuous measurements. Fortunately most of the available software for doing meta-analysis provides such methods, and readers are referred elsewhere for the details of the properties of the various alternative statistical methods (DerSimonian and Laird, 1986; Littenberg and Moses, 1993; Cooper and Hedges, 1994; Rothman and Greenland, 1998).

8.3.4 Generalizability and heterogeneity

The variation between studies is often considered a weakness of a systematic review but, if approached correctly, it can be a considerable strength. If

Table 8.3. Methods of meta-analysis for different types of questions

Question	Major quality issues	Databases	Usual goal of synthesis	Common synthetic methods
Intervention effectiveness	1. Randomization of groups 2. Adequate follow-up ($>80\%$) 3. Blind and/or objective assessment of outcomes	Cochrane Library	a. RRR b. Mean difference	a. Mantel–Haenszel estimator of RRR b. Weighted mean
Frequency or proportion (e.g., pretest probabilities)	1. Random or consecutive sample 2. Adequate ascertainment ($>80\%$) 3. Diagnostic gold standard	MEDLINE	Proportion	Pooled proportion
Diagnostic accuracy	1. Random or consecutive sample 2. Independent reading of test and reference standard 3. Adequate verification ($>80\%$ or adjustment for sampling) 4. Adequate reference standard	MEDLINE, Best Evidence	Summary ROC	Log odds ratio plot back-transformed to ROC
Prognosis	1. Random or consecutive sample 2. Patients at first presentation (or other defined time-point) in disease 3. Adequate ($>80\%$) follow-up 4. Adequate measurement of outcomes	MEDLINE, Best Evidence	Proportion or duration	Weighted average
Multivariable prediction rules (prognostic or diagnostic)	As per question	MEDLINE, Best Evidence	Multivariable rule	Requires individual patient data or variance–covariance matrix from each study

RRR, relative risk reduction; ROC, receiver operating characteristic.

the results are consistent across many studies, despite variation in populations and methods, then we may be reassured that the results are robust and transferable. If the results are inconsistent across studies then we must be wary of generalizing the overall results – a conclusion that a single study cannot usually reach. However, any inconsistency between studies also provides an important opportunity to explore the sources of variation and reach a deeper understanding of its causes and control.

The causes of variation in results may be due to population factors such as gender or genes, disease factors such as severity or stage, variation in the precise methods of the intervention or diagnostic test, or, finally, to differences in study design or conduct such as duration and completeness of follow-up or the quality of measurements. If the meta-analysis can adjust for the variation of these various factors across studies (through meta-regression) and any residual variation is thought to be due to limited sample size of the studies, then some fixed underlying true value is assumed to exist and we refer to such a model as a fixed effects model. When residual variation is due to both limited sample size of studies and due to residual heterogeneity (after adjustment) across study populations, we speak of a random effects model (DerSimonian and Laird, 1986).

8.3.5 Question-specific methods

In addition to the general issues that have been described, there are additional issues and methods specific to the different types of questions: intervention, frequency, diagnostic test accuracy, risk factors and etiology, and prognosis. The principles of finding, appraising and synthesizing apply to each, but specific literature search methods, appraisal issues, and methods of synthesis are needed. Table 8.3 outlines some of these specific issues. For example, column two lists some of the important quality issues relevant to each type of estimate. For further background on the appraisal for each type, we recommend the JAMA User's Guides series (Guyatt et al., 1993, 1994).

There are various software packages available to perform the calculations and plots. None of these is comprehensive and most packages focus on a single question type. Even for addressing a single question more than one package may be required to provide all the needed calculations and plots.

8.4 Subjective estimates

Sometimes it is not possible to assess a probability from 'hard' data. Even if we are comfortable in assuming that the patient at hand is representative of some well-defined population, we may not have any data available on what proportion of individuals in that population have experienced the event of interest. For example, the intervention being considered may be too new for any reliable studies to have been published. Moreover, it can be argued that each patient and each circumstance is unique. Therefore, while data on other patients might help us to assess each individual situation, a physician must often rely on personal judgment. A probability based on a judgment as to one's strength of belief that an event will occur is called a *subjective probability* (or *personal probability* or *judgmental probability*). Subjective probability is a judgment, belief, or opinion ('the chances are...') but we do not restrict the use of the word 'probability' to events for which true, underlying frequencies exist. Finally, subjective probabilities, as we have defined them, should obey all of the laws of objective probabilities, such as the summation principle. Subjective probabilities (a) should add to 1 for a mutually exclusive and exhaustive set of possibilities, and (b) are combinable by multiplication using the laws described in Chapter 3. If so, they are logically and mathematically equivalent to objective probabilities, and one can be unhesitatingly substituted for the other in decision trees, expected utility calculations, or Bayes' formula.

8.4.1 Why use subjective probabilities in decision analyses?

When the probabilities used in a decision analysis are based on objective evidence, we may have confidence in using such an analysis to help guide decision making. In effect, the decision analysis provides a structure for the information you want to take into account in reaching a decision. The analysis incorporates this information and the structural assumptions in a systematic fashion so that conclusions may be drawn.

When all of the required probabilities cannot be estimated from objective data, however, and subjective probabilities are used, the decision analysis continues to produce a quantitative conclusion that one strategy is better than another. By the nature of the method, however, the conclusion drawn is no more than a synthesis of the information that enters into the analysis. Therefore, if the probabilities are based on incomplete evidence or unsubstantiated personal judgment, then why bother with a formal analysis? This is a serious question and one that requires a serious answer, because many probabilities that are needed for decision analyses are not available from the medical literature. Here we offer a brief response to this question.

Most important is the observation that decisions must be made with or without decision analysis. Consider the following scenario. Suppose that you structure a decision analysis for a problem you face but find that one key probability cannot be estimated objectively. You agonize over this situation, but in the end you are unwilling to base your decision on an analysis into which is built a 'best guess' of this unknown probability. Since you have to make a decision, you do so based on your best intuitive judgment. In effect, you are discarding the entire analysis because of one weak link, this unknown probability. Now, suppose that you were to use the decision analysis, but instead of inserting your 'guess' for the unknown probability, you perform a threshold analysis that will indicate over what range of this probability your intuitive decision would be optimal. You find that your intuitive decision would be optimal only if the unknown probability is greater than 0.9. Therefore, in effect, your decision is consistent with an implicit belief that this probability is greater than 0.9. Whatever your beliefs about this unknown probability, *you have acted as if the probability were greater than 0.9.* If, in fact, you are quite confident that the probability, while unknown, is less than 0.5, you have acted inconsistently. Would it not have been better to make a subjective assessment of the probability, if only so that you could take advantage of the rest of the analysis? Then, when you find the result, you can always go back and do a sensitivity analysis with respect to that probability.

The point here is that decisions must be made and are implicitly based on judgments about probabilities of uncertain events. Why not be as explicit as possible about your strength of belief if you are going to act implicitly on that strength of belief in any case?

8.4.2 Decision making versus truth

Many physicians and public health professionals object to the use of subjective probabilities and utilities because they are viewed as 'unscientific.' Some might also view subjective adjustments to objectively estimated probabilities, or syntheses of estimates from different data sources, as unscientific. Agreed, if your purpose is to state a scientific conclusion that one treatment is better than another, then subjective probabilities have no role to play. If you want to know the truth, then a 'best guess' is not acceptable, and you are right to insist on unimpeachable evidence, low P-values, and complete objectivity. If, however, you want to prescribe decisions *that have to be made* one way or another, then decision analysis is a tool for incorporating evidence, beliefs, and values in a systematic way. A careful decision analyst couches all conclusions as *conditional upon the assumptions*, and performs extensive sensitivity analyses to back up that outlook. A scientist in search of truth states conclusions as unconditional: $E = mc^2$, the earth is round. If Columbus and his peers had demanded unimpeachable evidence, the discovery of the New World by Europeans might have been delayed until the advent of satellite imagery!

In the following section, we consider some techniques designed to improve a clinician's skill in probability assessment and to permit several clinicians to pool their opinions in a structured way.

8.4.3 Integrating the evidence and subjective probabilities

What do you do when the literature doesn't quite fit your patient or target population? Over the past decade hundreds, perhaps thousands, of studies have been conducted and published which provide relevant and useful data for decision making. These include scores of studies of clinical outcomes, both randomized and non-randomized clinical trials, studies of new technologies, new drugs, clinical prediction rules, and so forth.

So, all things considered, whether a decision concerns choosing a treatment or assessing the usefulness of a diagnostic procedure, a clinician searching for relevant evidence is far more likely to find published evidence now than 20 years ago. Still, situations do arise when the literature doesn't quite fit and has to be somehow 'adjusted'. For example:

1 Your patient is not precisely the same as those in the sample used in any published study. In many randomized clinical trials, patients with co-morbidities are rigorously excluded, so that the effect of the experimental treatment on the index disease can be assessed with minimal confounding. Hence, patients in RCTs are less likely to have confounding co-morbidities. Your patient, on the other hand, may not match those who were enrolled. Your patient may be younger or older, sicker or healthier, and have more or different co-morbidities. The same problem may arise if you want to extrapolate the findings from a clinical study to the general population.

2 Of the studies bearing on your problem, the study whose sample most closely resembles your patient or target population appears to be the

least trustworthy, perhaps due to flaws in the research plan, small sample size, or simply being older and perhaps out of date.

Given what we have said about possible errors in estimating subjective probabilities and the poor fit between your patient and the findings reported in the literature, we seem to have a dilemma: on the one hand, one must treat subjective probabilities cautiously, and on the other hand, one cannot avoid using them if the evidence in the literature really does not apply to your problem.

What can be done in these situations? There are a number of possible routes out of this dilemma:

1 Determine if the clinical situation, as you see it, is sensitive to variations in the plausible range of relevant probabilities. For example, your subjective estimates of the probabilities of various outcomes may be different from the frequencies provided in the literature, but in a simple decision tree, a threshold analysis may show that both estimates are on the same side of the treatment threshold. A related point is that sensitivity analysis and threshold analysis are always available as ways of improving your confidence in the conclusions of a decision analysis. We will return to the role of sensitivity analysis in the context of subjective probabilities shortly.

An important advantage of pursuing the analysis, even with subjective probabilities, is that it permits a more focused discussion of a clinical problem among physicians or policy makers. We believe that clinical and policy discussions are much more productive when the source of the disagreement over a decision can be isolated than when the discussion ranges unsystematically from issues of treatment efficacy to issues of valued outcomes to issues of treatment options. It is helpful to be able to focus on a subjective probability (or a utility value) as the source of dispute. The evidence pertaining to this probability can then be marshalled and, if a consensus cannot be reached, at least the parties to the discussion may be able to agree as to the reasons for their disagreement.

2 If the different estimates lie on opposite sides of the treatment threshold, reflect on possible reasons for the discrepancy between the literature and your views:

  (a) Is your clinical impression based on audit or retrospective analysis of 30 or 50 or 150 local cases? Or is it based on three or fewer memorable cases? Memorable cases are likely to be unusual (due to the availability bias) and may be an unreliable guide to future experience.

  (b) Is your preferred line of action driven by regret minimization rather than by expected utility maximization? Are you really willing to forgo a fairly sizeable gain to avoid a very small chance of causing serious harm? Recall what we said in the opening chapter: the fundamental assumption of decision analysis is that the decision maker wishes to maximize expected utility. The techniques we have discussed in this book are designed to reach that goal. Regret minimization is sometimes a powerful motive, but it is not what decision analysis generally aims to achieve although methods to include regret could theoretically be developed.

(c) Ask if your subjective estimates are overly optimistic. If surgery is being considered for your patient and your estimates of the probability of a good outcome are substantially better than what is reported in the literature, consider this: Is it probable that local outcome experience is substantially better than the pooled outcome data in a series of published studies? If you believe it is, what kind of data can be reviewed to support this claim? In other words, try to put your subjective estimates to the test of local evidence.

3 Go with a literature-derived composite and ignore personal and local experience. Limited personal clinical experience with the problem at hand, especially compared to the sample sizes reported in the literature, argues for this strategy. Also, this strategy may help you persuade others that your conclusion applies more broadly, an important consideration if you want to get your analysis published.

4 Ignore published literature and go with personal experience. It is tempting to do this because it will circumvent the prescriptive-descriptive issue. But this strategy is unwise if you expect to publish your work or convince others of its merits.

5 Combine estimates. The following approach should help to minimize undesirable effects of anchoring and adjustment:
  (a) Anchor on your personal or local experience and adjust your estimate in the light of the evidence.
  (b) Repeat this process, except now anchor on the evidence and adjust in the light of your clinical experience and beliefs.
  (c) Split the difference between these estimates, weighting for the likely differences in the sample sizes behind each.

6 Formally revise a prior probability distribution on the unknown quantity. Formal Bayesian approaches may be helpful here. For example you may assess a subjective prior probability distribution for the quantity of interest. Then, using the evidence, revise your probability distribution using Bayes' theorem.

To illustrate the 'fully Bayesian' approach, suppose that you want to estimate a frequency, P, such as the prevalence of disease in your local clinic. You aren't sure what the value of P is, but you assess a distribution, assigning probabilities to the range of possible values of P from 0 to 1. The family of β distributions is often convenient for this purpose. Next, specify the likelihood of the observed data in the literature, conditional upon each possible true value of P. Data generated from a proportion p are usually modeled according to the binomial distribution, so it is possible to write down the binomial probabilities for the observed data. Finally, use Bayes' theorem to revise your prior distribution on p. This can be done with software designed to perform Bayesian probability revision, such as WIN-BUGS. If your prior distribution was a β distribution, the posterior distribution will also be a β distribution. Useful distributions for continuously valued quantities include the normal (Gaussian) distribution, the lognormal distribution, and the γ distribution. (For details, see a textbook on Bayesian statistics, such as Gelman et al., 1995.)

8.4.4 Probability assessments by groups of experts: the Delphi method

Subjective probabilities may not be perfectly accurate, but often in clinical medicine they are the only ones available and have to be used, either implicitly or explicitly, because a decision must be made. Clinicians can learn to appreciate the human tendencies toward error and thus improve the accuracy of their probability assessments. Sometimes a probability is crucial to a policy decision but there is no direct evidence available, e.g., what are the chances that a vaccine will be developed within 5 years for a particular infectious disease, such as HIV or malaria? One approach to obtaining such probability assessments for policy decisions is to poll a group of experts. The premise in doing so is that, by interacting with each other, the group members will not be as prone to bias. Formal methods for obtaining group assessments are most likely to be useful in situations in which it is desirable to convince others of the validity of the decision analysis, objective estimates are not available, the personal opinions of a single decision maker will not suffice, and sensitivity analysis indicates that the conclusion is especially sensitive to a particular probability assessment.

One method for obtaining the consensus of a panel of experts is called the Delphi method. Under this method each member of the group of experts is asked for an assessment of the probability in question, along with the reasons for the assessment. Then, the results of this round of assessments are fed back to the members of the group, but in a way that preserves the anonymity of the assessors. Thus, they might be told that five assessors gave a probability between 0.2 and 0.25, 10 assessors gave a probability between 0.25 and 0.30, and so forth. Then another round of assessments is solicited, and the process of feedback is repeated. The process continues until some specified level of consensus is reached or until a certain number of rounds have been conducted, whichever happens first. The theory behind the Delphi method is that the interaction of opinions still leads toward a consensus and will help eliminate individual biases. It is also held that the anonymity of responses will prevent the participants from reaching an agreement simply because of peer pressure. The method has been applied in studies of medical decisions and convergence was achieved.

A possible serious drawback of the Delphi method is that the tendency toward consensus may reinforce, and not eliminate, the biases that underlie some of the participants' probability assessments. Moreover, there is no guarantee that an assessment is accurate just because a group of experts can be made to agree on it. Caution should therefore be exercised in interpreting the probability assessments derived from a Delphi procedure. Sensitivity analysis should always be used, just as for individual assessments, and there should be no misconceptions that a Delphi study of expert opinion is a substitute for a well-designed clinical study. For purposes of a clinician's own decision making group assessment methods are generally impractical, although they can be used in certain hospital and group practice settings as part of a program of clinical rounds or, in particular, for developing guidelines.

8.4.5 A definition of 'subjective probability'

Leaving the medical world temporarily, suppose that you are asked to estimate the probability that the next president of the United States will be a Republican. One approach might be to look at the record over the past century; if 13 of the last 25 elections had been won by Republicans, you might estimate the probability as 13/25, or 0.52. These are useful background data, but because times have changed, this might now be viewed as a poor estimate. An alternative approach would be to marshal all the information at your disposal to answer subjectively questions of the following kind:

'Do you think it more or less likely that a Republican will be elected than that a flip of a coin, whose sides are equally weighted, will come up heads?'

DEFINITION

Suppose that a person believes that an event E is just as likely to occur as another event whose probability of occurrence is defined objectively as $P*$. Then $P*$ is this person's *subjective probability* that event E will occur.

An answer of 'more likely' indicates that:

$P*$ [Republican] > 0.5

where the asterisk reminds us that this is a subjective probability. (Once we are accustomed to the notion of subjective probability, we will do away with the asterisk.) An answer of 'less likely' means that:

$P*$[Republican] < 0.5

Suppose that your subjective answer is 'less likely,' so that $P*$ is less than 0.5. Then you might proceed by answering the following question:

'Do you think it more or less likely that a Republican will be elected than that the roll of a six-sided dice will come up with one or two dots?'

An answer of 'more likely' narrows the range further. Now:

$1/3 < P*$ [Republican] $< 1/2$

We could continue to narrow the range by analogy to 'known' probabilities until we settle on a point estimate.

This process will lead to a probability assessment between 0 and 1, as long as the probability assessor is careful to be consistent with the principle of transitivity; that is, if event A is thought to be more likely to occur than event B, and event B is thought to be more likely to occur than event C, then event A is thought to be more likely to occur than event C. This procedure of probability assessment can be used, for our purposes, as a definition of subjective probability.

In many clinical decision problems, it is not important to reduce the assessment to a point estimate; a range of probability (e.g., $0.3 < P < 0.4$) may suffice, depending on the results of sensitivity analysis.

8.5 Sensitivity analysis revisited

How precise do our estimates of probability and values need to be? There is no single answer to this question. Rather it depends on whether and how changing a particular parameter changes the optimal decision. This in turn will depend on three things: how influential the parameter is in the analysis, its range of uncertainty, and how close the decision is to a particular threshold.

The influence of a probability or value depends on its overall contribution to the expected value, or more precisely, its contribution to the *difference* in expected value of different decision options. Some parameters may have little influence on a decision, even if they appear to be a large component. For example, if two drugs have similar toxicity profiles then

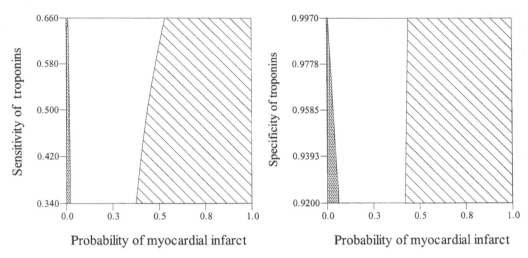

Probability of myocardial infarct   Probability of myocardial infarct

Figure 8.4   The two-way sensitivity analyses for the probability of acute myocardial infarction and for the sensitivity and specificity of troponin. Dotted area, wait; unshaded area, troponin; hatched area, immediate thrombolytic.

the choice of drug will be insensitive to the values placed on those toxicities. However, the decision to use a drug at all may be very sensitive to those values. A better understanding of the influence of different probabilities and values may be gained through a series of sensitivity analyses.

Ideally, a sensitivity analysis should be done for each parameter over its range of uncertainty. If you have good external relevant data, then the confidence interval may be used for the range of uncertainty. If there is only a subjective estimate then a subjective range may be needed.

Recall the example in Chapter 6 of the man with chest pain and suspected myocardial infarction. Important uncertainties in the decision to use the serum troponin (a blood test suggestive of whether or not a patient has had a myocardial infarction) were the uncertainty about the sensitivity and specificity of troponin, and the probability of a myocardial infarction. Based on the Antman et al. data (1995) the 95% confidence for the sensitivity is 34% to 66%; the 95% confidence interval for the specificity is 92% to 99.7%. The two-way sensitivity analyses for the probability of acute myocardial infarction and for the sensitivity and specificity of troponin respectively are shown in Figure 8.4. This demonstrates that for certain ranges, the decision is not sensitive to the exact probability of myocardial infarction. For example, within the ranges of uncertainty of the troponins' sensitivity and specificity, above a probability of myocardial infarction of 0.50 the optimal decision is immediate thrombolytic. Similarly, between 0.05 and 0.40, testing with troponin appears optimal. Provided we believe that the probability of myocardial infarction lies within one of these ranges, then the exact value does not matter.

If the sensitivity analysis shows that the decision is particularly sensitive to one or two parameters, then you should devote more care to how these were estimated. For example, you may consider doing a systematic review to obtain a combined estimate for a probability that is crucial to the decision. You may even consider that you need to initiate further research to obtain better values for future similar decision problems. Decision analysis is not just a tool for making an individual decision or policy, but is also helpful in identifying what information is most needed to improve decision making. We would strongly recommend conducting a decision analysis before undertaking any new research so that the study can be designed to gather information on the most relevant parameters.

8.6 Summary

The merit of a decision analysis depends on both the overall structuring of the problem and on the accuracy of the individual probabilities and values used. It is therefore important to access the best available information for these parameters. Some probabilities and values will come from external data. When there are several potential sources, we would ideally find a systematic review. However, a systematic review or meta-analysis is considerable work, and hence to make the analysis practical you may need to focus on the best single source available (using appraisal methods such as those described in Chapter 2). In choosing a source there may be a trade-off between the quality of the source (internal validity) and its relevance to your particular situation (external validity). There is no perfect 'objective' data, as there is always some degree of mismatch between the available data and your requirements, and hence a subjective adjustment may be needed. If there is no external data, we still need to make a decision, and hence subjective probabilities may be needed. Whether the probabilities are objective or subjective, you should undertake sensitivity analysis to check the robustness of any conclusions.

Exercises

Exercise 8.1

Intermittent claudication is a common complaint in the elderly; about 2% of the population suffer from claudication. Characteristic symptoms are

Table 8.4

Authors	Reference	Sensitivity (%)	Specificity (%)	D	$1/SE(D)$
Adamis et al. (1995)	*Radiology*, **196**, 689–95	99	85	6.06	0.69
Hany et al. (1997)	*Radiology*, **204**, 357–62	96	97	6.52	1.24
Ho et al. (1998)	*Radiology*, **206**, 683–92	92	98	6.47	1.64
Ho et al. (1998)	*Radiology*, **206**, 673–81	91	93	4.87	1.60
Laissy et al. (1998)	*J. Magn. Reson. Imag.*, **8**, 1060–5	100	96	8.73	0.69
Poon et al. (1997)	*Am. J. Radiol.*, **169**, 1139–44	96	99	8.28	0.49
Quinn et al. (1997)	*J. Magn. Reson. Imag.*, **7**, 197–203	98	98	8.20	0.61
Rofksy et al. (1997)	*Radiology*, **205**, 163–9	96	96	6.40	1.04
Snidow et al. (1996)	*Radiology*, **198**, 725–32	98	95	6.90	0.67

D, natural logarithm of the diagnostic odds ratio, a measure that is used in a summary receiver operator characteristic analysis; SE, standard error.

pain, cramp, or fatigue in the muscles of the lower extremity caused by walking, which are completely relieved after a few minutes of rest. Over time patients may develop more severe symptoms such as ischemic rest pain, ulcers, or gangrene, known as critical limb ischemia. These symptoms are explained by impaired blood flow to the lower extremity caused by atherosclerotic obstructive disease in the peripheral arterial system, known in the medical literature as peripheral arterial disease.

A diagnostic test to evaluate disabling claudication and critical ischemia is gadolinium-enhanced magnetic resonance angiography (MRA). It is a relatively new imaging modality with excellent diagnostic performance. For a decision model evaluating the diagnostic workup of peripheral arterial disease you would like to have an estimate of the sensitivity and specificity of gadolinium-enhanced MRA. You decide to do a systematic review of the medical literature.

(a) Think about a search strategy to find studies on gadolinium-enhanced MRA for detecting peripheral arterial disease. Optional: perform your own search strategy.

In a meta-analysis on gadolinium-enhanced MRA (Visser, K. & Hunink, M.G.M. (2000) Peripheral arterial disease: gadolinium-enhanced MR angiography versus color-guided duplex US – a meta-analysis. *Radiology*, **216**, 67–77) the tabulated studies were found in the period between January 1990 and November 1998 (Table 8.4).

(b) On which criteria could you judge the quality of the individual studies? Would you make an overall quality score?

(c) Make a funnelplot for MRA using the D (natural logarithm of the diagnostic odds ratio) from the table. What is your conclusion about publication bias?

(d) Plot the true and false positive rates in ROC space. What do you notice?

(e) For decision analysis you want a 'pooled' sensitivity and specificity based on the individual studies that takes into account the different cutoff values used by the individual studies. Describe how you can obtain these values.

REFERENCES

Antman, E.M., Grudzien, C. & Sacks, D.B. (1995). Evaluation of a rapid bedside assay for detection of serum cardiac troponin T. *J.A.M.A.*, **273**, 1279–82.

Cooper, H. & Hedges, L.V. (1994). *The Handbook of Research Synthesis*. New York: Russell Sage Foundation.

DerSimonian, R. & Laird, N. (1986). Meta-analysis in clinical trials. *Control. Clin. Trials*, **7**, 177–88.

Detsky, A., Naylor, C.D., O'Rourke, K., McGreer, A.J. & L'abbe, K.A. (1992). Incorporating variations in the quality of individual randomized trials into meta-analysis. *J. Clin. Epidemiol.*, **45**, 255–65.

Dickersin, K., Min, Y.I. & Meinert, C.L. (1992). Factors influencing publication of research results: followup of application submitted to two institutional review boards. *J.A.M.A.*, **267**, 374–8.

Gelman, A., Carlin, J.B,, Stern, H.S. & Rubin, D.B. (1995). *Bayesian Data Analysis*. London: Chapman & Hall.

Guyatt, G.H., Sackett, D.L. & Cook, D.J. (1993). Users' guide to medical literature. *J.A.M.A.*, **270**, 2598–601.

Guyatt, G.H., Sackett, D.L. & Cook, D.J. (1994). Users' guides to the medical literature II. How to us an article about therapy or prevention. *J.A.M.A.*, **271**, 59–63.

Haynes, R.B., Wilczynski, N., McKibbon, K.A., Walker, C.J. & Sinclair, J.C. (1994). Developing optimal search strategies for detecting clinically sound studies in Medline. *J. Am. Med. Inf. Assoc.*, **1**, 447–58.

Littenberg, B. & Moses, L.E. (1993). Estimating diagnostic accuracy from multiple conflicting reports: a new meta-analytic method. *Med. Decis. Making*, **13**, 313–21.

Mahoney, M.J. (1977). Publications prejudices: an experimental study of confirmatory bias in the peer review system. *Cogn. Ther. Res.*, **1**, 161–75.

McManus, R.J., Wilson, S., Delaney, B.C. et al. (1998). Review of the usefulness of contacting other experts when conducting a literature search for systematic reviews. *Br. Med. J.*, **317**, 1562–3.

Mulrow, C.D. & Oxman, A. (1997). *Cochrane Collaboration Handbook* [updated Sept. 1997]. Oxford: The Cochrane Collaboration.

Rothman, K.J. & Greenland, S. (1998). *Modern Epidemiology*. Philadelphia: Lippincott-Raven.

Schulz, K.F., Chalmers, I., Hayes, R.J. & Altman, D.G. (1995). Empirical evidence of bias: dimensions of methodological quality associated with estimates of treatment effects in controlled trials. *J.A.M.A.*, **273**, 408–12.

Simes, R. (1987). Confronting publication bias: a cohort design for meta-analysis. *Stat. Med.*, **6**, 11–29.

Towler, B., Irwig, L., Glasziou P. et al. (1998). A systematic review of the effects of screening for colorectal cancer using the faecal occult blood test, hemoccult. *Br. Med. J.*, **317**, 559–65.

Towler, B., Irwig, L., Glasziou, P., Weller, D. & Kewenter, J. (2000). Screening for colorectal cancer using the faecal occult blood test, hemoccult. *Cochrane Database Syst. Rev.*, **2**, CD001216. http://www.health.library.mcgill.ca/database/cochran2.htm.

Tramer, M.R., Reynolds, D.J.M., Moore, R.A. & McQuay, H.J. (1997). Impact of covert duplicate publication on meta-analysis: a case study. *Br. Med. J.*, **315**, 635–40.

Visser, K. & Hunink, M.G.M. (2000). Peripheral arterial disease: gadolinium-enhanced MR angiography versus color-guided duplex US – a meta-analysis. *Radiology*, **216**, 67–77.

9

Constrained resources

There is no question that financial and medical effects will both be considered when making health care decisions at all levels of policymaking; the only question is whether they will be considered well.

Elaine J. Power and John M. Eisenberg

9.1 Introduction

Medical care entails benefits, risks, and costs. Until this chapter our approach has involved weighing benefits against risks for individuals and groups of patients and choosing the actions that provide the greatest expected net benefit. Now we extend our analysis to consider expressly the economic costs of health care.

As with all economic goods and services, the provision of health care consumes resources. Hospital beds, medical office facilities, medical equipment, pharmaceuticals, medical devices, and the time of physicians, nurses, other health-care workers, and family members all contribute to health care. The consumption of these resources constitutes the economic costs of health care.

Sometimes the word *cost* is used to refer to any negative effect of an action; for example, we might refer to the side-effects of a drug as a 'cost' of treatment. In this chapter, however, we use *costs* only in the specific economic sense of resources consumed, whether materials or time.

Resources available for health care are limited in supply. This means that whenever resources are used for one activity, they are not available for other activities. An hour of a physician's time spent with one patient is unavailable for another, and an intensive care bed occupied by one patient cannot be used that day for another. Resources devoted to a smoking cessation campaign cannot be spent to increase seat belt use. Society can add to the resources devoted to health care by training more nurses, building more clinics, or launching new outreach programs. But even in the longer term, resources available for health care will be finite. Any medical decision or policy decision that entails the use of resources implicitly excludes those resources from alternative possible uses.

Health resources are consumed in order to produce health benefits.

Given the limited availability of resources, we are led naturally to ask questions about their most efficient use: is this particular expenditure of health resources worthwhile, given the alternative uses to which they might be put?

Our aim in this chapter is to introduce the conceptual and analytic issues surrounding decisions that involve the allocation of health resources. We will begin by considering a type of decision concerning the allocation of resources that busy clinicians face every day: the allocation of their time. Then we will introduce the principles underlying the efficient allocation of limited resources and discuss the major elements of cost-effectiveness analysis (CEA). Next we will focus on the correct calculation of incremental ratios for comparing the cost-effectiveness of interventions, describe current guidelines for the conduct of CEAs, and review methodological and ethical concerns. By the end of the chapter, you should know the rationale underlying CEAs, be able to assess them critically, and appreciate the potential for different conclusions about preferred interventions and programs when resource costs are ignored versus when they are included.

9.2 The efficient allocation of constrained resources

9.2.1 An example: time as a constrained resource for the clinician

Physicians and other clinicians know they cannot spend as much time with every patient as might be ideal. The constraints on time, which may have been pressing in years past, are even more pronounced in the current, more competitive health-care environment. Time spent addressing one health concern is time that is not spent in addressing another.

Let us say that the clinician's objective is to maximize the overall health benefits to patients, given a limit, for example, of 20 min of contact time with a patient during an annual physical. Suppose that the clinician has estimated the impact of care on each patient in terms of the expected number of days of disability prevented. (Note that this 'expected' benefit would not accrue to every patient but would accrue on average over the long run.) Each intervention consumes a certain amount of the limited time available. Hypothetical information of this kind is given in Table 9.1. The physician time estimates presented in this table are intended to represent time taken to explain the procedure, carry it out (if it is conducted by the physician), and, if needed, discuss the results. The estimates would vary depending on the patient. For example, the expected health benefit of clinical breast examination and discussion of mammography

Table 9.1. Hypothetical health benefits and physician time requirements for clinical preventive services, listed in order of expected health benefit

Intervention (for adult women)	Expected health benefit (days of disability prevented)^a	Time required (min)^a
Papanicolaou smear	50	5
Blood pressure	50	1
Total blood cholesterol	47	2
Clinical breast exam and discussion of mammogram	45	2
Height and weight	35	1
Counseling on limiting fat and cholesterol	25	2
Fecal occult blood test and/or sigmoidoscopy (≥ 50 years)	22	2
Counseling on tobacco cessation	22	4
Counseling on regular physical activity	20	2
Counseling on lap/shoulder belts	17	1
Counseling on adequate calcium intake	14	2
Screening for problem drinking	12	1
Screening for rubella serology or vaccination	9	2
Counseling on smoke detectors	5	1
Counseling on safe storage of firearms	5	2
Counseling on bicycle helmets	4	1
Counseling on prevention of sexually transmitted diseases	3	2
Counseling on regular visits to dentist	2	1
Chest X-ray for lung cancer	0	3

^{a}These examples are for illustrative purposes only; they are not based on actual data.

would be higher for a 50-year-old woman with a familial history of breast cancer than for a 40-year-old woman with a negative history, based on her risk profile.

In order to maximize total benefit, the clinician should allocate time to interventions according to the amount of benefit provided per unit of time required, or 'time-effectiveness.' Thus, in the table the most time-effective use is the allocation of the clinician's time to blood pressure screening, which results in an expected benefit of 50 days of disability prevented but consumes only 1 min of physician time. The next most time-effective use is the allocation of time to height and weight, which has a time-effectiveness ratio of 35.

The best decision rule for the clinician to follow in meeting the objective is to establish priorities according to this ratio and choose interventions in decreasing order of priority (in descending order of the effectiveness/time ratio until the available time is exhausted; Table 9.2).

Table 9.2. Hypothetical health benefits and physician time requirements for clinical preventive services in order of effectiveness/time ratio

Intervention (for adult women)	Expected health benefit (days of disability prevented)^a	Time required (min)^a	Effectiveness/time ratio (E/T)
Blood pressure	50	1	50.0
Height and weight	35	1	35.0
Total blood cholesterol	47	2	23.5
Clinical breast exam and discussion of mammogram	45	2	22.5
Counseling on lap/shoulder belts	17	1	17.0
Counseling on limiting fat and cholesterol	25	2	12.5
Screening for problem drinking	12	1	12.0
Fecal occult blood test and/or sigmoidoscopy ($\geq$ 50 years)	22	2	11.0
Papanicolaou smear	50	5	10.0
Counseling on regular physical activity	20	2	10.0
Counseling on adequate calcium intake	14	2	7.0
Counseling on tobacco cessation	22	4	5.5
Counseling on smoke detectors	5	1	5.0
Screening for rubella serology or vaccination	9	2	4.5
Counseling on bicycle helmets	4	1	4.0
Counseling on safe storage of firearms	5	2	2.5
Counseling on regular visits to dentist	2	1	2.0
Counseling on prevention of sexually transmitted diseases	3	2	1.5
Chest X-ray for lung cancer	0	3	0.0

^{a}These examples are for illustrative purposes only; they are not based on actual data.

Note that some clinical preventive services that offer significant benefit but which are also very time-consuming will be excluded. In our example, screening for rubella serology is one of these. It will be selected as a lower priority than other interventions, such as counseling on smoke detectors, which, although offering less total benefit, require much less of the physician's time. Some interventions, such as chest X-ray for lung cancer, confer no benefit and will never be selected. But in general, the physician must draw the line for which interventions to administer well above these no-benefit procedures, omitting some which confer real benefit because of the limits on his or her time.

Other examples of this sort of allocation that physicians regularly perform include triage in an emergency room and the allocation of intensive care unit beds. Although the constrained resources in these examples include skilled nursing care and intensive care unit beds, the same principles of ranking in terms of resource-effectiveness and choosing according to the order of greatest efficiency apply.

9.2.2 Analytic tools for resource allocation: an overview

The analytic methods we present in this chapter are premised on a desire to use available resources to gain the most health benefit. We begin with the proposition that it is not possible to provide all beneficial health services to all people. In many countries, there is a fixed budget for health care; limited resources like hospital beds and specialized medical procedures are allocated by eligibility rules and waiting lists. Patients and clinicians alike are cognizant of the reality of resource limits. In the US, where there is no fixed budget for health care, the pressures of competing demands for tax dollars and employee compensation, and of price competition among insurers and providers, none the less constrain health-care spending.

There are several ways to control health-care costs. We can eliminate inefficiency in the delivery of care. Thus, many hospital services that can be provided on an outpatient basis with no loss in quality have been shifted to the lower-cost setting in recent years. We can weed out interventions known to be ineffective, saving the resources devoted to these interventions for productive purposes. Some have argued that investing resources in preventive services will save on future costs of chronic illness, although this proposition is not true in many cases.

Figure 9.1 categorizes health interventions in terms of their cost (on the x-axis) and their health effect (on the y-axis). For interventions that can improve health and save money at the same time (upper left quadrant), there is no need for analysis; they should be adopted. Similarly, there is no question that interventions that decrease health and cost money (lower right quadrant) should be discontinued if currently used and not adopted if new. Interventions falling into the other two quadrants, however, require choices if health benefit is to be maximized subject to available resources. These are interventions that improve health yet cost money – the majority of effective interventions. In addition, actions that save money although at some loss of health outcome should be considered. These decisions apply to effective interventions currently in place that achieve less benefit with the resources they require than would a different use of these resources.

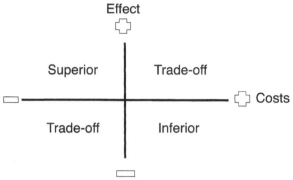

Figure 9.1   Cost-effectiveness space, with costs on the *x*-axis and effectiveness on the *y*-axis.

There are several related but distinct approaches to the assessment of health practices, which allow comparisons among interventions so that decision makers can trade off opportunities for health-care investments falling in one of these two quadrants. These are included under the general heading of *economic evaluation*. The first, *cost-minimization analysis*, compares interventions based solely on their net cost. This method applies when alternative options have (or are assumed to have) the same effectiveness. The measure used for comparison is the net difference in resource costs. Because health benefits, which are often difficult to quantify, do not enter into the calculation, cost-minimization analysis is generally simpler to undertake than other methods of economic analysis. But this restriction also limits its applicability.

Cost-effectiveness analysis compares interventions based on a common measure of their costs and a common measure of their health effectiveness. The measure used for health effectiveness may be cases of a disease prevented, cases cured, lives saved, or years of life saved. It may also be a preference-based measure such as quality-adjusted life years (QALYs) gained, discussed in Chapter 4. Analyses using health measures that are expressed in quality-adjusted units are sometimes referred to as *cost–utility analyses*. Here, we use the term CEA to include this subset of analyses. CEA can be used when alternative options have different costs and, when a common metric such as the QALY is used, different types of health consequences; by definition, however, all interventions compared must affect health.

Cost–benefit analysis requires that all effects of alternative interventions, as well as all costs, are valued in monetary terms. It can be used to compare very different interventions, including health and nonhealth investments of resources. Alternatives are considered on the basis of their net benefit:

options with a positive net benefit should be implemented while those with a negative net benefit should not. Cost–benefit analysis is used less frequently in health care than CEA, because many people are uncomfortable valuing health effects, such as human lives and the quality of life, in monetary terms. Objections are both technical, concerning the validity of methods used to assign a value to health effects, and ethical.

Because the concerns regarding cost–benefit analysis have led to a preference for CEA in the realm of health care, our focus in this chapter is on CEA. However, cost–benefit analysis is used in a sizeable fraction of economic analyses concerning health, particularly those examining environmental programs and other interventions that have important effects in nonhealth domains as well as affecting health.

9.2.3 Perspectives for analysis

Resource allocation decisions are often made in the context of diverse views and preferences. Although there is sometimes an identifiable decision maker, such as a patient facing a decision regarding her own choices of therapy, often there is not. Many health and medical policies seem to 'emerge' or follow a tradition. More often than not, decisions made are the result of complex processes involving many protagonists.

Although actual decisions may involve a mix of perspectives and interests, CEA, as a normative decision-making tool, begins with the specification of the decision-making perspective – the perspective of the analysis. The explicit specification of perspective is essential to economic evaluation generally and CEA in particular. An explicit perspective provides a framework for analysts in conducting an analysis and for users of that analysis, in making judgments about its validity. For example, in deciding whether to offer a particular screening program, a health maintenance organization (HMO) would consider more than its costs to run the program and the potential health benefits to current enrollees. Factors such as the attractiveness of the program to desirable enrollees, its attractiveness to the medical staff, and the likelihood of those benefiting remaining enrolled would also be part of the equation. When the perspective of the analysis is clear, it is also clear what properly belongs in the analysis.

It is generally the consideration of resources in health and medical decisions that makes perspective a critical issue. If we consider only risks and benefits of health-care decisions, we usually encounter no conflicts of interest affecting these decisions. A notable exception involves communicable diseases, for which the actions of some individuals may affect the health of others: preventing or curing infection may reduce the risk of transmitting infection to others, and vaccination may reduce community risk through herd immunity. But in most cases, when cost is disregarded, the decision belongs to the patient and family, even when health-care providers and patients have different information about an intervention or different values concerning the outcomes.

Once concerns about health resources are introduced, however, the different perspectives invariably come into play. The owners of these differing perspectives have different goals for the allocation of resources. In addition, they experience different costs and different effects of interventions. For example, the benefit of successful knee surgery may be very different to a surgical practice or hospital, or to the health benefits manager of a professional sports franchise, than to an employer of computer programmers or the benefits manager of a symphony orchestra. The cost of a follow-up visit for a child's ear infection will be different for an uninsured patient facing a billed amount, an HMO patient with a per-visit charge, or a private pediatrician, whose cost would reflect her own time and her office expenses.

Resource allocation issues arise whenever decision makers face budget constraints. In the health-care arena, a range of decision makers confront these decisions. These include hospitals, clinics, private insurers, government entitlement programs, patients, and managed-care organizations in addition to clinicians.

The societal perspective
Although CEAs intended to assist patients, clinicians, and administrators with a specific decision will generally take the perspective of the individual or institution making the decision, many decisions require a broader analysis conducted from the societal perspective. The societal perspective is the most comprehensive perspective for a CEA. It considers all ramifications of a decision: all costs, regardless of who experiences them, and similarly, all health benefits. The societal perspective is that of society at large – the sum of all individuals in society.

The societal perspective is prescribed for analyses that consider programs affecting the distribution of societal resources. In health care, however, many if not most decisions have implications for broader resource allocation. Societal implications are perhaps most obvious in decisions regarding government health policies and public health: programs financed by taxes for disease prevention, food and drug regulation, and

> **DEFINITION**
>
> The *societal perspective* is the one that considers everyone affected by an intervention and all significant effects and resource uses of the program.

publicly financed health care. But decisions in much more local contexts may also have implications for societal resource allocation. Choices concerning medical education and the practice of medicine may have a localized effect in the context of any particular patient but have a significant influence on society when they establish patterns of medical practice.

Because a prime benefit of CEA is to allow decision makers to compare and make choices among programs, it is important that there be a bank of comparable CEAs. For this reason, analysts sometimes choose to conduct an analysis from the societal perspective instead of, or in addition to, an analysis from the patient, provider, or organizational perspective.

9.2.4 The cost-effectiveness analysis model

As described earlier, the underlying premise of CEA in health problems is that, for any given level of resources available, the decision maker wishes to maximize the aggregate health benefits conferred to the population of concern. Alternatively, a given health benefit goal may be set, the objective being to minimize the cost of achieving it. In either formulation the analytic methodology is the same. First, health benefits and health resource costs must each be expressed in terms of some unit of measurement. Health resource costs are usually measured in monetary terms but might equivalently be expressed in units of hospital days or hours of clinician time. Health effectiveness (or health benefit) is expressed in terms of some unit of output, such as the number of cases of cancer detected or in terms of a measure of ultimate outcomes, such as the number of lives or years of life saved. The use of QALYs has the advantage of incorporating changes in survival and morbidity in a single measure.

The cost-effectiveness measure is the ratio of costs to benefits and is expressed, for example, as the cost per year of life saved or the cost per QALY saved. Alternative programs or services are ranked from the lowest value of this cost-per-effect ratio to the highest, and then they are selected starting with the highest-ranked program or service until available resources are exhausted. The cost-per-effect ratio at which one is no longer willing or able to pay the price for the benefits achieved becomes the cutoff level of permissible cost per unit of effectiveness. For example, the level of blood pressure at which antihypertensive treatment is recommended might be based on some number of dollars per QALY. The application of this procedure insures that the maximum possible expected health benefits will be realized, subject to whatever resource constraint is in effect.

The cost-effectiveness formulation

The cost-effectiveness ratio contains the net increase in health-care costs for an intervention as compared to an alternative in the numerator, and the net increase in health effect in the denominator. This ratio ($\Delta C/\Delta E$) can be summarized as follows:

$$\Delta C/\Delta E = (\Delta C_{Prog} + \Delta C_{Ind} + \Delta C_{Morb} + \Delta C_{SE} + \Delta C_{Prog\Delta LE})/\Delta E \qquad (9.1)$$

where: ΔC_{Prog} = the cost of the program or intervention; ΔC_{Ind} = the cost or savings for procedures induced or avoided as a result of the program; ΔC_{Morb} = the cost or savings for morbidity averted; ΔC_{SE} = the cost of treating side-effects and complications; $\Delta C_{Prog\Delta LE}$ = the cost of health care in added years of life; ΔE = the change in QALYs or other measure of health benefit.

These components of cost and health benefit are explained further in the sections on costs and effectiveness below.

CEA has been approached from more than one disciplinary direction. Cost-effectiveness research is conducted by economists, psychologists, physicians, and policy analysts. In this book, we present CEA in the context of a broader discussion of decision analysis. Decision analytic concepts and methods are frequently used to perform CEA. CEAs often contain important areas of uncertainty; as a result, the calculation of net health benefits and net costs on the basis of a complex set of possible events and the probabilities associated with them is a primary challenge of the analysis. The methods described in this book – the construction of decision trees, Markov modeling, and the valuation of health outcomes – are central to CEA, although these elements may also be found in a variety of other analytical approaches. Other tools, including epidemiological analyses, spreadsheet programming, and simulation modeling, may also be employed to calculate the net costs and net health benefits in the cost-effectiveness ratio.

9.3 Costs

When health-care resources are limited, the consumption of resources by one patient means that somewhere, sometime, resources are unavailable for some other health-care purpose. It is thus the consumption of resources that constitutes the cost of care. The measure of cost is the value that is forgone when resources are used for one purpose rather than for the next preferred use. This amount – the value of resources in the next best use – is known as the *opportunity cost* of the resource.

DEFINITION

The *opportunity cost* of a resource consumed in the provision of a good or service is the value of that resource in its next best alternative use.

The perspective of a CEA plays an important role in determining the opportunity cost of a resource. According to economic theory, the price of a good being sold in a competitive market should equal its opportunity cost. For a health-care institution that pays this price, the price is indeed the opportunity cost; this is the amount that could be spent on the next best alternative if it were not used in this purchase. From the perspective of an insured patient, however, the cost of a drug may be equal not to its price but to the 20% co-payment the patient pays. From the societal perspective, opportunity cost may also be difficult to ascertain, since impediments to perfect competition may push the price up or down relative to true opportunity cost. Some practical approaches to the calculation of cost from the societal perspective are discussed in the next section.

It is important to note that real resource consumption is different from the transfer of resources from one party to another. The distribution of costs is an important but separate issue. If the government sends a check to a pharmacist as reimbursement for a Medicaid prescription, this in itself does not constitute a resource cost from the societal perspective, because the resource pool is in no way depleted. From the societal perspective, the cost occurs when the drug is produced, because resources put to this use cannot be put to another societal use. The cost is assigned to the patient who consumes the drug, because she is the end-user of the resource, and this cost is unaffected by whether the patient, an insurer, the hospital (through unreimbursed care), or the government actually pays for it. (Of course, if only the government's perspective were considered, the Medicaid payment would be a cost, because it would deplete the government's resources – the only resources of relevance in an analysis from this perspective. In CEA, the governmental perspective is different from the societal perspective.)

9.3.1 Components of cost in CEA

9.3.1.1 Types of costs

Several types of cost comprise the total resource use to be considered in comparing health-care interventions. The first category, *health-care resources*, is perhaps the most obvious. Health-care resources used to produce a dental appointment, an inpatient admission, an X-ray, a prenatal class, or other health-care service consist of supplies, pharmaceuticals, equipment and facilities, and tests. The time of health-care personnel – physicians, nurses, dieticians, and others – is often the most important health-care resource.

Nonhealth-care resources may also be required to produce a health-care service. For example, the transportation a patient needs to reach a clinic is a nonhealth-care resource, as is the television time used for a substance abuse prevention campaign. Costs associated with dietary changes or exercise routines taken up for health improvement purposes are other examples of nonhealth-care resources that are inputs to a health-care intervention.

The costs of time for the recipient of services are another resource used in the production of almost every health-care service. These *time costs* reflect the time required for transportation, for waiting in a clinician's office, and for receiving a service. They are distinct from the costs of health-care professionals' time, categorized as health-care costs, as described earlier. From the societal perspective, the value of an hour of the patient's time – the opportunity cost from the point of view of society – is assumed to be equal to the value of that time to the patient, and is assumed to be reflected in the patient's wage. From other perspectives, however, the patient's time cost may be very different. The physician or managed-care organization may value the patient's time at zero. The patient herself, receiving paid sick leave, might also assign a cost of zero to time spent in recovering from an illness.

A related category of resource use is *caregiver time*. Caregiver time includes the value of time spent by informal caregivers ministering to a patient, and which would otherwise have been devoted to other activities. These individuals may be volunteers or family members. (If caregivers are paid a market rate for their services, they are generally included in the category of health-care resources, rather than counted as 'caregiver time.') Perspective again plays a role in determining the value of caregiver time. From the perspective of a hospital or managed-care organization, the time of a family caregiver is free. From the societal perspective or the perspective of the patient's family, the caregiver's time has an opportunity cost.

Illness (and death) affect the individual's ability to do his or her normal activities. The lost or impaired ability to do work results in costs from the societal perspective. These costs are referred to as *productivity costs*. Since individuals trade off leisure and work based on their relative value, according to economic theory, productivity costs include the value of lost leisure as well. Productivity costs are in addition to time costs, which only account for the time the recipient of health care devotes to the health-care program or intervention. Productivity costs reflect the societal value of time spent sick or in reduced health, or of time lost through death.

In cost–benefit analysis, effects on longevity and impaired or improved productivity are translated into their monetary value. These productivity costs are combined with other types of costs and savings to obtain a summary measure of net benefit. In CEA, these same consequences are treated as 'effects' and placed in the denominator of the cost-effectiveness ratio, measured in terms of quality of life. Technically, it would not be incorrect to monetize part or all of these productivity effects and place them in the numerator. In fact, a number of analyses have used this approach. The only caveat is that an effect on productivity must not be double-counted by being placed in the denominator (e.g., as a reduction in QALYs) and in the numerator (as a dollar loss) at the same time. The economic value of productivity gains to individuals *other than* the patient – to employers, to taxpayers, and to the rest of society – should ideally be counted in the numerator, although this is not always done if the so-called 'external benefit' is small.

9.3.1.2 Sequence of costs

The cost of health-care resources, nonhealth-care resources, patient time, and informal caregiver time may be accrued in a single time period or in progressive stages associated with an intervention. Analysts generally calculate the net cost of an intervention by laying out the stream of events occurring with the intervention and the stream of events occurring without the intervention, and then comparing the costs associated with each scenario. This process of 'laying out' the scenarios can be done through a simple itemization of events, a decision tree, a Markov model, or a complex simulation of events.

The costs in the event streams fall into the categories of *initial costs, induced costs,* and *averted costs.* The *initial costs* are those associated with the intervention itself, such as the costs associated with a physician visit and pathology examination for cervical cancer screening. The *induced costs* are those that result from the intervention. In the case of cervical cancer screening, costs for the follow-up of a positive test are induced costs – for the investigation of false-positive as well as true-positive results. The costs of treatment for cases of cancer detected would also be induced costs. *Averted costs* are the costs associated with the stream of events that would have occurred in the absence of the intervention, but because of it did not occur. The cervical cancer screening program would detect some early-stage cases of cervical cancer, and by doing so, it would avert some cases that would have been detected in later stages. All costs associated with averted cases – costs associated with their future detection, diagnosis, and treatment and any costs associated with the morbidity they would have imposed – are included in the scenario that would have occurred without the intervention, and thus included in the calculation of *net* cost for a CEA.

9.3.1.3 Costs in added years of life

One of the outcomes that may ultimately result from a successful intervention is an increase in life span. Many health-related programs, including legislation requiring child safety seats and interventions such as antihypertensive medications, have been shown to increase longevity. Although these added years are part of the scenario that occurs with the intervention – and are included in the calculation of net *effectiveness* almost without exception – there is some debate about whether to include all of the *costs* associated with these added years of life.

The costs associated with *health-care interventions* during added years of life are typically included. Thus, if a drug regimen averts a fatal myocardial infarction at age 53, but a fatal stroke occurs at age 83, the costs of medical care for the myocardial infarction and the stroke are included in the respective scenarios. Most decision analysts and health economists include costs for health-care interventions whether these costs are related or unrelated to the specific disease spectrum at issue. For example, in this case, 'unrelated' health-care costs would include those for osteoporosis or accidents. Further details on this issue may be found in papers by Meltzer (1997) and Johannesson et al. (1997).

A more vexing question is whether *nonhealth-related* resource use for years of added life should be included in the treatment scenario. The nonhealth-related costs, for example for food and clothing, represent real resource use and theoretically should be included as costs associated with added years of life. However, some have argued that including costs of living as real 'costs' to society runs counter to the social objective of lengthening life. Others argue on a technical level that the consistent exclusion of these costs would simply result in consistently lower cost-effectiveness ratios, and therefore would not affect decisions made using CEA results. In practice, most CEAs have not explicitly included these costs.

9.3.1.4 The scope of costs associated with an intervention

The sequence of initial, induced, and averted costs reflects the timeline of costs that are included in a CEA. However, it is also important that an analysis reflect the breadth of costs associated with an intervention. These include costs associated with side-effects and complications of an intervention. The costs may be short-term, such as the costs of acetaminophen for a fever or soreness following a child's vaccination. They may also be long-term, such as the costs associated with treatment of chronic mental disorders or of long-term disability associated with stroke.

Events initiated by an intervention may also spill over to individuals other than those directly receiving the intervention. Preventing a human immunodeficiency virus (HIV)-infected blood transfusion may prevent infection in a spouse and future children. A smoking cessation program may prevent morbidity among household members as well as the smoker himself. In general, analysts decide on whether to include costs associated with these chains of events extending from an intervention based on their potential importance in the analysis. Large costs should be included, while relatively small ones can safely be ignored.

9.3.2 Measuring costs – health-care resources

From most analytic perspectives, the measurement of health-care resource costs – their opportunity cost – is relatively straightforward: it is the price the patient or health-care institution pays for a drug, an hour of physician time, or other resource. It is clear in this individual or institutional setting that the price reflects the value of resources that are no longer available for an alternative use. The measurement of such costs from the societal perspective is conceptually and practically more challenging; most of this section will be devoted to costs from this perspective.

Society's opportunity cost for a resource is also, in theory, equal to the market price for that good or service in a competitive market. In practice, however, opportunity cost may be much more difficult to establish. For one thing, the assumption that market price reflects opportunity costs implies that the marketplace meets the criteria set forth in welfare economics for a perfectly competitive market – or at least, that the market does not diverge too much from these criteria. But the health-care marketplace is noncompetitive in many respects. Because medical science is complex, the consumers of health care frequently are not the 'fully informed' buyers that consumers of commodities are assumed to be. In addition, the patient is frequently covered by insurance and therefore does not experience the full cost of a purchase. For these reasons and many others, the economic forces of supply and demand cannot be presumed to function in the same way as in the market for bananas or bicycles.

There are many other reasons why 'prices' in the health-care arena must be viewed with skepticism. Prices are often set administratively by an insurer or government program. Physicians, facing one set of administrative prices from Medicaid, may adjust their prices to recoup earnings from other payers, making it even more difficult to determine the 'real' price. Hospital charges may be inflated above cost by an arbitrary ratio, with the amount depending upon the purchaser. In public clinics and hospitals which have an annual budget, there may be very little accounting of the costs of clinician time and no way to determine costs in relation to specific patient diagnoses. Managed-care organizations, too, do not have prices for specific health-care services.

There are two general methods of developing cost estimates for health-care services that have multiple components, such as a hospital inpatient day, a clinic visit, or complete prenatal care. The first is to begin with an existing price or set of prices and adjust for known influences. This method, sometimes referred to as *gross-costing*, draws upon fee or payment schedules, such as the Medicare fee schedules for professional and ambulatory care or hospital payment schedules such as the diagnostic-related group (DRG) rates established for Medicare. Hospitals' fee schedules are also used, adjusted using cost-to-charge ratios that may be applied broadly or to specific cost centers. Adjustments for geographic price variations or practice variations may also be used.

The second method, *micro-costing*, involves enumerating the inputs to a service, collecting data on unit prices, and then compiling the cost estimate. For example, an HIV counseling and testing session might be broken down into many components, including the counselor's time, the nurse's time, the test supplies, other medical supplies, telephone time, and written materials (Farnham et al., 1996). Each of these components would be assigned a unit cost, for example, $2 for each 10 min of the counselor's time. The cost estimate would then be developed using the estimates of resource use and the unit cost estimates.

Some rules of thumb have been developed for pricing resources commonly used in health care. The cost of pharmaceuticals, for example, is often taken from the cost paid by government formularies in countries that have them. In the US, the average wholesale price, which approximates drug prices in discount pharmacies, is frequently used.

9.3.2.1 Long-run versus short-run resource costs

One important consideration in assessing the cost of a service is whether and how to include 'overhead' items such as telephone, rent, or office equipment and other 'fixed' costs. In assessing the cost-effectiveness of an intervention, fixed costs – those that are not affected by the decision under consideration – should not be included in the analysis. Thus, if a clinic is deciding whether or not to add an evening health education class that will use the facility during hours when it would otherwise be closed, the cost of running the class should not include an allocation of the clinic's rent. However, the initial start-up costs, such as for training volunteers or purchasing extra chairs, should be included. And if the class requires the clinic to add hours for their cleaning service, this incremental cost should also be included as a cost of the program. The costs that do vary as a result of the program are termed 'variable costs.'

The determination of whether a cost is fixed or variable depends to a great extent on the time frame of the analysis. The costs of implementing a community-based cancer screening program or developing a drug are variable when the decision is whether to undertake the program, but they are fixed once a program has been started, drug has been developed, or a large capital investment has been made. Costs for rent or for large pieces of equipment are typical examples. The marginal cost for one additional computed tomography (CT) scan examination may be low, and this is the appropriate cost to use in a short-run decision. The marginal cost of letting a patient remain in a hospital bed for an extra day when there is extra capacity on the hospital floor is also relatively low – presumably, it does not affect staffing levels, costs for heat or electricity, administration, or any other of the 'fixed' costs of running the hospital.

However, costs that are fixed in the short run are generally variable over the longer term. Utilization levels over time will determine decisions regarding staffing levels, the purchase of additional equipment, and construction of additional capacity over the long term. As a result, equipment such as the CT scanner, items included in 'overhead,' and other seemingly fixed costs should be included in any analysis that has general policy implications or implications for health care practices over the long term. As a general rule, CEA should employ *long-run marginal costs*.

When the decision has been made to include the cost of a relatively long-lasting resource, there are a variety of methods for spreading the cost over the life of the investment – a process known as *depreciation*. The simplest method of depreciation is to divide the purchase cost (less the residual value at the end of useful life) by the number of years the resource will be used. This gives the yearly cost of the capital investment. If a new piece of diagnostic equipment is purchased for $2 million and is fully depreciated over 10 years, its cost could then be calculated as $200 000 per year. This method is known as *straight-line depreciation*.

The annual cost can also be calculated using an amortization formula. The amortized annual cost is the amount that would have to be paid during each year of the useful life of the capital investment in order to repay the principal plus interest on a loan (e.g., mortgage) to purchase the investment. Since construction and capital equipment are often financed through borrowing, amortization frequently approximates the actual timing of expenditures. If the annual interest rate is i, the term (useful life) is N years, and the purchase price is P, then the amortized annual cost M (i.e., the annual mortgage payment for payments incurred at the beginning of the year) is given by the formula:

$$M = P \cdot i \cdot \frac{(1+i)^{N-1}}{(1+i)^N - 1} \tag{9.2a}$$

If the mortgage payments are incurred at the end of each year, the formula is:

$$M = P \cdot i \cdot \frac{(1+i)^N}{(1+i)^N - 1} \tag{9.2b}$$

From the societal point of view, the amortized value is more accurate than the straight-line value, because money invested in equipment cannot be used productively elsewhere to yield the normal rate of return. Therefore, the imputed annual cost should reflect not only the purchase price but also the forgone interest.

9.3.2.2 Adjustments to prices

Inflation

Most of us are accustomed to the idea that $20 today can buy less than $20 years ago, say in the 1950s. These differences in purchasing power result from inflation. Because of inflation, expenditures or savings occurring in different years cannot simply be added together. They must first be converted to a common year by adjusting for inflation.

Inflation-adjusted amounts represent real resource costs in the chosen year. Dollar amounts that are inflation-adjusted are said to be in *constant dollars* or *real dollars*.

Analysts generally adjust for inflation using the Consumer Price Index (CPI). The CPI, published annually by the Bureau of Labor Statistics, is derived by evaluating the changes in price for a given market basket of goods. Although this index may be subject to error if the composition of the market basket is not reflective of purchases generally, the CPI is an accepted standard for price adjustment.

DEFINITION

Inflation is a fluctuation in the value of a currency resulting in an increase in prices unrelated to changes in the value of commodities.

The CPI is available for all items and for various categories of goods and services, such as medical care, medical care commodities, and dental services. The component indices are more accurate than the general CPI for categories of goods or services experiencing a different rate of inflation than the overall economy. Health economists do not agree on whether the overall CPI or the Medical Care CPI should be used in health-related CEA. While it would seem silly to factor in price inflation for items having little to do with the production of health care, there are inevitable limitations in the way price inflation is measured for health care that render it questionable. For example, the quantity and quality of health services, such as a hospital day, are hopelessly intermingled, leaving open to question whether the Medical Care CPI really measures the relative prices of a fixed market basket of health-related items.

Cross-national conversions
To compare cost-effectiveness results across national boundaries or to use cost estimates from different countries, currencies must be converted to the same metric, for example Canadian dollars or Japanese yen. This can be done simply by applying current currency conversion rates – or rates for another base year. Those conducting such comparisons, however, must use caution, because analyses from different countries may contain many assumptions that affect cost-effectiveness results. For example, the relative rates for physician labor and prices for pharmaceuticals often differ sharply depending on the country. More significantly, the actual quantities of resources used for a service may differ widely from country to country. In a CEA of hypertension treatment, for example, it would be incorrect to apply the averted costs for stroke and heart disease in the US and simply convert the currencies, if the practice patterns and interventions for treating cardiovascular disease differ markedly across countries.

9.3.3 Measuring time and other resource costs

9.3.3.1 Time
According to economic theory, the value of patient and caregiver time, like the value of health-care commodities, is equal to the opportunity cost of these resources. Although the opportunity cost of medical supplies, drugs, and other direct health-care resources may be indicated by its market price, this measure does not exist for patient and caregiver time.

To assign a value to patient and caregiver time from the societal perspective, analysts generally look to the market price – wage – for an hour of time of employed people with similar characteristics. Thus, the opportunity cost for the value of the time of a 45-year-old, college-educated woman caring for an elderly parent at home would be estimated using the average hourly wage of similar women in her geographic area.

One dilemma in using wages is how narrowly to define the group for which the wage is assessed. For example, if a patient is a 20-year-old Hispanic woman, should her time cost be approximated using an average wage for all 20-year-olds? All 20-year-old women? All Hispanic 20-year-old women? Narrower definitions can produce more accurate estimates of the individual's true opportunity cost. However, a broader definition may be preferred if it captures relevant characteristics and omits spurious ones.

9.3.3.2 Measuring productivity costs

As noted earlier, productivity costs may be included as monetary costs in the numerator of a CEA or subsumed in the QALY measure in the denominator. Even when the patient's valuations of productivity changes are subsumed in the QALYs, there is still a need to value the productivity-related benefits to others, such as employers and taxpayers.

As stated earlier, the economic theory of competitive labor markets suggests that earnings reflect the value of an individual's productivity. Economic theory holds that this valuation also applies to leisure time, as long as the individual has the opportunity to adjust hours worked in response to opportunities. Physicians call it moonlighting, professors call it consulting, laborers call it overtime, but these are all examples of this phenomenon. The implication for CEA is that, if one chooses to measure the value of productivity in monetary terms, the wage is a good place to start.

However, some special issues arise when considering the value of productivity to parties other than the patient. Employers who have to replace workers in the short run incur replacement costs. These costs may already be reflected in the 'sick pay' and 'vacation pay' they consider part of the full cost of retaining an employee. But if an employee is lost for the long term, there are costs of recruitment, training, and waiting for the new employee to reach the same place on the 'learning curve' as the former employee. These costs are called *friction costs*, and they may be substantial. In addition, workers who continue to work at a lower level of productivity after an illness impose costs on their employers which may not be reflected in the QALYs if the individual continues to experience the same level of well-being and compensation. While friction costs and costs of reduced productivity are not routinely included in CEA, they should be included if their magnitude is important compared to the other costs in the analysis.

9.3.3.3 Valuing outcomes in cost–benefit analysis

In cost–benefit analysis, all resource use and all health benefits are monetized, so effects on both health and productivity are always expressed in monetary terms. The classic approach to valuing these outcomes in cost–benefit analysis is called the *human capital* method. The human capital approach equates the value of health to earnings. Thus, the value of lost years of life is estimated as the value of projected future earnings, taking into account such factors as the age, gender, and education of the individual. Some who have taken this approach use the *net* value of earnings, subtracting the individual's anticipated consumption from expected earnings. This approach implies that the individual's value is only what he or she contributes to the rest of society, excluding himself or herself. Others use the *gross* present value of earnings, effectively counting the individual as one of the intended beneficiaries of his work.

The other main monetary method for valuing added years of life and improved functioning is the calculation of the amount an individual is willing to pay for these improvements. The *willingness-to-pay* method takes into account subjective values associated with health and life. We introduced the willingness-to-pay method in the context of valuing health states, and in this regard it functions much like a utility scale. When the values from a population are aggregated, willingness to pay provides a measure of the societal value attached to a given health benefit.

Estimates of willingness to pay can be obtained either by looking at revealed willingness to pay – actual purchases or risk trade-offs – or by eliciting willingness to pay from individuals. For in vitro fertilization, for example, revealed willingness to pay could be determined by looking at the amounts paid by couples not covered by health insurance. (This would provide an upper-bound estimate, as couples who are willing to pay a lower amount would be unable to purchase the service.) Willingness to pay could also be elicited by presenting couples with various scenarios concerning their probability of becoming pregnant with and without in vitro fertilization, and asking their willingness to pay for the intervention.

Like the human capital approach, willingness to pay has important limitations as a measure. A person's willingness to pay varies according to the initial likeliness of death or illness and by the amount the intervention reduces the risk. However, since these variations do not have a linear relation to risk changes, willingness to pay cannot easily be inferred across a range of initial probabilities, posing a daunting task for a researcher requiring willingness-to-pay information for a broad range of possible risk scenarios. Furthermore, willingness to pay can assign higher values to life-saving interventions and quality-of-life improvements for the affluent, since willingness to pay increases with wealth. On a practical level, it may also be difficult for subjects to contemplate how much they would be willing to pay for changes in low-probability risks.

9.4 Effectiveness

As discussed earlier, health benefits in CEA are described using non-monetary measures. A wide variety of measures have been used. These include both single measures and combined measures of health benefit.

9.4.1 Single measures of health outcome

The outcomes of programs and interventions are frequently multidimensional, but in some instances an analyst may be interested in only one dimension of a health outcome. Single measures of health effect include, for example, the number of cases of polio prevented, number of cases of breast cancer detected, or a reduction in average number of cigarettes smoked per day. These measures are appropriate for very targeted analyses, where an immediate goal has been identified and the objective of the analysis is to determine efficient ways of reaching this goal. Because the outcome measure is an initial or intermediate outcome, the analysis will not be able to contribute to assessing longer-term goals of health care, quality-of-life improvement or longevity.

Data collected for a CEA very often will focus on a short-term outcome. For example, a study of a smoking cessation program would collect data on outcomes reflecting the amount of smoking and the length of time smoking cessation or reduction is maintained. The study would be unlikely to collect data on morbidity or longevity long-term. However, the CEA, if it is to contribute to broad resource allocation decisions, can and should link these initial outcomes to long-term outcomes, using data from other studies to model length and quality-of-life effects. A careful ascertainment of the links between initial and longer-term outcomes is essential to insure that the initial outcome is in fact meaningful in terms of its real implications for health.

Single measures of health effect can also be measures of long-term outcomes. Number of lives saved and number of life-years saved are measures of health benefit that are frequently used alone. Their drawback is that they are usually incomplete measures of the effect of interventions, which generally influence quality of life over a span of time as well as length of life. Furthermore, the notion of 'saving a life' is really meaningless, since lives cannot be saved, only extended. It is possible for a single intervention in an individual patient to 'save' the same life many times over! For interventions that primarily extend life, however, the measure of life-years gained may be adequate.

9.4.2 Combined measures of health outcome

For interventions where both effects on quality of life and length of life are important – or where the timing of quality-of-life effects is important – the preferred outcome measure is the QALY, which combines measures of length and quality of life. As described in Chapter 4, QALYs are calculated by using a scale to value the quality of life in a particular health state, multiplying by the amount of time in the health state, and then summing these weighted values.

Two important methodological concerns in developing QALY estimates for CEA concern the appropriate type of weight to be used for adjusting life years and the appropriate source of the weight.

9.4.2.1 Preference-based measures vs. health status measures

The measures of quality of life used in CEA are preference-based. *Preference-based measures* are those that reflect the value an individual attaches to a health state. Thus, these measures do not simply characterize a state of health but demonstrate people's preferences for these states. Preference weighting gives meaning to QALY measures in that results can be interpreted to reflect the relative desirability of health outcomes (Chapter 4).

Preference-weighted measures are distinct from the health status measures that currently abound in the field of health services research. *Health status measures* are systems for defining and describing health states. These measures define a set of domains of health, such as physical health, mental health, and role functioning, and describe health status based on an instrument that assesses health in each domain. The result is a numerical score, such as obtained by the Medical Outcomes Study SF-36 (Ware and Sherbourne, 1992) or the Sickness Impact Profile (SIP; Bergner et al., 1981).

Health status measures can be used as part of the process of estimating QALYs, describing the health states to which preferences are applied. However, they are not in themselves preference-weighted measures – in fact, they are not weighted at all, either using preferences or other weights. Their preferred use is in assessing health status in population surveys or clinical trials, rather than in CEA. So, for example, the SF-36 has been used in studies monitoring health status for patients with diabetes, cancer, and other conditions, and examining the outcomes of medical and surgical interventions.

Preference-based measures fall into two categories: those derived from utility theory, such as the standard gamble and time trade-off, and psychological scaling methods such as the rating scale. As pointed out in Chapter 4, however, there is no justification for using the numerical values from a rating scale in calculating quality-adjusted life expectancy, because there is no indication that these reflect either preferences under uncertainty, or trade-offs between longevity and quality of life, let alone both. For this reason, many analysts prefer utility-based methods for assigning weights to be used in CEA.

Utility-based methods include the standard gamble and time trade-off. These methods involve comparisons of hypothetical choices between the certainty of time in a health state and a gamble between a better and a worse option. Respondents' preferences are used to reveal their utility for a health outcome, a preference that satisfies the axioms of utility theory. These preferences are theoretically suitable for computation of expected utilities to represent preferences among alternatives with uncertain outcomes. The main disadvantage of utility-based measures is that they can be conceptually difficult for respondents, as discussed in Chapter 4.

9.4.2.2 Sources of preferences for CEA: community vs. patient preferences

An important consideration in determining QALYs is the source of preferences to be used in an analysis. In an analysis from the patient's perspective, the patient is clearly the appropriate source. In an analysis from the societal perspective, the choice is less evident. Patients and their families have the most experience with a given health state and are most familiar with implications for quality of life. However, people's views about illness and disability change based on their experience, and from an *ex ante* perspective, it is perhaps the general population that has claim to the more 'objective' point of view.

Use of patient preferences is often preferred when an analysis is designed to compare different interventions for the same patient group. For example, in a CEA comparing two drug therapies for coronary artery disease, preferences could be solicited from cardiac patients without introducing concerns regarding the relative valuation of health states that are cardiac disease-related vs. those that are not. The advantages of using patient preferences in this type of analysis include convenience – the patient population is likely to be more available and more interested in a survey of preferences than a general population sample – and the feasibility of obtaining a more sensitive outcome measure, because of the patients' ability to discriminate among a variety of states they have experienced. The main disadvantage to using the patients' preferences is that this analysis would not be as comparable to analyses using general population preferences.

General population preferences (often referred to as *community preferences*) are preferred for CEA designed to inform broader resource allocation decisions. From the societal perspective, which is intended to represent the public interest rather than the interests of any particular group, these preferences are the most defensible choice. The ideal source of preferences would be an unbiased, broad community sample of people who are well informed about the health states in question. This sample would probably include people who had some experience with the illness or condition under study, in proportion to its occurrence in society. Those with no experience would be giving their views about the health state without knowing whether they would, in the future, experience the condition. From behind this so-called 'veil of ignorance,' a construct used by health ethicists to judge principles for resource allocation, these respondents would evaluate the relevant health states from an *ex ante* perspective in terms of their relative desirability compared with other possible health states.

9.4.2.3 Approaches to obtaining health-state utilities

Preferences are frequently assessed by presenting respondents with holistic vignettes, describing all domains of health that comprise a particular health state. So, for example, for a scenario describing mild arthritis, the vignette would describe the patient's role function, mental health, cognitive functioning, and other domains, whether or not they are affected by the condition, giving a full picture of the health state. The respondent would then provide preferences for the state as a whole. This contrasts with elicitation of preferences that are based on descriptions – possibly more detailed – that focus on the problems specific to the illness. For example, the arthritis example would be comprised of scenarios characterizing the joint pain and mobility directly associated with the condition.

The health status scales to which preferences are assigned can be either disease-specific (or condition-specific) or generic. Disease-specific scales, such as in the examples above that use either the problem-specific or holistic vignette approach to getting utilities for arthritis, gather data for scenarios where a condition or a disease is explicit in the description. An example of such a scale is the Q-tility index developed to obtain utilities for health states associated with cancer (Chapter 4).

Disease-specific scales contrast with generic measures, which characterize the domains of health (for example, ability to do self-care, mobility, sensory function, aspects of social function, and health perceptions) without relating them to any particular illness. Generic scales provide an important level of convenience and standardization in the derivation of QALYs. Community or patient preferences can be obtained for health states comprised of the various levels of each health domain. An analyst studying a particular illness can then 'map' health states associated with that illness on to the generic scale. Given this type of assessment – which is usually much easier to accomplish than elicitation of preferences – the analyst can look up the population preferences that have already been surveyed.

Well-known examples of generic scales used to compute QALYs include the Health Utilities Index (HUI; Feeny et al., 1995), the 5-Item EuroQOL Scale (EQ-5D; EuroQol Group, 1990), and the Quality of Well-Being (QWB) Scale (Kaplan and Anderson, 1988). The HUI, developed in Canada, is a multiattribute (multiple domain) scale that has been used in clinical studies, cost-effectiveness studies, and population health surveys. Preferences have been elicited for its health states for a general population sample of Canadians, using the standard gamble, and applying methods of multiattribute utility theory to infer utilities for the complete set of states from elicited utilities for a subset. The EQ-5D, which also combines multiple domains, contains approximately 250 health states. Preferences were elicited using the time trade-off from a general population in the UK. Preferences for the QWB were obtained for a general population sample of Americans. This scale differs from the HUI and EQ-5D in that preferences were assessed for it using a category scaling method (a psychological scaling approach) rather than a utility-based approach. Work on a preference-weighted utility scale based on a six-item subscale of the SF-36 is also underway (Brazier et al., 1998a, b).

The disadvantage to using a generic health-state classification system is that, if it is general enough and simple enough to apply to health states across diseases, conditions, and interventions, it may not be sensitive enough to the variations in health status associated with a particular disease. As a result, depending on the analysis, disease- or condition-specific measures may be preferred.

9.4.2.4 A note on disability-adjusted life years (DALYs)

In 1993, the World Bank published a report on the global burden of disease using the disability-adjusted life year (DALY) as the measure of health (Musgrove, 1993; World Bank, 1993). This measure deserves mention in any discussion of measures of health benefit. The DALY is a combined measure of health like the QALY, incorporating both length and quality of life. Disabilities are categorized as falling into one of six levels of severity, with each level having an assigned weight. For example, about half of the cases of pelvic inflammatory disease examined in the World Bank study fell into class 4, which has a severity weight of 0.22; other cases of this disease fell into categories associated with higher and lower levels of disability and corresponding severity weights. In addition to an adjustment using disability weights, years of life in the DALY are adjusted based on age. The age weights reflect a higher valuation of years of life for a young or middle-aged adult than for a child or an elderly person. The first and last years of life are given a very low weight, while the highest weight is given to a year at age 25.

The DALY is not generally used in CEA, because it is not a preference-weighted measure. (The disability weights used to adjust life years were chosen by a panel of experts.) The DALY's preferred uses to date are in describing the impact of morbidity and mortality, particularly in the developing world (Murray and Lopez, 1997a, b).

9.4.2.5 Calculating life expectancy in cost-effectiveness models

So far in this section, our discussion has focused on the measurement of the quality-of-life benefits of health interventions. Life years are the base unit to which quality weights are applied in the QALY. In addition, as noted earlier, measures of life expectancy are sometimes used as the single measure of outcome. Differences in survival in CEA capture the life-saving and life-extending benefits of interventions, while in the QALY, the differences in weighted life years capture the duration of health effects.

Most CEAs that use long-term measures of health benefit (length and quality of life) model the full life expectancy for the target population of the analysis with and without the intervention, comparing the two results to obtain differences in costs and health outcome to calculate the cost-effectiveness ratio. Calculations of life expectancy can be based on age-specific mortality rates derived from population life tables, adjusted for mortality differences attributable to specific procedures or illnesses under study. These calculations are typically done using Markov models and using methods for survival analysis described in Chapter 10.

9.5 Discounting costs and health outcomes

DEFINITION

Discounting is a process for computing how much a quantitative measure of resource cost or health outcome at some point in the future is worth today. The *present value, or value today, of a future dollar or QALY depends on how far into the future it is obtained and on the rate at which it is discounted, or its *discount rate*.

Leaving aside issues of inflation, alternative programs that require the same total investment over the life of the project may differ in their requirement for funds from year to year. Consider, for example, three programs that each consume $100 000 worth of resources over 5 years, but program A entails uniform investment each year, B requires more resources in the early years, and C is weighted more heavily in the later years. If these programs produce identical benefits, should we be indifferent among them? There is general agreement that future costs should be weighted less heavily than present ones. Although somewhat more controversial, there is also general agreement that future health consequences should be weighted less heavily than present ones. In this section we discuss the reasons for such time preferences and describe a method, *discounting*, to quantify the magnitude of this preference. Discounting enables us to compare future costs and health consequences with those in the present.

9.5.1 The mechanism of discounting

One dollar invested at an interest rate of 3% will bring $1.03 a year from now. We use discounting, the reverse of this 'interest' process, to compute the *present value (PV)* of a dollar that we will obtain a year from now. The PV is the amount of money that, if invested, will yield $1 1 year from now, so PV × 1.03 = $1.00. Doing the division, we find that PV = $0.97. At a 3% discount rate, then, the present value of $1.00 next year is 97 cents.

In the same way, we can calculate that the value of a dollar spent or received *2 years* from now has a present value of 94 cents:

$1.00 2 years from now is worth $1.00/1.03 = $0.97 1 year from now
$0.97 1 year from now is worth $.97/1.03 = $0.94 today

The general formula for present value is:

Table 9.3. Current cost and discounted cost (amounts are assumed to be incurred at the end of each year)

	Current cost or income (2001$)	Discounted (3%) cost or income (2001$)
Year 0	− 50 000	− 50 000
Year 1	− 4500	− 4369
Year 2	5000	4713
Year 3	10 000	9151
Year 4	10 000	8885
Year 5	10 000	8626
Total		− 22 994

$$PV = \frac{FV}{(1+r)^t} \tag{9.3}$$

where PV is present value, FV is the future value, r is the discount rate expressed as a decimal fraction (e.g., $r=0.03$), and t is time (such as 2 years in the previous example). Using this formula, the present value of a $500 check that will be received 10 years from now, given an 8% discount rate, is $PV = \$500/(1+0.08)^{10} = \$232$.

When costs or income are incurred in different amounts over a stream of years, they are discounted according to when they occur, and then summed as shown in Table 9.3. Note that Table 9.3 indicates the currency year in which *all* the dollars are reported (as it always should be), i.e. '2001$.' This has nothing to do with discounting; instead it tells the reader the value of the currency considering inflation.

In Table 9.3, there is a 3-year period during which the income stream is $10 000 per year. There is a shortcut method of calculating present value for a constant amount of money, $\$C$, spent or received in each of the next N years:

$$PV = \frac{C}{r} \cdot [1 - (1/(1+r)^N)] \tag{9.4}$$

This formula can be derived from the standard formula for the sum of a geometric series, with the geometric proportion equal to $1/(1+r)$.

In the example above, the present value of the 3-year stream can be calculated by recognizing that it is the difference between a 5-year stream and a 2-year stream, each beginning at time zero. The value of the 5-year stream is:

$$PV_5 = 10\,000/0.03 \times (1 - 1/1.03^5) = 45\,797$$

The value of the 2-year stream is:

$$PV = 10\,000/0.03 \times (1 - 1/1.03^2) = 19\,135$$

For the value of the 3-year stream beginning in year 3, we subtract the value of the 2-year stream from the value of the 5-year stream: $26 662. This method is handy for estimating present values or double-checking other methods.

Note that the assumption underlying the present-value calculations in Table 9.3 is that all dollar amounts are incurred at the end of each year, and that the present value is calculated as of the end of year 0 (which is the beginning of year 1). In discounting costs, it matters whether costs are counted at the beginning or the end of the year. If $10 000 payments are received at the beginning of the year for 5 years, the first payment should not be discounted. The calculation of present value would look like this:

$$PV = 10\,000 + 10\,000/(1.03) + 10\,000/(1.03)^2 + 10\,000/(1.03)^3$$
$$+ 10\,000/(1.03)^4 = \$47\,171$$

In contrast, if each payment is received at the end of the year, the present value calculation should reflect this difference in timing. The first payment is discounted for the first year, the second payment for the second, etc.:

$$PV = 10\,000/(1.03) + 10\,000/(1.03)^2 + 10\,000/(1.03)^3$$
$$+ 10\,000/(1.03)^4 + 10\,000/(1.03)^5 = \$45\,797$$

Note that the formula above discounts the first payment in the stream – it makes the assumption that costs are received at the end of each year.

If costs are spread evenly over the year, or if they occur in the middle of the year, a half-cycle correction may be used. This approach 'corrects' for the underestimate in present value that would result from assuming the payments were received at the end of each year and the overestimate that would result from assuming they were received at the beginning of each year. The calculation of present value with a half-cycle correction looks like this:

$$PV = 10\,000/(1.03)^{0.5} + 10\,000/(1.03)^{1.5} + 10\,000/(1.03)^{2.5}$$
$$+ 10\,000/(1.03)^{3.5} + 10\,000/(1.03)^{4.5} = \$46\,479$$

with 0.5 year of discounting for the first payment, 1.5 years for the second payment, and so forth. Tables for calculating present values are available in textbooks, and present values can also be calculated easily using spreadsheet software. Financial calculators can also be used.

9.5.2 The rationale for discounting

One reason for discounting future costs is that a dollar that is not spent today can be invested productively to yield a larger number of real dollars in the future. Investment occurs through building factories and equipment, research and development, and training of personnel. The simplest evidence that investors can earn returns on resources over time is that you can take a dollar to the bank and deposit it in a money market account that pays, for example, 5% interest, and get $1.05 a year from now. The bank's interest rate reflects not only the anticipated rate of inflation but also the real value of investments – the opportunity cost of money – in the national economy. A dollar's worth of resources in the national economy, if not spent this year, can be put to productive use to yield $1.05 worth of goods and services next year. If this includes 2% inflation, then the inflation-adjusted value would be $1.03, or a 3% return.

A second reason for discounting is that you may prefer to have the goods and services a dollar can buy now rather than to wait. This may be true either because you genuinely prefer immediate gratification, or because of potential risks – such as the failure of the bank holding your money – associated with delay. If neither of those motivations applies, then the fact that you could have earned interest from an investor – who can earn a return on your money – would lead you to demand interest from the bank. For any of these reasons, you demand a premium in the form of interest if you must postpone consumption.

The arguments for discounting health outcomes differ somewhat from the rationale for discounting costs. Clearly, there is no 'bank' for health benefits and no interest rate to demonstrate differences between present and future value. Arguments for discounting health benefits are generally made on the basis of normative theory, which specifies that the discount rate should be positive, and on the basis of people's observed time preferences for health, although studies investigating these have found discrepancies with theory on a number of variables (Redelmeier and Heller, 1993; Chapman and Elstein, 1995; Lipscomb et al., 1996).

There are, in addition, two frequently-cited 'proofs' of the need to discount health benefits, the Keeler–Cretin paradox and Weinstein and Stason's consistency argument (Weinstein and Stason, 1977; Keeler and Cretin, 1983). Keeler and Cretin use an example which shows that a logical paradox develops if one discounts costs and health benefits at different rates. The paradox is that, if a program's costs and effectiveness are discounted at different rates, it is possible to improve the program's performance (health benefit per dollar spent) simply by delaying its implementation. As a result, it is always preferable to wait rather than begin the program.

Weinstein and Stason's consistency argument holds that the basic reason for discounting future health benefits is because they are being valued relative to dollars that could be invested to yield even more dollars in the future. They show that it is equivalent (a) to calculate the future value of a stream of dollars for comparison with a future health benefit and (b) to calculate the present value of a stream of QALYs for comparison with a present cost. Since (a) is clearly correct, the equivalence of (a) and (b) proves that discounting of QALYs is required for consistency.

Several arguments have been advanced against discounting health benefits. Most rest on distaste for the implications of discounting. One of the more compelling arguments, for example, is that discounting discriminates against programs which offer future health benefits to children – an argument which is, however, countered by arguments (and data) noting individuals' revealed preference for health benefits sooner rather than later. Notwithstanding the objections to discounting, the discounting of both costs and health effects – and at the same rate – is standard practice in CEA.

9.5.3 The discount rate

Because the purpose of the discount rate is to account for the opportunity cost of money, it is appropriate to choose a market-based rate for discounting. There are other considerations, however. When possible, it is important for analysts to choose a rate that is consistent with other analyses in the field and consistent over time, in order to facilitate the comparability of analyses.

Over the past two decades, discount rates used in economic evaluation have ranged from as low as 1 or 2% to 10%. Perhaps the most common discount rate in CEA has been 5%; however, this rate was initially used when market-based interest rates were significantly higher than they were around the turn of the century. As of 2001, we recommend a lower rate of 3% to reflect the trend toward lower interest rates and to be consistent with published guidelines (Gold et al., 1996). Many analysts include the 5% rate when conducting sensitivity analyses on the discount rate, in order to facilitate comparability with older analyses. It is recommended that analysts follow the literature for current recommendations on the choice of a discount rate.

9.6 Incremental cost-effectiveness analysis

All health applications of CEA involve a comparison between at least two alternatives. For example, CEA might be used to compare two drug regimens for patients following myocardial infarction. As discussed earlier, the main use of CEA is in situations when one alternative is both more costly and more effective than the other (upper right quadrant of Figure 9.1). The cost-effectiveness ratio describing this alternative is the ratio of the difference in net cost to the difference in net health effectiveness, compared to the other choice. Notice that the ratio is a ratio of differences – an incremental ratio.

This paradigm of alternatives is always embedded within the basic cost-effectiveness model. In our example of physicians' choice of clinical preventive services, each clinical service on the 'menu' could either be performed or not performed. The clinician's problem is to decide which combination of services to perform, and which ones not to perform. The yes/no decisions for each option can be made independently, so as to maximize health benefit given a budget constraint.

In many health applications of CEA, however, the choices involve two or more interventions that, by definition, cannot be selected at the same time – not just a yes/no choice for each alternative. The choice among four strategies for breast cancer screening, each involving a different screening interval, is such a choice among mutually exclusive, or *competing choices*. Another is the choice between two different surgical procedures. This situation contrasts with the choice facing a public health agency of whether to implement an antismoking campaign and/or a skin cancer screening program, since the decision to perform one service does not inherently preclude a decision to perform the other one (although the budget might constrain the decision).

The basic difference between these situations is that in competing choice situations such as that among breast cancer screening methods, the alternatives are not independent. In other words, the choice of the first alternative influences the benefit to be gained (or the cost incurred) by the second. In a noncompeting situation – such as the public health agency with a financial budget or the clinician with a time budget – the benefits of each program can be added. In the competing choice situation, they cannot. The benefit of Program A – annual mammogram – clearly will depend on whether the alternative is no mammogram, biannual mammogram, or mammogram every 5 years.

Table 9.4. Noncompeting programs: a 'shopping spree' problem

Program	QALYs gained	Cost ($)
A	100	1 800 000
B	100	5 000 000
C	500	1 000 000
D	100	2 200 000
E	100	1 200 000
F	500	2 000 000
G	100	10 000 000
H	200	1 200 000
I	150	4 500 000
J	50	800 000
K	250	2 000 000

QALYs, quality-adjusted life years.

The decision algorithm for using CEA differs in these two situations. We provide an example of each below.

9.6.1 The shopping spree problem

The shopping spree problem is an example of the basic (noncompeting choice) cost-effectiveness model. In this problem, there are a number of available programs, for which net costs and net effectiveness have been evaluated, relative to the alternative of no program. There is a limited budget; that is, the total net cost of the programs that are selected cannot exceed a specified amount. The decision maker's objective is to maximize the total net effectiveness (health benefit) of the programs selected.

Program alternatives in this problem are assumed to be independent. Any combination of programs is feasible – limited only by the budget constraint. Neither the net cost nor the net effectiveness of any program depends on what other programs are selected. Programs are also assumed to be divisible, with proportional costs and effectiveness. (In other words, a program that costs $1.0 million and saves 500 QALYs can be partially implemented, such as at the $500 000 level, and the benefit achieved will be proportional (250 QALYs).)

The programs in this problem are given in Table 9.4.

In the shopping spree problem, the decision maker first rules out any programs that cost money but have negative effectiveness. These programs,

Table 9.5. Noncompeting programs in order of cost-effectiveness

Program	Cost ($)	QALYs gained	C/E
C	1 000 000	500	2000
F	2 000 000	500	4000
H	1 200 000	200	6000
K	2 000 000	250	8000
E	1 200 000	100	12 000
J	800 000	50	16 000
A	1 800 000	100	18 000
D	2 200 000	100	22 000
I	4 500 000	150	30 000
B	5 000 000	100	50 000
G	10 000 000	100	100 000

QALYs, quality-adjusted life years; C/E, cost-effectiveness ratio.

which would fall into the lower right quadrant of Figure 9.1, are said to be *dominated* by their alternative of no program. No $/QALY threshold can make such programs cost-effective; they would not be selected under any scenario. Similarly, the decision maker would select any programs that are cost-saving and offer some benefit. Because they do not require resources, these programs can be selected regardless of the specified budget. Furthermore, their net cost savings could be added into the budget, thus increasing the resources available for other programs on the list. Neither of these types of programs (dominated or cost-saving) appears in Table 9.4.

The other programs, those with positive cost and positive effectiveness, are ranked in ascending order of their cost-effectiveness ratio in Table 9.5. (Alternatively, the programs could be ranked in descending order of their effectiveness-to-cost ratio.) Programs are then selected from the least to the most expensive until the budget is expended. The final array of programs selected will depend on the budget constraint. In Table 9.5 with a $3.0 million budget, only Programs C and F could be selected. A total of 1000 QALYs would be gained and the $3.0 million budget limit would be reached. Also note that if the budget is $3.0 million, the last program selected, F, has a cost-effectiveness ratio of $4000 per QALY. The significance of this 'marginal cost-effectiveness ratio' associated with a budget constraint will become clear when we turn to the competing choice situation. If the budget were instead $10.0 million, the decision maker would again begin with Programs C and F, but could also add Programs H, K, E, J, and A before reaching the budget ceiling. With the $10.0 million budget, the marginal cost-effectiveness ratio (for Program A) is $18 000 per QALY.

Not surprisingly, programs with higher (less desirable) cost-effectiveness ratios can be adopted as more resources are added to the budget.

9.6.2 The competing choice problem

In the competing choice problem, there are again a number of available programs. As with the shopping spree problem, the programs are assumed to be divisible. The decision maker's objective is the same: to maximize the total net effectiveness of programs selected subject to a limited budget.

In the competing choice problem, however, a subset of the available programs are mutually exclusive: if you select Program M1 you cannot select Program M2. For example, M1 and M2 might be two dosages of the same drug; if you chose to administer M1, which requires giving 5 mg of Drug A per day, you could not at the same time implement M2, 10 mg of Drug A. By definition, one of these choices (in this case presumably M2) is more effective but more costly than the other, and the decision between the two depends on whether the extra benefit is worth the extra cost.

Because the choices are mutually exclusive, it becomes necessary to look at the incremental cost-effectiveness ratio as a basis for decisions, rather than at average cost-effectiveness ratios such as those calculated for each option in Table 9.5. This is exactly what we were doing in the shopping spree, although we may not have recognized it, but in the shopping spree, each program was being compared to a null alternative. Now we have two or more active alternatives for some of the options, in addition to the null option. The incremental cost-effectiveness ratio gives the added cost per unit of added benefit of an option, relative to the next less expensive choice. Use of the incremental cost-effectiveness ratio permits the decision maker to account for the fact that there was a less expensive option when making her selection of programs.

For example, consider two programs, M1 and M2 (Table 9.6). Option M1 yields 10 QALYs at a cost of $100 000. Its average cost-effectiveness ratio is $10 000 per QALY. The second program, M2, costs $10 000 more. It is also more effective, but the difference in effectiveness between the two programs is tiny: 0.001 QALY. Its incremental cost-effectiveness ratio is $10 000/0.001 = $10 000 000 per QALY.

If the decision maker were to use Option M2's average cost-effectiveness ratio of $10 999 in making program selections, M2 would be selected in a line-up of programs before Program E in the previous example, with its cost-effectiveness ratio of $12 000.

Table 9.6. The distinction between average and incremental cost-effectiveness ratios

Program alternative	Effectiveness	Cost	Average cost-effectiveness ratio (C/E)	Incremental cost-effectiveness ratio ($\Delta C/\Delta E$)
M1	10	$100 000	$10 000/QALY	$10 000/QALY
M2	10.001	$110 000	$10 999/QALY	$10 000 000/QALY

QALYs, quality-adjusted life years.

Table 9.7. Total quality-adjusted life years (QALYs) gained: a check on selection of competing choice M1 vs. M2
Original choice:

Program	Program cost ($)	QALYs gained	C/E	Cumulative QALYs	Cumulative program cost
C	1 000 000	500	2000	500	1 000 000
F	2 000 000	500	4000	1000	3 000 000
H	1 200 000	200	6000	1200	4 200 000
K	2 000 000	250	8000	1450	6 200 000
E	1 200 000	100	12 000	**1550**	7 400 000

Choose M2:

Program	Program cost ($)	QALYs gained	C/E	Cumulative QALYs	Cumulative program cost
C	1 000 000	500	2000	500	1 000 000
F	2 000 000	500	4000	1000	3 000 000
H	1 200 000	200	6000	1200	4 200 000
K	2 000 000	250	8000	1450	6 200 000
M2	**110 000**	**10.001**	10 999	1460.001	6 310 000
E (partial)	1 090 000	90.833	12 000	**1550.834**	7 400 000

Choose M1:

Program	Program cost ($)	QALYs gained	C/E	Cumulative QALYs	Cumulative program cost
C	1 000 000	500	2000	500	1 000 000
F	2 000 000	500	4000	1000	3 000 000
H	1 200 000	200	6000	1200	4 200 000
K	2 000 000	250	8000	1450	6 200 000
M1	**100 000**	**10**	10 000	1460	6 300 000
E (partial)	1 100 000	91.667	12 000	**1551.667**	7 400 000

But is that really a good choice? A check of the potential QALYs gained shows that it is not. If $1.2 million were spent on Program E, 100 QALYs would be gained (Table 9.7). This is in fact less than would be gained if the decision maker purchased M2 and then used the remaining funds on Program E. But this calculation overlooks M1, which we know will yield almost as many QALYs as M2. If we select M1, we would gain slightly fewer QALYs than if M2 were chosen, but the remaining funds spent on Program E would purchase more QALYs. The final total of QALYs gained with the $7.4 million would be greater if we chose M1 rather than M2.

The calculation of incremental cost-effectiveness (Table 9.6) gives the true ratio of cost-effectiveness for mutually exclusive programs, allowing us to 'see' the relative worth of programs that we arrived at in the example of M1 and M2. This calculation gives the ratio of *additional* cost per unit of *additional* benefit when programs are mutually exclusive. The incremental cost-effectiveness ratio of Program M2 reveals that, although the dollar and QALY amounts do not differ radically in the context of the programs A through M2 in our examples (Table 9.7), the decision maker is actually paying $10 000 000 per QALY in selecting M2 over M1. Even though it yields more total QALYs than M1, M2 should not be selected over M1 until all programs which yield health benefit at a rate less expensive than $10 000 000 per QALY have been exhausted.

9.6.3 Extended dominance

The consideration of mutually exclusive programs reveals a final pitfall in comparing programs. This is that a program may look like a reasonable choice on the basis of its incremental cost-effectiveness ratio *only* if a more expensive but more efficient option has not yet been considered. Once all options are considered, this program can be shown to cost more per additional unit of benefit than another option, and thereby be ruled out by *extended dominance*. Extended dominance differs from simple dominance described earlier, because with simple dominance, a program is less advantageous on two dimensions than its alternative – that is, it is more costly and yields less benefit. This is not true in extended dominance, where the program is more costly but yields more benefit. The problem is simply that it doesn't yield as much *extra* benefit as a third option.

Consider Programs L1, L2, L3, L4, and L5 shown in Table 9.8. These are mutually exclusive programs. To calculate their incremental cost-effectiveness, the programs are arranged in the order of increasing cost and

Table 9.8. Incremental cost-effectiveness with dominance and extended dominance

Program	QALYs	Cost ($)	Incremental cost-effectiveness ratio ($\Delta C/\Delta E$)
L1	10	50 000	5000
L2	15	150 000	20 000
L3	20	450 000	60 000
~~L4~~	~~35~~	~~800 000~~	
L5	40	750 000	15 000

QALYs, quality-adjusted life years.

Table 9.9. Recalculation of incremental cost-effectiveness program eliminated by extended dominance

Program	QALYs	Cost ($)	Incremental cost-effectiveness ratio ($\Delta C/\Delta E$)
L1	10	50 000	5000
L2	15	150 000	20 000
L5	40	750 000	24 000

QALYs, quality-adjusted life years.

increasing effectiveness. A dominated program, L4, with higher cost but lower effectiveness than L5, can be eliminated immediately. This leaves Programs L1, L2, L3, and L5. The incremental cost and incremental effectiveness are calculated for each program relative to the preceding program. Then the incremental cost-effectiveness ratio for each option compared to the next most effective option is calculated.

At this point, Program L3 can be ruled out by extended dominance. It stands out in Table 9.8 because its incremental cost-effectiveness ratio, $60 000, is higher than that of Program L5. We reason as follows: 'If we are willing to spend additional resources at a rate of $60 000 per QALY for L3, then surely we would spend more resources to pay for L5, which can buy QALYs more cheaply than L3.' Removing this program and recalculating the incremental cost-effectiveness ratios (Table 9.9) confirms that L5 indeed achieves additional benefit at a lower per-unit cost than L3 did.

A graph illustrates both forms of dominance. Costs vs. effectiveness for the five competing programs L1 to L5 have been plotted in *cost-effectiveness space* (Figure 9.2). Some recommend presenting cost-effectiveness space with costs on the *x*-axis and effectiveness on the *y*-axis (Figure 9.2a; Gold et al., 1996). In this plot, dominated and extended dominated programs

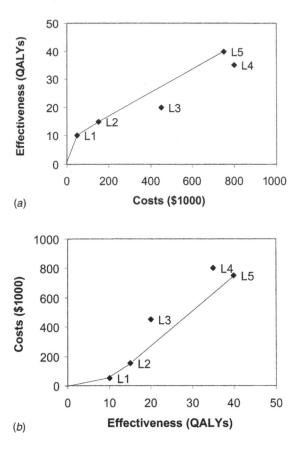

(a)

(b)

Figure 9.2   Costs vs. effectiveness for five competing programs L1–L5 plotted in cost-effectiveness space. L4 is inferior by simple dominance and L3 is ruled out by extended dominance. (a) In cost-effectiveness space, with costs on the x-axis and effectiveness on the y-axis, (extended) dominated programs fall below the line representing the efficiency frontier. This plot demonstrates the diminishing marginal returns of programs as you go up the efficiency frontier. The Panel on CEA recommends presenting results with this plot. (b) In cost-effectiveness space, with effectiveness on the x-axis and costs on the y-axis, (extended) dominated programs fall to the left and above the line representing the efficiency frontier. In this plot the slope of the line connecting a program with the next best program equals its incremental cost-effectiveness ratio. QALYs, quality-adjusted life years.

(L4 and L3 respectively) fall below the line of optimal programs (also known as the *efficiency frontier*) and the graph demonstrates the diminishing marginal returns of programs as you go up the efficiency frontier. Many analysts use the reverse plot (Figure 9.2*b*; Drummond et al., 1997) in which costs are plotted on the y-axis and effectiveness on the x-axis. In the latter plot (extended) dominated programs fall to the upper left of the line representing the efficiency frontier and the slope of the line connecting a program with the next best program equals its incremental cost-effectiveness ratio.

Another trap is revealed by the correction of the incomplete analysis in Table 9.8, before taking into account the extended dominance of the extravagant L3 option. At this stage, it might appear that L5 has an incremental cost-effectiveness ratio of $15 000/QALY. If the cutoff is $18 000/QALY, then L5 might seem to be cost-effective. But it is not! After eliminating L3, the true incremental cost-effectiveness ratio of L5 is revealed to be $24 000 per QALY. Evidently, Option L1 is the cost-effective option if we can only afford up to $18 000 per QALY. Option L5 would be most cost-effective only if our next best uses of the resources cost more than $24 000 per QALY gained.

The issue of extended dominance highlights an important analytical concern in CEA. A suboptimal program can be made to look reasonable if better options are omitted. For this reason, it is important that cost-effectiveness analysts carefully consider the choice of program options to be included in an analysis. In particular, the best available option and the most widely used option should always be considered.

9.6.4 Combining the shopping spree and competing choice problems

To review the steps in selecting among programs, let us look at the full array of programs we have considered in this section, including some that are not mutually exclusive (Programs A–K) and some that are (L1, L2, and L5). To select among these programs, the decision maker first rules out any dominated programs, and selects any programs that save money and yield positive effectiveness. (If we have been lucky enough to have cost-saving options, we can add the money saved to the budget before selecting from the remaining programs.) The next step is to rank the independent programs (those that are not mutually exclusive) in the order of their cost and effectiveness and calculate their cost-effectiveness ratios (Table 9.5). Looking at the list of programs, we can do a preliminary selection of programs, establishing which programs our budgeted amount of funds will cover. The cost-effectiveness ratio of the final (marginal) program demonstrates the opportunity cost of resources.

At this point, we arrange the competing programs in the increasing

Table 9.10. Noncompeting and competing programs in order of cost-effectiveness

Program	Cost ($)	QALYs gained	Incremental cost-effectiveness ratio ($\Delta C/\Delta E$)
C	1 000 000	500	2000
F	2 000 000	500	4000
L1	**50 000**	**10**	**5000**
H	1 200 000	200	6000
K	2 000 000	250	8000
E	1 200 000	100	12 000
J	800 000	50	16 000
A	1 800 000	100	18 000
L2–L1	**100 000**	**5**	**20 000**
D	2 200 000	100	22 000
L5–L2	**600 000**	**25**	**24 000**
I	4 500 000	150	30 000
B	5 000 000	100	50 000
G	10 000 000	100	100 000

QALYs, quality-adjusted life years.

order of their cost, and calculate incremental cost-effectiveness ratios. We exclude options that are ruled out by extended dominance, and then recalculate the incremental cost-effectiveness ratios for the remaining options (Table 9.9). With this new set of ratios, it may again be necessary to rule out options that are dominated by extended dominance. Once the options are in increasing order of incremental cost-effectiveness ratios, this step is complete.

The final selection of programs from among both the independent and the mutually exclusive options will depend on the overall budget that is available. The decision maker will begin with Program C and continue selecting until the budget is exhausted. L1, L2, or L5 will be selected in the order they appear in the table; however, because these programs are mutually exclusive, only one of them may be included in the final package of programs.

In Table 9.10, we use the notation 'L2–L1' to denote the *substitution* of L2 for L1, thus adding its *incremental* QALYs relative to L1 but absorbing its *incremental* cost in the budget. The cost-effectiveness ratio for this transaction is the ratio of the incremental cost to incremental QALYs: $20 000/QALY.

9.6.5 Comparing cost-effectiveness studies

The hypothetical examples above demonstrating incremental CEA make use of tables presenting various program or intervention alternatives and their respective cost-effectiveness ratios. These tables became known in the UK as *league tables* – a reference to listings of soccer teams and their performance – and the name has stuck. The 'textbook' case for using CEA for resource allocation indeed implies the use of such tables for making decisions across alternative uses of resources.

CEAs have traditionally referenced other cost-effectiveness studies as points of comparison for cost-effectiveness ratios presented. For example, a cost-effectiveness study of a new drug to decrease mortality from myocardial infarction might provide cost-effectiveness ratios obtained for a widely used antihypertensive medication as a point of reference. A widely used benchmark in the US is the cost-effectiveness ratio for dialysis for end stage renal disease, the first and only intervention for many years to have been singled out for coverage under the Medicare program for citizens of all ages.

As the field of CEA has grown, tools to facilitate comparisons among interventions in health and medicine are becoming more available. Some projects have devoted a great deal of effort to developing league tables, dissecting and adjusting analyses to assure their comparability. An example is a study of CEA of breast cancer screening by Brown and Fintor (1993). Other projects have developed databases of studies to make cost-effectiveness information more accessible and to assess the studies' quality. The most comprehensive efforts of this type are the National Health Service Economic Evaluation Database compiled in the UK, an ongoing database which analyzes approximately 400 cost-effectiveness studies annually, and a database compiled at the Harvard School of Public Health, Boston (Chapman et al., 2000).

9.7 Handling uncertainty in cost-effectiveness analysis

In modeling and calculating the changes in discounted costs and health benefits needed for a cost-effectiveness study, there are many areas where uncertainty can enter the analysis. The most evident of these is uncertainty surrounding the various estimates that are used as inputs to the analysis – estimates of the size of a treatment effect or the cost of an hour of a practitioner's time, for example. Uncertainty of this type includes sampling variability around a central estimate of a parameter's value, uncertainty about the generalizability of estimates obtained from a particular sample, and uncertainty caused by lack of data on which to base certain estimates. A range of assumptions also underlies the structure of cost-effectiveness models – their methods of combining various data – and this is another source of uncertainty in calculations of cost-effectiveness.

All CEAs should contain sensitivity analyses that test the robustness of results given plausible ranges for important parameter values. Sensitivity analyses may examine high and low values, specific alternative values, or they may be threshold analyses that determine the value of a parameter that would change a decision.

Methods for exploring the parameter uncertainty around CEAs involve assigning explicit probability distributions to the uncertain parameters. These distributions may be estimated from parametric sampling distributions of empirical data, from bootstrap analyses of data from clinical trials and databases, or from Bayesian and meta-analytic approaches that combine data with subjective prior distributions. Analysis and presentation of uncertainty in CEA will be discussed in more detail in Chapter 11.

9.8 Guidelines for the conduct of cost-effectiveness analysis

The standardization of methods has been an important concern in the cost-effectiveness field. Guidelines provide analysts and users of CEA with benchmarks for insuring the quality of analyses. Equally important, standardization promotes the comparability of analyses, a feature central to the usefulness of CEAs, taken as a group, for assessing the relative value of programs and interventions.

Early guidelines for CEA were published by individual authors and by the Office of Technology Assessment. These guidelines tended to be somewhat general, and a lack of quality and consistency persisted in the field. The US Public Health Service took an important step in addressing these issues during the 1990s. It convened the Panel on Cost-Effectiveness in Health and Medicine, a group of experts in cost-effectiveness and related fields, to develop guidelines with the input of US federal agencies that fund and use CEA in the health arena. The Panel developed a set of consensus recommendations referred to as the Reference Case to serve as a point of reference for analysts seeking comparability with other analyses in the literature (Gold et al., 1996; Russell et al., 1996; Siegel et al., 1996; Weinstein et al., 1996).

The Reference Case is comprised of recommendations concerning the nature and limits of CEA, components to be included in the numerator and denominator of the cost-effectiveness ratio, measuring terms in the numerator, estimating effectiveness of interventions, valuing health consequences, discounting, handling uncertainty, and reporting the analysis. These recommendations are included in the appendix to this chapter. Although the Panel based its recommendations on theoretical grounds when possible, many recommendations reflect the practical constraints (and budget limitations) facing analysts, and others are somewhat arbitrary, generated for the purpose of establishing a consistent convention in the field.

The Reference Case analysis is recommended for analyses intended to inform broad resource allocation decisions, and, for this reason, it takes the societal perspective. The Panel recommends that a Reference Case be included in other analyses as well, to contribute to the pool of studies using a comparable methodology and to serve as a point of comparison between perspectives.

9.9 Distributive justice and equity issues in cost-effectiveness analysis

CEA is not an ethically neutral methodology. It contains assumptions that, although defensible, influence the results of analyses and may raise moral questions as a result. The ethical implications of CEA may conflict with important values that decision makers hold or adopt with respect to decision making in the public interest.

Some important critiques derive from the assumption in CEA that years of life are equal – apart from distinctions reflecting quality of life. Although this approach seems 'fair,' it can be argued that society may or should value years of life differently based on a variety of factors. Thus, some may argue with a CEA that finds an intervention that saves 5 years of life for a healthy 80-year-old to be of equal value as an intervention saving the same number of QALYs for a healthy 50-year-old. Similarly, it is not clear that an intervention that confers small benefits on many people is equally desirable to one that confers large benefits on a few individuals, even if the total QALYs conferred by each is identical. Or that a health gain of 1 QALY conferred on a seriously ill person is equivalent to the same gain given to a mildly ill person, from society's point of view.

Another issue in the valuation of health benefits enters with the use of weights to determine QALYs. There are strong arguments against using lower values of quality of life for those with disabling conditions. If a year of life in a wheelchair is given a quality weight of 0.8, interventions that save a year of the life of the wheelchair-bound person will be worth less than interventions that save a year of life for a nondisabled person – a disturbing result. Yet, if analyses do not assign a lower quality weight to a year of life with a disability, an intervention to prevent or cure that disability will appear to have no value. Analysts have used a variety of approaches to address this dilemma, but ethical objections or logical inconsistencies seem to persist.

CEA can inadvertently insert existing patterns of social inequality and health risk into resource allocation recommendations. For example, the analysis that examines a successful HIV prevention intervention for intravenous drug abusers will find that the intervention is less cost-effective than a successful intervention for another population subgroup, because the intravenous drug users have a higher mortality from other causes. Similarly, on the cost side, an analysis that uses women's average wage rate to determine the opportunity cost for family caregivers in a study of prostate cancer will have assigned a lower value to time than if an overall average rate were used, because of the gender-based discrepancy between women's and men's wages.

It is important that analysts and users of CEA be cognizant of its assumptions, including those of CEA generally and those that are specific to a given analysis. A good cost-effectiveness study will present sensitivity analyses on variables that may be problematic, as well as discussing the effect of the assumptions on the results and implications of the analysis.

9.10 Using cost-effectiveness analysis

Cost-effectiveness assists a decision maker or contributes to a policy discussion by summarizing large amounts of information and by clarifying the decision-making process. It provides information concerning the relative worth of an intervention per unit of cost. Although CEA can make a significant contribution, it is far from sufficient for most decisions regarding health and medical interventions.

The appropriate use of CEA depends on the recognition of what this tool provides. A cost-effectiveness ratio, as distinct from a measure like that of net benefit found in cost–benefit analysis, does not give an absolute measure of value that can be used in a decision of whether or not to undertake a program. The cost-effectiveness ratio alone cannot determine whether the benefit of an intervention is worth its cost. Instead, 'cost-effective' is a relative term reflecting the 'price' of additional units of benefit. An intervention can only be cost-effective as compared to another use of resources or as compared to some recognized standard. Annual cervical cancer screening for 50-year-old women can be more cost-effective – cost less per unit of health benefit – than annual cervical cancer screening for 40-year-old women. It can also be incrementally cost-effective compared to semiannual screening for 50-year-old women. However, the decision about which intervention is appropriate must be made on the basis of available resources and the values associated with the decision context.

Misinterpretations of cost-effectiveness information are frequently evident in the way cost-effectiveness results are communicated. One often hears statements that, 'Program X is cost-effective.' This general statement is technically without meaning, because it does not identify either the comparator or the $/QALY standard by which the cost-effectiveness ratio is judged. A program that costs $75 000 per life year saved might or might not be cost-effective – depending on what available alternatives exist for saving lives.

It is most accurate in describing cost-effectiveness results to state the full comparison that is being made, for example, that 'Program X has an incremental cost-effectiveness of $40 000 per QALY saved as compared with Program Y.' The user of general claims about cost-effectiveness may mean to imply that Program X is a cost-effective use of resources compared to available or widely used alternatives. Although an argument of this type may sometimes serve in a political context, it is rarely appropriate in a research or decision-making forum.

Although it can be an important aid to decision making, CEA is not intended to be a decision-making algorithm. Decisions must be made within the context of the decision makers' values and considering a variety of influences and inputs, of which CEA may be one. Values and goals relevant to a decision – political, social, religious, and ethical – are often excluded from a CEA. This is particularly the case for decisions at the societal level, since, in decisions at the patient level, the patient's values can be directly incorporated into the QALY or other measure of health outcome, while outcomes in societal level analyses are aggregates. The methods of CEA do not of themselves prevent an analyst from trying to incorporate specific values into an analysis, for example, by adjusting the weights used to calculate a measure of health outcome or even weighting costs differently based on who ultimately pays them. However, the values entering into decisions are too complex – and not well enough known – to make their systematic incorporation into CEA a feasible practice. In addition, including them would make analyses less transparent, less consistent, and more difficult for users to understand and interpret.

Finally, in applying CEA, it is always important to be aware of the scope of other interventions to which a program is being compared. In a good-quality analysis, the analyst will take stock of the relevant alternatives and include them in the analysis. For example, a surgical cardiac procedure should be compared to available medical procedures, not only to other surgeries. However, because of space limitations, most cost-effectiveness reports will be unable to take a truly broad view, with the result that certain patterns of resource allocation are left unchallenged. It is left to users of CEA to bear in mind that there may be important preventive approaches to the same problems that are in search of cures, and that interventions in the arenas of public health, medicine, education, criminal justice, and environmental safety may have widely different cost-effectiveness. Similarly, from the standpoint of good policy, it may sometimes be better to challenge a budget constraint than to ration resources within the constraint.

Appendix

Summary Recommendations of the Panel on Cost-Effectiveness in Health and Medicine

These framing propositions and recommendations are compiled from the report of the Panel on Cost-Effectiveness in Health and Medicine (Gold et al., 1996). They are classified as follows: framing propositions (F) describe the nature and limits of CEA and serve as basic starting points in defining CEA. Reference Case recommendations (R) are intended for use in a Reference Case analysis as defined by the Panel, which seeks to improve comparability for analyses that will be done to inform resource allocation. Guidance recommendations (G) are intended to improve the conduct of analyses, but are not explicitly required for a Reference Case analysis. An 's' notes instances when a sensitivity analysis would be of particular importance. Additional recommendations, including recommendations for future research, may be found in the Panel's report.

I. The Nature and Limits of CEA and of the Reference Case

1 Cost-effectiveness analysis (CEA) is a methodology for evaluating the outcomes and costs of interventions designed to improve health. F

2 CEA evaluates a given health intervention through the use of a 'cost-

effectiveness ratio.' In this ratio, all health effects of the intervention (relative to a stated alternative) are captured in the denominator, and changes in resource use (relative to the alternative) are captured in the numerator and valued in monetary terms. F

3 CEA is an aid to decision making, not a complete procedure for making resource allocation decisions in health and medicine, because it cannot incorporate all the values relevant to such decisions. F

4 CEA, cost-consequence analysis, and cost–benefit analysis are complementary, rather than mutually exclusive, forms of analysis. The use of one does not preclude the use of any of the others in a given study. F

5 When a CEA is intended to contribute to decisions on the broad allocation of health resources, a Reference Case analysis should be done to enhance comparability across studies. The Reference Case includes not only the associated baseline computation but also a meaningful set of sensitivity analyses. F

6 The Reference Case is based on the societal perspective. This perspective requires that an analysis consider all health effects and all changes in resource use. R

   6.1 Evaluation of effectiveness should incorporate both benefits and harms of alternative interventions. R

   6.2 The boundaries of a study should be defined broadly enough to encompass the range of groups of people affected by the intervention and all types of cost and health consequences. R

   6.3 The time horizon adopted in a CEA should be long enough to capture all relevant future effects of a health care intervention. R

   6.4 Decisions about costs and health effects to include in a CEA, such as the precision with which costs and effects are measured, the time horizon of the study, and the definition of the study boundaries, should strike a reasonable balance between expense and difficulty, and potential importance in the analysis. R

7 The Reference Case analysis should compare the health intervention of interest to existing practice (the 'status quo'). If existing practice appears not to be a cost-effective option itself, relative to other available options, the analyst should incorporate other relevant alternatives into the analysis, such as a best-available alternative, a viable low-cost alternative, or a 'do-nothing' alternative. R

   7.1 When varying levels of program intensity are relevant, alternative program options (e.g., as defined by variation in duration or frequency of the intervention) should be included in the analysis and compared using the incremental cost-effectiveness algorithm. R

8 The estimates of resource consumption and effects of relevance for a CEA are those for the population or group that is actually affected by the health intervention. R

II. Components Belonging to the Numerator and the Denominator

1 The major categories of resource use that should be reflected in the numerator of a C/E ratio include costs of health care services; costs of patient time expended for the intervention; costs associated with caregiving (paid or unpaid); other costs associated with illness such as childcare or travel expenses; and costs associated with nonhealth impacts of the intervention (e.g., on the education system or the environment). R

2 Effects of a health intervention on length of life are incorporated in the denominator of the C/E ratio. A monetary value should not be imputed for lost life years and should not be included in the numerator of the C/E ratio. R

3 For a Reference Case analysis, health-related quality of life should be captured by an instrument that, at minimum, implicitly incorporates the effects of morbidity on productivity and leisure. Effects of a health intervention on subsequent morbidity, including the full value of morbidity time to patients, are incorporated in the denominator of the C/E ratio. R

   3.1 Effects of lost productivity borne by others (e.g., employers, co-workers) including 'friction costs,' when significant, should be included in the numerator. R

4 Time spent seeking care or undergoing an intervention is a resource and a component of the intervention. It should be valued in monetary terms and incorporated in the numerator of a cost-effectiveness ratio. R

   4.1 In some instances (e.g., when recuperating from surgery), time could be categorized either as morbidity time (valued in the denominator) or as input to the intervention itself (costed out in the numerator). As a general rule, in a Reference Case analysis, this time should be considered as morbidity time. G

   4.2 In some instances, time may be a clear input to a health intervention, but the intervention will, in addition, produce a significant impact on health status. When relevant to a Reference Case analysis, the impact on health status should be captured in the denominator, leaving the time component (costed out) in the numerator. G

III. Measuring Terms in the Numerator of the C/E Ratio

1 Changes in the use of resources caused by a health intervention should be valued at their opportunity cost. R

   1.1 Costs should reflect the marginal or incremental resources consumed. R

   1.2 Resource consumption should be assessed from a long-term perspective. R

2 To the extent that prices reflect opportunity costs, they are an appropriate basis for valuing changes in resources. R

   2.1 When prices do not adequately reflect opportunity costs because of market distortions, they should be adjusted appropriately. R

   2.2 When substantial bias is present in prices, and adjustment is not feasible, more suitable proxies for opportunity costs should be considered. G

3 In aggregating resource costs across time, CEAs should be conducted in constant dollars that remove general price inflation. If the prices of the goods in question change at a rate different from general price levels, this variation should be reflected in the adjustment used. R

4 'Transfer payments' (e.g., cash transfers from tax payers to welfare recipients) associated with a health intervention redistribute resources from one individual to another . While administrative costs associated with such transfers are included in the numerator of a C/E ratio, the transfers themselves are not since, by definition, their impact on the transferor and the recipient cancel out. R

5 For individuals in the labor force, wages are generally an acceptable measure of time costs. Wages corresponding to the target population should be used to approximate time costs. In general, age- and gender-specific wage estimates will provide adequately specific estimates. R

   5.1 Use of group-specific wages may influence the conclusions of the analysis in ways that are ethically problematic. In these instances, sensitivity analysis should be conducted to explicitly indicate the nature of this influence. R s.

   5.2 The wage rate generally does not adequately reflect the value of time for persons engaged primarily in leisure or in activities for which they are not compensated. For individuals not engaged in compensated employment, wages, used as proxies, must be adjusted to reflect the full opportunity cost of time. R

6 In theory, the numerator of a C/E ratio should include the net costs of health care and nonhealth consumption during years of life added by the intervention. However, because of problems in measuring these costs,

and because of unresolved issues concerning the role of nonhealth costs in CEA, the Reference Case may either include or exclude health care costs associated with diseases other than those affected by the intervention, in added years of life. R

6.1 Whenever the inclusion or exclusion of health care costs of unrelated diseases makes a significant difference to the analysis, a sensitivity analysis should be performed to assess the effect on the C/E ratio. R s

IV. Measuring Terms in the Denominator of a C/E Ratio

1 For a Reference Case analysis, incorporation of morbidity and mortality consequences into a single measure should be accomplished using QALYs. R

1.1 In general, since lives saved or extended by an intervention will not be in perfect health, a saved life year will count as less than 1 full QALY. R

2 To satisfy the QALY concept, the quality weights must be preference-based, interval-scaled, and measured or transformed onto the interval scale where the reference point 'death' has a score of 0.0 and the reference point 'optimal health' has a score of 1.0. C

3 A CEA should be based on a health-state classification scheme which reflects domains (attributes) that are important for the particular analysis. R

3.1 If the CEA is intended for Reference Case use, the preference measure used should be a generic one, or be capable of being compared to a generic system. R

4 In general, community preferences for health states are the appropriate ones for use in the Reference Case analysis. R

4.1 When adequate information is unavailable regarding community preferences, patient preferences may be used as an approximation, but the manner in which they might differ from community preferences should be discussed and, where relevant, sensitivity analyses that reflect likely differences should be included. R s

4.2 If distinct subgroup preferences are identified that will markedly affect a C/E ratio, the study should provide this information and conduct sensitivity analyses that reflect this difference. R s

5 The health-related quality of life of those whose lives have been saved or extended by a health intervention may be influenced by characteristics such as age, gender, or race. This may affect the Reference Case analysis in ways that are ethically problematic. In these instances, sensitivity

analyses should be conducted to indicate explicitly how the results are affected by these characteristics. R s

6 When designing primary data collection efforts, or deriving the necessary probability estimates from secondary data sources for estimation of effectiveness in a CEA, outcome probability values should be selected from the best designed (and least biased) sources that are relevant to the question and population under study. G

7 Evidence for estimation of effectiveness may be obtained from: randomized controlled trials, observational data, uncontrolled experiments, descriptive series, and expert opinion. G

   7.1 Good quality meta-analysis and other synthesis methods can be used where any one study has insufficient power to detect effects, or where results conflict. G

   7.2 Expert judgment should only be used to fill in values where no adequate data sources exist, or when the parameter is of secondary importance in the analysis. G

8 Where direct primary or secondary empirical evaluation of effectiveness is not possible (e.g., in important subpopulations or in differing time frames), the use of modeling to estimate effectiveness is a valid mode of scientific inquiry for CEAs. G

V. Discounting

1 Costs and health outcomes should be discounted to present value. R

2 Costs should be discounted to present value at a rate consistent with the shadow-price-of-capital (SPC) approach to evaluating public investments. This rate (often termed the *social rate of time preference*) can be approximated by the real rate of return on long-term government bonds. R

3 Costs and health outcomes should be discounted at the same rate. R

   3.1 A real, riskless discount rate of 3% should be used. R

   3.2 Because of the large number of CEAs that have adhered to a discount rate of 5%, analysts should perform sensitivity analyses using 5% as well as a reasonable range of rates (drawn from 0% to 7%). R s

   3.3 The discount rate should be subject to review, and possible revision, over time in light of significant changes in the underlying economic data. However, to retain comparability with other analyses, both 3% and 5% should continue to be used in analyses for at least the next 10 years. R s

VI. Uncertainty

1 At a minimum, univariate (one-way) sensitivity analyses should be conducted in order to determine where uncertainty or lack of agreement about some key parameter's value could have substantial impact on the CEA's conclusions. R

2 Analysts should conduct multivariate (multiway) sensitivity analyses for important parameters. R

3 Where possible, where parameter uncertainty is a major concern, a reasonable confidence interval or credible interval should be estimated based on either statistical methods or simulation. G

VII. Reporting guidelines
(For a summary of reporting guidelines see Siegel et al., 1996)

1 We encourage analysts to document cost-effectiveness studies in two parts, a *journal report* and a more comprehensive *technical report*, making the latter available on request to readers requiring more detail concerning the analysis. G

2 For the specific purpose of journal review, we recommend that editors request and authors submit a concise *technical addendum* with the journal report to assist reviewers assessing the study's methodology. This material may or may not be published along with the journal report. G

3 If a cost-effectiveness analysis is intended to allow comparisons among the interventions studied and health care interventions broadly, the report should highlight the Reference Case results. Key sensitivity analyses should be conducted with respect to the Reference Case. R

4 The perspective(s) of the analysis should be explicitly identified in a cost-effectiveness report. R

5 The following information comprises a basic set of results in the journal report: total costs, total effectiveness, incremental costs, incremental effectiveness, and incremental cost-effectiveness ratios, both discounted (at the Reference Case rate of 3%) and undiscounted. G

6 An appropriate number of significant figures should be used to report C/E results, generally two significant figures unless the precision of the data warrants a greater number. G

7 In reporting incremental cost-effectiveness ratios, options ruled out because of dominance or extended dominance should be excluded. Among undominated options, incremental C/E ratios should be reported in increasing order of cost and effectiveness, starting with the lowest-cost option considered (generally the status quo or 'do nothing' option). R

Table 9.11.

	Cost-effectiveness	
Perspective	$	QALY
Societal		
No drug treatment	0	10.2105
Sildenafil treatment	3970	10.5624
Third-party payer		
No drug treatment	0	10.2105
Sildenafil treatment	3950	10.5624

$, United States dollars; QALY, quality-adjusted life years.

8 C/E ratios should be compared to available C/E ratios for other interventions that compete for resources with the intervention under study. Such interventions may be drawn from health care broadly if the decision context is broad, or from restricted areas, such as particular diseases or intervention modalities. G

Exercises

Exercise 9.1

What is the discount rate if you know that $100 6 years in the future are worth $80 today?

Exercise 9.2

Sildenafil (for example, Viagra) is used for the treatment of erectile dysfunction. It is an effective treatment, but costly, and may lead to serious illness and death when used by men with cardiac disease. Since erectile dysfunction is not a life-threatening illness, some have questioned the appropriateness of insurance coverage for sildenafil given its costs and side-effects.

An analysis was performed to address the costs and effectiveness of using sildenafil for the treatment of erectile dysfunction (Smith, K.J. & Roberts, M.S. (2000). The cost-effectiveness of sildenafil. *Ann. Intern. Med.*, **132**, 933–7). Sildenafil treatment was compared with no treatment for two different perspectives, namely the societal perspective and the third-party payer perspective.

(a) What is the societal perspective and what is the third-party payer perspective?

The tabulated results were available from the article (Table 9.11).

(b) Would you calculate the (incremental) cost-effectiveness ratio by using the 'shopping spree problem' approach or by using the 'competing choice problem' approach? Explain your answer.

(c) Calculate the (incremental) cost-effectiveness ratio based on the table (use the approach from question b). What is your conclusion?

(d) Try to redo the CEA by making a Markov model with the data and assumptions supplied in the original article. (Optional; you will first need to study Chapter 10.)

Exercise 9.3

Read the following abstract (Bosch, J.L., Haaring, C., Meyerovitz, M.F., Cullen, K.A. & Hunink, M.G.M. (2000). Cost-effectiveness of percutaneous treatment of iliac artery occlusive disease in the United States. *Am. J. Roentgenol.*, **175**, 517–21.)

Cost-Effectiveness of Percutaneous Treatment of Iliac Artery Occlusive Disease in the United States

Objective. The costs of percutaneous transluminal angioplasty and stent placement for iliac artery occlusive disease in the United States were assessed and the cost-effectiveness was evaluated.

Materials and methods. Lifetime costs and quality-adjusted life expectancy were estimated using a Markov decision model for a hypothetic cohort of patients with life-style-limiting claudication caused by an iliac artery stenosis for whom a percutaneous intervention was indicated. Various percutaneous treatment strategies were evaluated, each consisting of an initial intervention followed by a secondary intervention. Procedures considered were angioplasty alone and angioplasty with selective stent placement.

Results. From the perspective of the interventional radiology department, angioplasty with selective stent placement costs more than angioplasty alone ($2926 versus $2106). Taking into account follow-up costs and procedures for long-term failures, the cost differential was reduced because of a lower failure rate of selective stent placement ($13 158 versus $12 458, respectively). Treatment strategies using angioplasty with selective stent placement (as an initial procedure or including reintervention) dominated treatment strategies using angioplasty alone (incremental cost-effectiveness ratio was $7624–8519 per quality-adjusted life-year gained).

Table 9.12.

Treatment strategy	QALE[a]	Lifetime costs[a]
Angioplasty followed by no revascularization	8.46	10 048
Angioplasty and repeated angioplasty	8.73	12 458
Initial and repeated angioplasty with selective stent placement	8.89	13 158
PTA followed by PTA with selective stent placement	8.79	12 830
No revascularization	7.79	4531
PTA with selective stent placement followed by no revascularization	8.63	10 903

QALE, quality-adjusted life expectancy; PTA, percutaneous transluminal angioplasty. Lifetime costs are 1998 US$.
[a]Both costs and QALE were discounted.

Conclusion. Angioplasty with selective stent placement is a cost-effective treatment strategy compared with angioplasty alone in the treatment of intermittent claudication in the United States.

(a) Based on the abstract, from which perspectives were the costs calculated? Which costs should these perspectives include?

The tabulated results were available from the paper (Table 9.12).

(b) In the results section it was stated that strategies using angioplasty with selective stent placement dominated all other strategies. Can you recalculate the mentioned incremental cost-effectiveness ratios? (The calculated ratios will not exactly match the ratios in the abstract because of rounding.)

(c) Calculate the net health benefits (NHB) for each strategy using:

NHB = effectiveness − cost/G
where G = 20 000 and 50 000/QALY gained.
Which strategy is best? Does this correspond with the analysis based on incremental CE ratios?

Exercise 9.4

An analysis was performed to address the costs and effectiveness of screening for anal squamous intraepithelial lesions and anal cancer in homosexual and bisexual men (Goldie, S.J., Kuntz, K.M., Weinstein, M.C., Freedberg, K.A. & Palefsky, J.M. (2000). Cost-effectiveness of screening for anal squamous intraepithelial lesions and anal cancer in human

Table 9.13.

Screening strategy	Undiscounted quality-adjusted life expectancy (years)	Discounted incremental quality-adjusted life expectancy (months)	Discounted lifetime costs ($)
No screening	47.59		4130
Every 3 years	48.06	1.79	5178
Every 2 years	48.14	0.32	5583
Every 1 year	48.22	0.38	6676
Every 6 months	48.26	0.17	8744

immunodeficiency virus-negative homosexual and bisexual men. *Am. J. Med.*, **108**, 634–41). The tabulated results were available from the article (Table 9.13).

(a) Determine, using incremental cost-effectiveness ratio calculations, which screening strategy you would choose if you were prepared to pay US$50 000 per QALY gained (use the discounted quality-adjusted life expectancy).

(b) In your opinion and in your setting, how much should society be prepared to pay to increase a patient's life expectancy with 1 life year in full health (= gain of 1 QALY)?

(c) Do you think it is unethical to tag a price on a life year? Assume someone says that the highest priority should be given to treating the patient and extending life expectancy and that the costs are of no importance. With what estimate of society's willingness to pay would this correspond?

Exercise 9.5

Pick a recently published CEA in your area of interest and read it carefully. Take the list of recommendations from the Panel on Cost-Effectiveness in Health and Medicine and check to what extent the analysts have followed the recommendations.

REFERENCES

Bergner, M., Bobbit, R.A., Carter, W.B. & Gilson, B.S. (1981). The Sickness Impact Profile: development and final revision of a health status measure. *Med. Care*, **19**, 787–805.

Bosch, J.L., Haaring, C., Meyerovitz, M.F., Cullen, K.A. & Hunink, M.G. (2000). Cost-effectiveness of percutaneous treatment of iliac artery occlusive disease in the United States. *Am. J. Roentgenol.*, **175**, 517–21.

Brazier, J.E., Harper, R., Thomas, K., Jones, N. & Underwood, T. (1998a). Deriving a preference based single index measure from the SF-36. *J. Clin. Epidemiol.*, **51**, 1115–29.

Brazier, J.E., Deverill, M., Roberts, J., Ware, J. & Gandek, B. (1998b). The estimation of a utility based algorithm for the Short Form 36 health survey. *Qual. Life Res.*, **7**, 574–5.

Brown, M.L. & Fintor, L. (1993). Cost-effectiveness of breast cancer screening: preliminary results of a systematic review of the literature. *Breast Cancer Res. Treat.*, **25**, 113–18.

Chapman, G.B. & Elstein, A.S. (1995). Valuing the future: temporal discounting of health and money. *Med. Decis. Making*, **15**, 373–86.

Chapman, R.H., Stone, P.W., Sandberg, E.A., Bell, C. & Neumann, P.J. (2000). A comprehensive league table of cost–utility ratios and a sub-table of 'panel-worthy' studies. *Med. Decis. Making*, **4**, 451–67. Corresponding database: www.hsph.harvard.edu/organizations/hcra/cuadatabase/intro.html.

Drummond, M.F., O'Brien, B.J., Stoddart, G.L. & Torrance, G.W. (1997). *Methods for the Economic Evaluation of Health Care Programmes*, 2nd edn. New York: Oxford University Press.

EuroQol Group (1990). EuroQol – a new facility for the measurement of health-related quality of life. The EuroQol Group [see comments]. *Health Policy*, **16**, 199–208.

Farnham, P.G., Gorsky, R.D., Holtgrave, D.R., Jones, W.K. & Guinan, M.E. (1996). Counseling and testing for HIV prevention: costs, effects, and cost- effectiveness of more rapid screening tests. *Public Health R*ep., **111**, 44–54.

Feeny, D.H., Furlong, W., Boyle, M. & Torrance, G.W. (1995). Multi-attribute health status classification systems. Health utilities index. *PharmacoEconomics*, **7**, 490–502.

Gold, M.R., Siegel, J.E., Russell, L.B. & Weinstein, M.C. (eds) (1996). *Cost-effectiveness in Health and Medicine*, 1st edn. New York: Oxford University Press.

Goldie, S.J., Kuntz, K.M., Weinstein, M.C., Freedberg, K.A. & Palefsky, J.M. (2000). Cost-effectiveness of screening for anal squamous intraepithelial lesions and anal cancer in human immunodeficiency virus-negative homosexual and bisexual men. *Am. J. Med.*, **108**, 634–41.

Johannesson, M., Meltzer, D. & O'Conor, R.M. (1997). Incorporating future costs in medical cost-effectiveness analysis: implications for the cost-effectiveness of the treatment of hypertension. *Med. Decis. Making*, **17**, 382–9.

Kaplan, R.M. & Anderson, J.P. (1988). A general health policy model: update and applications. *Health Serv. Res.*, **23**, 203–35.

Keeler, E.B. & Cretin, S. (1983). Discounting of lifesaving and other nonmonetary effects. *Manage. Sci.*, **29**, 300–6.

Lipscomb, J., Weinstein, M.C. & Torrance, G.W. (1996). Time preference. In: *Cost-effectiveness in Health and Medicine*, ed. M.R. Gold, J.E. Siegel, L.B. Russell & M.C. Weinstein, pp. 214–46. New York: Oxford University Press.

Meltzer, D. (1997). Accounting for future costs in medical cost-effectiveness analysis. *J. Health Econ.*, **16**, 33–64.

Murray, C.J. & Lopez, A.D. (1997a). Global mortality, disability, and the contribution of risk factors: Global Burden of Disease Study [see comments]. *Lancet*, **349**, 1436–42.

Murray, C.J. & Lopez, A.D. (1997b). Regional patterns of disability-free life expectancy and disability- adjusted life expectancy: global Burden of Disease Study [see comments]. *Lancet*, **349**, 1347–52.

Musgrove, P. (1993). Investing in health: the 1993 world development report of the World Bank. *Bull. Pan Am. Health Org.*, **27**, 284–6.

Redelmeier, D.A. & Heller, D.N. (1993). Time preference in medical decision making and cost-effectiveness analysis [see comments]. *Med. Decis. Making*, **13**, 212–17.

Russell, L.B., Gold, M.R., Siegel, J.E., Daniels, N. & Weinstein, M.C. (1996). The role of cost-effectiveness analysis in health and medicine. For the Panel on Cost-Effectiveness in Health and Medicine. *J.A.M.A.*, **276**, 1172–7.

Siegel, J.E., Weinstein, M.C., Russell, L.B. & Gold, M.R. (1996). Recommendations for reporting cost-effectiveness analysis. Panel on Cost-Effectiveness in Health and Medicine. *J.A.M.A.*, **276**, 1339–41.

Smith, K.J. & Roberts, M.S. (2000). The cost-effectiveness of sildenafil. *Ann. Intern. Med.*, **132**, 933–7.

Ware, J.E. Jr & Sherbourne, C.D. (1992). The MOS 36-item short-form health survey (SF-36). I. Conceptual framework and item selection. *Med. Care*, **30**, 473–83.

Weinstein, M.C. & Stason, W.B. (1977). Foundations of cost-effectiveness analysis for health and medical practices. *N. Engl. J. Med.*, **296**, 716–21.

Weinstein, M.C., Siegel, J.E., Gold, M.R., Kamlet, M.S. & Russell, L.B. (1996). Recommendations of the Panel on Cost-effectiveness in Health and Medicine [see comments]. *J.A.M.A.*, **276**, 1253–8.

World Bank (1993). *World Development Report 1993: Investing in Health. Community Disease Report CDR: Weekly*, vol. 3, p. 137. Washington, DC: International Bank for Reconstruction and Development.

Recurring events

Everything flows and all changes are cyclic.

Heraclitus, Greek philosopher

10.1 Introduction

In previous chapters we have seen several applications of decision trees to solve clinical problems under conditions of uncertainty. Decision trees work well in analyzing chance events with limited recursion and a limited time horizon. The limited number of sequential decision or chance nodes allows one to capture all the necessary information to maximize expected utility. However, when events can occur repeatedly over an extended time period, the decision tree framework can become unmanageable. Many decision situations involve events occurring over the lifetime of the patient, thus extending far into the future. Life spans vary, but conventional trees require us to specify a fixed time horizon. The probabilities and utilities of these events may change over time and must be accounted for. This is the case for most chronic conditions. Examples include heart disease, Alzheimer's disease, various cancers, diabetes, asthma, osteoporosis, human immunodeficiency virus (HIV), inflammatory bowel disease, multiple sclerosis and more. This chapter offers a methodology for dealing with recurring events and extended (variable) time horizons.

Example | Consider a patient with peripheral arterial disease (PAD: obstruction of the arteries to the legs) for whom a decision has to be made for either bypass surgery or percutaneous transluminal angioplasty (PTA: balloon dilatation). We assume that conservative treatment through an exercise regimen has been ruled out. A very simplified decision tree is presented in Figure 10.1. Following the choice of treatment, the patient may die as a result of the procedure (captured in the 'mortality' branches) or survive the procedure. If the patient survives, treatment may fail and the patient returns to the preprocedure prognosis, or treatment may be successful and the patient is relieved of symptoms. If we consider some fixed time horizon like a year or 5 years, we can assign utilities to the three possible outcomes (success, failure, death) and

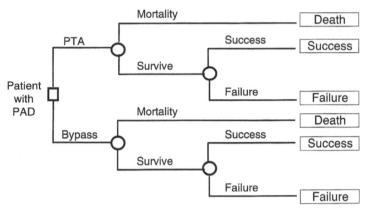

Figure 10.1	Decision tree for peripheral arterial disease (PAD). PTA, percutaneous trans-luminal angioplasty.

calculate expected utilities to choose a preferred treatment. In the current structure, there is no explicit allowance for the time horizon we are considering, nor for the timing of the various events. Even if we consider a fixed time horizon of, say, 5 years, there surely is a different implication for prognosis if failure occurs in the first year versus the fifth year.

To overcome the timing of events, we could break the problem into individual sequential years. Figure 10.2 depicts a partial tree with a 3-year breakdown. In this tree we can see that events can occur at different time points. For example, failure can occur during the first year, or in the second year, or in the third. Similarly, the patient can die during the first year, or second or third. We can similarly proceed and expand the depth of the tree to include many more years into the future. If we were to allow for such events as a stroke or a myocardial infarction (MI or 'heart attack'), these can occur repeatedly and not only once and we must accommodate these possibilities. Even if we have a fixed time horizon of, say, 20 years, the tree becomes very 'bushy' and unmanageable. The problems compound if we want to consider the 'lifetime' of the patient without having to specify a fixed time horizon. One clearly sees that the conventional decision tree approach has certain limitations, and we need a more complex model.

Another reason to adopt a type of decision framework having a more flexible time horizon is that some decision problems lend themselves to using life expectancy or quality-adjusted life expectancy as the outcome measure. This is especially true in cost-effectiveness analyses, in which a common outcome measure is needed to compare the benefits of different

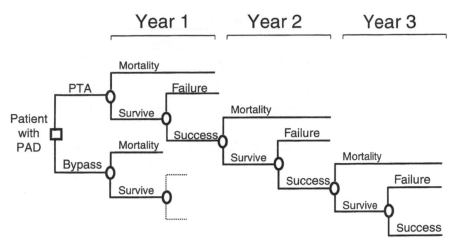

Figure 10.2　　Decision tree for peripheral arterial disease (PAD) with a 3-year time horizon. PTA, percutaneous transluminal angioplasty.

interventions to prevent or treat different conditions. The methodology offered in this chapter will enable such calculations.

There is another valuable contribution of the recursive models developed in this chapter. We often need survival curve data in modeling the choice among alternatives in a decision analysis. While it would be ideal to have such survival curve data for the alternative interventions being considered, this is usually not possible for several reasons. First, such data may not exist at all, e.g., we may have data for only a single time point such as 2-year follow-up. Second, even if we have some survival curve data, there is often the need to extrapolate the results further into the future. Finally, the population in which the data were acquired may be somewhat different from the population to whom we wish to apply them. Therefore we need some general means of modeling events over time. This chapter will describe the simplest and most useful technique, Markov models (Kemeny and Snell, 1976; Beck and Pauker, 1983; Sonnenberg and Beck, 1993).

10.2　Markov models

Markov models are most useful when the decision problem involves risk over time, when the timing of events is important, and when events may happen more than once. These models differ from decision trees in that, instead of modeling uncertain events at chance nodes, the uncertain events are modeled as transitions between defined health states. In mathematical representations of Markov models, these transition probabilities are

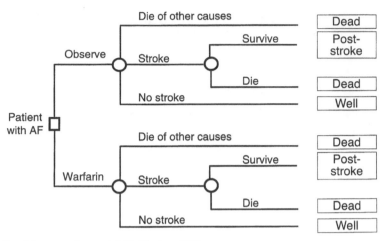

Figure 10.3 Decision tree for atrial fibrillation (AF).

typically represented in terms of matrix algebra, but we will not need this formal representation in this book. Instead, we discuss the conceptual structure of state-transition models, including more general structures that permit us to model transition probabilities that depend on individual patient characteristics and histories. We will build on the following example.

Example

Atrial fibrillation is a major public health problem, as it is the cause of 10–15% of all strokes. It is an irregularity of the heart rhythm that can lead to the formation of small blood clots (emboli) in the circulation. If these clots reach the brain, then a stroke occurs. Several trials have now demonstrated that anticoagulation with warfarin (a rat poison!) dramatically reduces this risk of stroke. The dilemma is that it also increases the risk of bleeding, the most serious form of which is a bleed into the brain (i.e., a stroke). Thus the decision problem is whether the reduced risk of embolic stroke from using warfarin is worth the increased risk of bleeding. Clearly this depends on the risk of emboli – the higher the risk the greater the payoff from anticoagulation. But how high does the risk need to be to make it worthwhile? One way to approach this is to draw the simplified decision tree in Figure 10.3. The uncertainty in this problem relates to what event the patient may experience (stroke, death, no event), which then translates into one of three possible outcomes (poststroke, dead, well). We have made some implicit simplifying assumptions that the poststroke state is the same following a bleed or an embolus, and that dead is the same regardless of how the patient dies. We can then assign utilities to the various outcomes and resolve the tree. As in the previous example, a stroke or bleed can occur repeatedly during the lifetime of the patient, so we must

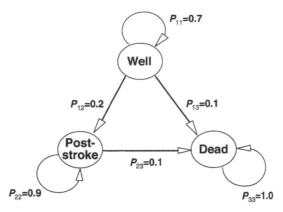

Figure 10.4   State-transition diagram. Well, poststroke, and dead represent the three Markov states. P_{ij}, transition probability from state i to state j.

model the entire uncertain life span of the patient, and allow for repeated uncertain events. Similarly, we have to allow for death to occur at any time point. The following development will relate to this example and present the Markov model.

In this problem, the patient must be in one of three mutually exclusive and collectively exhaustive *states*: well, poststroke, or dead. The well state includes patients who are asymptomatic, but in whom the atrial fibrillation continues. Their physical functioning is normal and let's assume they have a normal quality of life in spite of the increased risk of stroke; we assume that the risk of death from all other causes is similar to the rest of the population. The poststroke state relates to patients who have survived a stroke. They have a reduced quality of life and an increased base risk of further stroke (and hence require treatment with warfarin).

The time horizon of the analysis is divided into equal time intervals (e.g., year, month), referred to as cycles. All events of interest are modeled as *transitions* from one state to another. Figure 10.4 presents a *state-transition diagram*. The arrows represent possible transitions among the states. Notice that it is possible for a patient to remain in a given state in successive time periods. This is represented by an arrow leading from a state into itself. Also notice that some transitions are not possible (e.g., from dead to well). The model also assumes that in any given cycle, only one transition is possible.

The length of the cycle can vary; it is chosen to reflect a time interval which is clinically meaningful. If the decision problem considers the entire life span of the patient, and if critical events are not especially frequent,

Table 10.1. Probability transition matrix

		State of next cycle		
		Well	Poststroke	Dead
State of current cycle	Well	0.7	0.2	0.1
	Poststroke	0.0	0.9	0.1
	Dead	0.0	0.0	1.0

then a cycle of 1 year may be appropriate. For shorter time horizons, or if critical events tend to occur frequently we may choose shorter cycles, such as 1 month. It is important to choose the cycle so that we can expect events to occur only once during a cycle (one transition per cycle). Another factor influencing cycle length is the availability of data. If we have only annual survival data, it is natural to use a cycle length of 1 year, although it is fairly straightforward to convert transition probabilities from one cycle length to another, provided that we are willing to assume that the instantaneous transition *rate* doesn't change within a cycle.

The numbers written beside each transition arrow in Figure 10.4 represent the probabilities of making that transition in one cycle. They are called the one-cycle *transition probabilities*. P_{ij} represents the probability of going from state i to state j in one cycle. For example, the probability that a well patient moves into the poststroke state is 0.2. (We are using hypothetical numbers for this example to make the calculations more intuitive.) In any given cycle, the patient must be in one and only one of the states. Hence the sum of the probabilities over all arrows leading out of every state must equal 1.0.

The probabilities in Figure 10.4 can also be represented in matrix form, as in Table 10.1. The rows of the table represent the current state, and the columns represent the state of the next cycle. The probabilities in each *row* must add to 1.0. This is called the one-cycle *transition matrix*, or the *P-matrix*. In a model with many states, it is convenient to present the states and transition probabilities in matrix form.

The one-cycle transition probabilities may be constant throughout many cycles or may depend on time and thus change from cycle to cycle. If they are the same for every cycle, the Markov model is said to be a *stationary Markov model*, or a *Markov chain*. In most health applications, however, the assumption of stationarity is seldom met, if only because the probabilities of transition to 'dead' tend to increase with age and, therefore, with time. Markov chains will be useful to evaluate situations that do not evolve over a long time horizon, or situations where mortality is not involved and the patient moves among various other states. An example of this situation is psoriasis, where treatment is evaluated not on patient survival but on a patient's transitions among various symptomatic stages of the disease.

Each state may be associated with a different quality of life and may involve different resource costs. Hence we can assign a different utility to being in each state. Our modeling will enable the calculation of life expectancy, quality-adjusted life expectancy, expected utility, and expected resource costs.

Any process evolving over time with associated uncertainty is referred to as a *stochastic process,* and models of such processes are called stochastic models or, equivalently, probabilistic models. If an additional restriction is applied, the process is referred to as a Markov process. This restriction states that the behavior of the process subsequent to any cycle does not depend on the history prior to that cycle. This is known as the *Markovian property* and reflects a 'lack of memory' for the process. In other words, prognosis in the above example depends only on the current state and not on how the patient reached the current state. If the patient is now in the poststroke state it doesn't matter if he or she has already spent several cycles in that state or has reached this state for the first time this cycle.

Obviously, in reality this 'memorylessness' property in Markov models does not always hold. However, we will still be able to use Markov models even for situations where the prior history or length of time spent in a state does matter. For example, the prognosis of a patient may depend on how many MIs or strokes the patient had. The trick is to create additional states to correspond to different past histories leading to the current state. This will be dealt with later in the chapter.

10.3 Evaluating Markov models

Defining a Markov process requires several steps: define the states, determine the cycle length, consider possible transitions among states, assess transition probabilities, and assess utilities (and, if you are using the model for a cost-effectiveness analysis, the costs) associated with being in each state for one cycle. Now it is time to consider the evaluation and calculation process involved with the model.

There are three basic methods to evaluate a Markov process:

1 Fundamental matrix solution (section 10.3.1)

2 Cohort simulation (section 10.3.2)

3 Monte Carlo simulation (section 10.3.9)

10.3.1 Fundamental matrix solution

The fundamental matrix solution can be used only for Markov chains, when the transition probabilities are constant over time. It requires some basic knowledge of matrix algebra which is beyond the scope of this book. This method generates values for the expected time spent in each state, yielding estimates for life expectancy in each state and overall. The duration in each state may be multiplied with a quality adjustment factor to yield quality-adjusted life expectancy. It also generates values for the standard deviation of the duration in each state. The matrix solution does not allow for changes in utility over time or for discounting of costs or life years. Details on the fundamental matrix solution may be found in Beck and Pauker's seminal paper (1983) on Markov models in health care.

10.3.2 Cohort simulation

Cohort simulation is a very intuitive representation of a Markov process. The simulation considers a hypothetical cohort of patients who are distributed among the possible states and follows their transition among the states from cycle to cycle based on the transition probabilities. In our stroke example, consider a hypothetical cohort of 10 000 patients who are all in the well state. The transition probabilities in Figure 10.4 (or Table 10.1) imply that there is a 0.7 chance the patient who is well will remain in the well state in the next cycle, a 0.2 chance the patient will go from well to poststroke in the next cycle, and a 0.1 chance of dying. Hence, after one cycle we can expect, on average, that 7000 of the 10 000 well patients will remain in the well state, 2000 patients will be in the poststroke state, and 1000 patients will be dead. This is represented graphically in Figure 10.5, which depicts the transitions through three cycles.

Table 10.2 presents the same information and extends the simulation for many more cycles until all (or nearly all) patients are in the dead state. The display in Table 10.2 is called the *Markov trace* for our example. The dead state is called an *absorbing state*, which means that once a patient enters that state, the probability of exiting from the state is zero. In the long run, all members of a Markov cohort end up in an absorbing state. For practical purposes, we are usually content to terminate the simulation when the

Table 10.2. Cohort simulation

Cycle	State		
	Well	Poststroke	Dead
0	10 000	0	0
1	7000	2000	1000
2	4900	3200	1900
3	3430	3860	2710
4	2401	4160	3439
5	1681	4224	4095
6	1176	4138	4686
7	824	3959	5217
93	0	1	9999
94	0	0	10 000

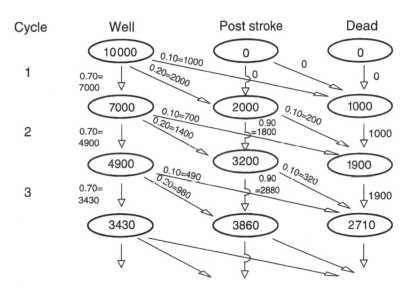

Figure 10.5   Cohort simulation.

fraction of the cohort remaining alive is below some small threshold (e.g., 1%).

10.3.3 Calculating life expectancy

Now that we have performed the cohort simulation we are ready for some calculations of life expectancy and quality-adjusted life expectancy. Let us calculate the total number of cycles (e.g., years) that the cohort of 10 000 lived. Every cycle where a patient is alive (either well or poststroke)

Table 10.3. Calculating life expectancy

Cycle	State			Cycle sum
	Well	Poststroke	Dead	
0	10 000	0	0	
1	7000	2000	1000	9000
2	4900	3200	1900	8100
3	3430	3860	2710	7290
4	2401	4160	3439	6561
5	1681	4224	4095	5905
6	1176	4138	4686	5314
7	824	3959	5217	4783
93	0	1	9999	1
94	0	0	10 000	0
Total	23 333	66 667		90 000

contributes one credit to this pool. In cycle 1 there are 7000 well patients and 2000 poststroke patients, contributing a total of 9000 cycle credits. Cycle 2 contributes 8100 (= 4900 + 3200) cycle credits, and so on. Table 10.3 presents the calculations in more detail. The fifth column of Table 10.3 presents the cycle sum for that cycle.

If we now look at the total of column 5, we obtain the total number of cycles lived by this hypothetical cohort of 10 000 patients. Dividing the total number of cycles by the number of patients yields the life expectancy of an individual patient, in this case 9.0 cycles. If all we need at some point of a decision tree is life expectancy, then we have just demonstrated how this is done.

Moreover, if we look at the totals of columns 2 and 3 we obtain the total number of cycles (e.g., life years) lived by cohort members in the well and poststroke states respectively. In this example we assumed that transitions occur at the beginning of each cycle and therefore we have not included the first entry of 10 000 in the sum. Dividing the sums by 10 000, we obtain an average duration of 2.333 cycles in the well state and 6.667 in the poststroke state. Obviously, the sum of these two numbers is the total average number of cycles lived by each patient (9.0).

In this example we have used constant transition probabilities. We could have easily used cycle-dependent probabilities as well. In both cases, stationary or time-dependent probabilities, the cohort simulation can easily be performed on any common spreadsheet.

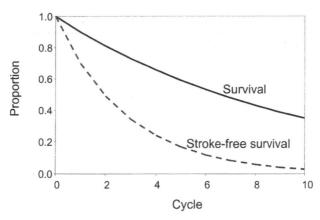

Figure 10.6   Markov survival trace.

10.3.4 Estimating survival curves

The cohort simulation presented in Table 10.3 can be used to plot the survival curve. This is presented in Figure 10.6 for a period of 10 cycles. On the vertical axis we have the percentage of patients surviving (i.e., alive) at the end of each cycle. On the horizontal axis we plot time in cycles. For example, in Table 10.3 we see that at the beginning of cycle 3 there are 2710 patients in the dead state, implying that 7290 patients are still alive, for a survival of 72.9%. This can be seen in Figure 10.6. This curve is also referred to as a *Markov trace*. Note that it contains the same information as in the dead column of Table 10.3. Thus, by means of a Markov trace we can visually model survival and use survival data for various needs. This is especially valuable for situations when we only have one or two points on a survival curve and we need more specific data for the analysis or need to project survival into the future to estimate life expectancy. The life expectancy calculated in the previous section can be viewed as the area under the Markov trace when we follow it until it approaches the horizontal axis. We will return to the Markov trace and its relation to the 'true' survival curve later in the chapter when we discuss some 'fine-tuning' of the model.

10.3.5 Estimating partitioned survival curves

We may be interested not only in overall survival, but also in disease-free survival. We can use the information in Table 10.3 to plot a 'stroke-free' survival curve for our hypothetical cohort. This curve, which lies below the overall survival curve, indicates the percentage of patients who remain well after each number of elapsed cycles. The disease-free (stroke-free in our

Table 10.4. Calculating expected utility

	State			
	Well	Poststroke	Dead	
Cycle	$U=1.0$	$U=0.6$	$U=0.0$	Cycle utility
0	10 000	0	0	
1	7000	2000	1000	8200
2	4900	3200	1900	6820
3	3430	3860	2710	5746
4	2401	4160	3439	4897
5	1681	4224	4095	4215
6	1176	4138	4686	3659
7	824	3959	5217	3199
93	0	1	9999	0
94	0	0	10 000	0
Total				63 331

example) survival curve is also part of the Markov trace, and is also shown in Figure 10.6.

10.3.6 Quality-adjusted life expectancy (expected utility)

As mentioned earlier, being in different states may imply a different quality of life for the patient. Let us assume that the quality of life in the well state has a utility of 1.0, dead has a utility of 0.0 and poststroke 0.6. The utility associated with spending one cycle in a particular state is referred to as *incremental utility*.

Table 10.4 presents the Markov trace for the cohort simulation in tabular form, but now with the utility calculations added. We will now assume that the cycle length is 1 year, so that each cycle spent in one of the 'alive' states contributes 1.0 year of life expectancy. Moreover, each cycle spent in the well state, whose utility is 1.0, contributes 1.0 quality-adjusted life year (QALY).

Column 5 now presents the sum of utilities (or QALYs) for the entire cohort for each cycle. For example, for cycle 1, 7000 well patients have a utility of 1 QALY, contributing a total of 7000 QALYs, and the 2000 poststroke patients contribute 1200 QALYs ($=2000 \cdot 0.6$), for a total of 8200 QALYs. If we now look at the total for column 5, we obtain the total expected utility for the cohort. Dividing by 10 000 we obtain an expected utility of 6.33 for an individual patient. This is equivalent to 6.33 QALYs, compared to a life expectancy of 9 years when there was no consideration of quality of life.

Life expectancy can also be visualized graphically as the area under the overall survival curve. This area represents the expected number of person years lived by the members of the cohort. The area *between* the overall survival curve and the stroke-free survival curve represents the expected number of person years lived in the poststroke state, and the area *under* the stroke-free curve represents the number of person years lived in the well state. Therefore, quality-adjusted life expectancy can be interpreted in Figure 10.6 as the weighted sum of the area *between* the overall survival and stroke-free survival curve (weighted by 0.6) and the area *under* the stroke-free survival curve (weighted by 1.0).

When we apply these types of results to cost-effectiveness analysis, we will want to weight each cycle by a factor that reflects how far it is in the future. This is called *time discounting*. If we want to discount life years and QALYs, then every figure in column 5 should be weighted by a *discount factor* before summing them to generate discounted QALYs. As we saw in Chapter 9, a typical discount factor for the nth cycle would be $1/(1.03)^n$. We will demonstrate this procedure presently in the cost calculation.

10.3.7 Cost calculations

Let us assume that the resource costs associated with being well are $100 per year, the costs for poststroke are $150 per year, and that being dead is costless. Table 10.5 presents the cohort simulation for the cost analysis. The first four columns represent the numbers of patients in each state for each cycle and are identical to the first four columns of Tables 10.3 and 10.4. Column 5 now represents the total costs for the respective cycle. For example, in cycle 1, 7000 patients have a cost of $100 each and 2000 patients accrue a cost of $150 each, for a total cost of $1 000 000. If we discount the costs from the nth cycle to the beginning of the simulation using a discount factor of $1/1.03^n$, then the present value of this sum is $970 874, and is presented in column 6. Each value in column 6 is obtained by dividing the amount in column 5 by $(1.03)^n$, where n is the cycle number. The total of column 6 gives us the discounted value of all costs during the lifetime of this process. Dividing this total by 10 000 patients, we get an average discounted cost of $932 for each patient.

As we saw in Chapter 9, the total discounted quality-adjusted cycles and

Table 10.5. Calculating expected (discounted) costs

	State				
	Well	Poststroke	Dead		Cycle PV
Cycle	$100	$150	$0	Cycle cost	(3%)
0	10 000	0	0		
1	7000	2000	1000	$1 000 000	$970 874
2	4900	3200	1900	$970 000	$914 318
3	3430	3860	2710	$922 000	$843 761
4	2401	4160	3439	$864 100	$767 742
5	1681	4224	4095	$801 700	$691 553
6	1176	4138	4686	$738 337	$618 346
7	824	3959	5217	$676 268	$549 868
93	0	1	9999	$83	$5
94	0	0	10 000	$75	$5
Total					$9 323 977

PV, present value.

the discounted costs data can be combined to yield cost-effectiveness ratios. In this example, $932/6.33 QALYs = $147/QALY.

10.3.8 Fine-tuning: the half-cycle correction

One of the basic assumptions underlying Markov models is that transitions can occur only once in each cycle. We are also assuming that the transition from state to state is instantaneous. However, we have not yet addressed the issue of when during a cycle these transitions take place. If we look at the cohort simulation of Table 10.2, we see that in cycle 1 there are 7000 patients in the well state, 2000 in the poststroke state and 1000 dead. Since this is cycle 1, it means that we have assumed that transitions occur at the beginning of the cycle, and membership in the cycle is counted at the end of the cycle. Alternatively, we could have assumed that transitions occur at the end of the cycle and then the accounting would have been different. In reality, though, transitions can occur at any time during the cycle along the continuous time axis. Thus, on average, we can assume that transitions occur halfway through the cycle. If this is the case, then the 10 000 patients make the transition in the middle of the first cycle rather than at the beginning. This means that each of them contributes an additional half-

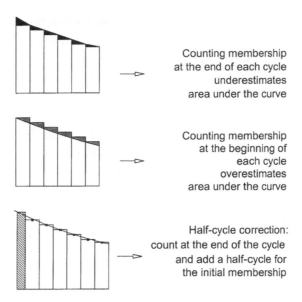

Counting membership at the end of each cycle underestimates area under the curve

Counting membership at the beginning of each cycle overestimates area under the curve

Half-cycle correction: count at the end of the cycle and add a half-cycle for the initial membership

Figure 10.7   Half-cycle correction.

cycle to the calculated life expectancy. We should add this 0.5 to the life expectancy of nine cycles which we had calculated earlier, yielding a corrected life expectancy of 9.5 cycles. We should also make this adjustment in the calculation of expected utility. Since all 10 000 started out in the well state, and if transitions occur in the middle of the cycle, we have to add 0.5 units to the expected utility, yielding an expected utility of 6.83 (i.e., 6.83 quality-adjusted cycles).

The above example showed that we have underestimated life expectancy by assuming that transitions occur at the beginning of the cycle. To correct this we have added 0.5 cycles to life expectancy. This is called the *half-cycle correction*. If our accounting had transitions occurring at the end of the cycle, we should subtract 0.5 cycles.

These approximations to life expectancy can be seen graphically in Figure 10.7. The continuous curve represents the 'true' survival curve. Allowing transitions in the beginning of each cycle is equivalent to counting membership at the end of the cycle, resulting in the underestimation of survival, as seen by the top graph in Figure 10.7. Life expectancy is the area under the survival curve. The rectangles represent the area calculated by the cohort simulation. Had we assumed transitions to occur at the end of each cycle, which is equivalent to counting membership at the beginning of the (next) cycle, we would have overestimated survival, as seen in the middle graph of Figure 10.7. The half-cycle correction is equivalent to moving the graph a half-cycle to the right to simulate that transitions occur halfway through the cycle. In a practical sense we count membership at the end of the cycle and add a half-cycle for the initial membership. This yields a better approximation to the true survival curve, as seen by the lower graph in Figure 10.7.

The half-cycle correction presented above is very appropriate for situations where we follow the process to absorption. There are also situations where we want to calculate 5-year survival, for example, or follow the process for a limited number of cycles. We must then make an additional correction for members of the cohort who are still alive at the end of the observation or simulation. We then subtract a half-cycle from these members in the final accounting.

10.3.9 Monte Carlo simulation

In cohort simulation, transitions are experienced by the proportion of persons in each state corresponding to the transition probabilities. In essence, this is the 'average' experience of the patients in the cohort. In Monte Carlo simulation, instead of proportions of patients making the transitions, individual patients are simulated going from cycle to cycle one at a time, based on their transition probabilities. The transition probabilities that govern each individual transition during each cycle are realized as a random event through computer-generated random numbers between 0 and 1. We will return to the mechanics of this random process shortly.

If a model involves an absorbing state, such as dead, then each patient is run through the process until he or she reaches that state. If the model does not have an absorbing state, then the simulation is run a predetermined number of cycles. The process is repeated for many patients (e.g., 100 000). The appropriate number of simulated patients depends on the magnitudes of the transition probabilities in the model (smaller probabilities of uncommon events necessitate more simulations), and on the size of the difference between intervention strategies that we are expecting to find. It is not uncommon for Monte Carlo simulations of Markov models to require 1 000 000 patients.

For each patient we keep track of the number of cycles spent in each state. The average times spent in each state other than dead can be summed to yield an estimate of life expectancy. Quality adjustments can be made to yield expected utilities, and expected costs for each state, and the whole process can be calculated.

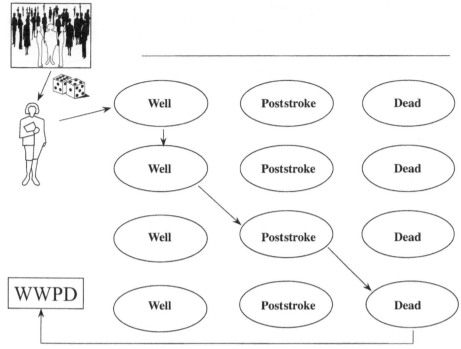

Figure 10.8　　Monte Carlo simulation for a single patient. WWPD, well, well, poststroke, dead.

Returning now to the atrial fibrillation example, Figure 10.8 depicts graphically the path of one patient from the well to the dead state. The patient remains in the well state for two cycles, moves to poststroke for one cycle and then moves to dead. This sequence of states is represented by WWPD. The dice represent the act of 'drawing probabilities' from an appropriate probability transition matrix. The technical side of performing the simulation will now be discussed.

Let us now go through a detailed example of how such a simulation is actually performed. We will use the transition probabilities of Table 10.1. To simulate each patient we need to 'simulate' the transition probabilities. This is achieved by drawing random numbers to represent the probabilities and guide transitions. Such random numbers can be found in tables of random numbers (usually found among statistical tables), but are usually generated by a computer when the simulations are run. Our example will only involve 10 patients, so it can easily be done by hand. Consider the following sequence of random numbers taken from an appropriate table:

10480 15011 01536 02011 81647 22368 46573 25595 85393 30995 24130 48360

Table 10.6. Monte Carlo simulation for 10 patients

Patient	Sequence of states	Number of cycles in W	Number of cycles in P	Number of cycles alive (W + P)	Lifetime utility
1	WWD	2	0	2	2
2	WWPD	2	1	3	2.6
3	WWWD	3	0	3	3
4	WWWD	3	0	3	3
5	WWWWWD	5	0	5	5
6	WWD	2	0	2	2
7	WWWPPPPPPPP PPPPPPPPPP PPPPPPPPD	3	26	29	18.6
8	WPPPPPPPD	1	7	8	5.2
9	WWPPPD	2	3	5	3.8
10	WWWWWW PPPPPPPP PPPD	6	11	17	12.6
	Total	29	48	77	57.8
	Mean	2.9	4.8	7.7	5.78
	Standard deviation	1.52	8.34	8.73	5.48

W, well: $U(W) = 1.0$; P, poststroke: $U(P) = 0.6$; D, dead: $U(D) = 0.0$.

Suppose that when we start a patient is in the well state. The probabilities of 0.2, 0.7, and 0.1 in Table 10.1 are simulated by referring to the first digit in the sequence of random numbers. The digits 1–7 represent the probability of 0.7 (remaining well), the digits 8 and 9 represent the probability 0.2 (transition to poststroke), and the digit 0 represents the probability 0.1 (death). For a patient in the poststroke state, the probability of 0.9 is captured by digits 1–9, and the remaining 0.1 is again captured by the digit 0. (If the probabilities were in 2-digit accuracy, we would have used pairs of random digits.) Drawing these numbers is like playing a lottery or a casino game, hence the name, *Monte Carlo simulation* (named after the famous casinos of Monte Carlo).

Table 10.6 presents the simulation results for 10 patients. Let us look at patient number 1, generated by the first two random digits above: the first digit is 1 so it represents a transition from well to well and the second digit is 0, representing transition to death. Hence the sequence WWD. The second patient is generated by subsequent digits: 4 represents transition to well, 8 to poststroke, 0 to dead, hence WWPD. Notice that patient number 2 is exactly the patient that is pictorially represented in Figure 10.8. Every time the sequence of digits reaches the digit 0, this indicates the death of the patient simulated.

Let us now examine Table 10.6. The second column represents the simulated sequence of states. Column 3 counts the number of cycles in well, column 4 the number of cycles in poststroke, column 5 is the total number of cycles alive (the sum of columns 3 and 4), and column 6 represents the total quality adjusted cycles for each patient (where $U(\text{well}) = 1.0$ and $U(\text{poststroke}) = 0.6$, as before). The row for 'Total' represents the sum of the 10 rows and is the aggregate value for the 10 patients. Taking the average (dividing the total by 10) we obtain the row for 'Mean.' Thus, the average duration in well is 2.9 cycles, in poststroke 4.8 cycles, for a total of 7.7 cycles. The average expected utility is 5.78 quality-adjusted cycles. We could similarly add a column for costs. All measures (number of cycles, costs, and quality-adjusted cycles) can and should be discounted in cost-effectiveness analyses.

The Monte Carlo simulation yields another important quantity that cannot be obtained via a cohort simulation, namely a measure of variation around the mean. The standard deviation for each distribution can be calculated, because we have all individual values. In the cohort simulation, the patients do not move individually but rather as a whole cohort and therefore we cannot observe individual variation. The fundamental matrix solution mentioned earlier can also provide us with exact values for the standard deviation.

If the above simulation had been performed a very large number of times (e.g., 10 000), the numbers in the totals and means would be very close to the figures in Tables 10.3 and 10.4. The reason for the discrepancy is the small sample size. The first 20 random digits contain six zeros, three times their expected number (i.e., 2). Hence the first six patients live rather short lives, because of 'bad luck.' Over a large number of simulations, these events should balance out to their expected frequencies.

10.4 Markov states

10.4.1 Temporary states

In the above examples, each state had an associated utility and cost per unit of time (i.e., per cycle). There are situations where the actual event that causes a transition from state to state involves a one-time cost or temporary change in quality of life. In the atrial fibrillation example consider the

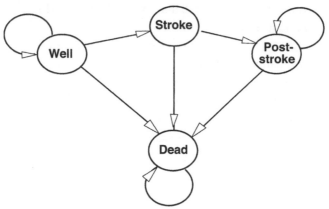

Figure 10.9　　Temporary state.

transition from well to poststroke as a result of a stroke. The stroke itself has certain morbidity and costs associated with the event: hospitalization, follow-up, recovery, etc. We cannot ignore these disutilities and costs in the utility and cost calculations.

These short-term effects can be incorporated by adding an additional state to the process, called a *temporary state*. This is depicted in Figure 10.9, where we added a state called 'stroke.' A temporary state is characterized by having transitions from it only to other states and not to itself. Thus, a patient can stay in this state for one cycle only and must move to another state for the next cycle. The presence of a temporary state enables the separate calculation of costs for that state or event and to consider the separate (usually lower) utility for the period in question. The poststroke state reflects all the years following a stroke after the patient has survived the year in which the stroke occurred. That specific year is captured in the (temporary) stroke state.

Another use of a temporary state is to be able to apply different transition probabilities following a short-term event. It is possible that the probability of dying during the months following a stroke is higher than the mortality probability a year or more after the stroke. By having stroke as a separate state, we can incorporate this temporarily different transition probability into our model.

10.4.2 Tunnel states

Recall that we said that a Markov model requires that transition probabilities may depend only on the current state, and possibly on time, but not on

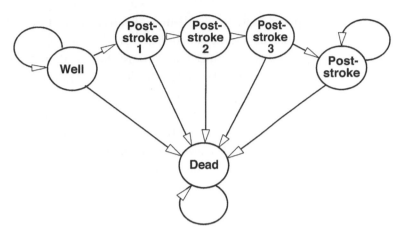

Figure 10.10   Tunnel states.

the history of prior states. This assumption has been implicit in our analysis of the atrial fibrillation example. There are situations where the history of the disease or the patient affects the transition probabilities. Fortunately, it is usually possible to modify a Markov model to incorporate this possibility.

In the atrial fibrillation example, let us assume that the annual probability of death is different in each of the first 3 years following a stroke. Starting from the fourth year, mortality remains constant. This can be handled by defining a series of temporary states, each leading into the next. This is depicted in Figure 10.10. The states poststroke 1, poststroke 2, poststroke 3 are temporary states and can only be visited in that particular sequence. This can be seen as analogous to passing through a tunnel and these states are indeed called *tunnel states*. Thus, using tunnel states is a simple 'trick' to model the impact of history on transitions. One can enter the poststroke 2 state *only* from the poststroke 1 state, etc. Note that the poststroke state is not a temporary state, as a patient can remain in this state for consecutive cycles.

10.4.3 Population heterogeneity

Another example where the addition of states can help is when we are dealing with population heterogeneity. If a patient's prognosis depends on other co-morbid conditions, then decomposing one heterogeneous state into separate states for each condition will enable us to treat each subgroup of patients separately with different transition probabilities. For example, suppose that, in a patient with atrial fibrillation, survival depends on whether or not the patient had a previous MI. Thus, the well state actually contains two distinct populations: those with and those without a prior MI. For the model to reflect the differential mortality and stroke probabilities, we must partition the well state into two separate states representing the two separate patient populations. A prior MI may also influence the poststroke patients, and this state may also require partitioning into two distinct states. Of course, the decision tree should then allow for an event MI to occur (which may require a temporary state). If we do not account for the occurrence of an MI in the model, then we can avoid the need for state partitioning by running the basic model separately on the two populations.

10.4.4 Absorbing states

The Markov models for both of our examples have a dead state. Once a patient reaches this state he or she will remain there forever. We have previously defined a state which has a transition only to itself (with probability 1.0) as an *absorbing state*, as the process is eventually totally 'absorbed' in this state. This is quite evident by the cohort simulation where all patients eventually end up in the dead state. Many chronic conditions in medicine fit such a model, and for such models the cohort simulation can be ended, for practical purposes, in a finite number of steps. These are the models usually used in published reports of decision analyses in the health and medical fields. However, there are situations where an absorbing state does not exist. If mortality is not involved we may want to follow the process for some time but may not be able to 'end' it. Models of this type are called 'nonabsorbing models.'

10.4.5 Nonabsorbing models

Consider the following example of a hypothetical skin disease which can either be acute or dormant. Let the cycle length be 1 month. The patient may bounce back and forth between the two states, as depicted in the state-transition diagram of Figure 10.11. A patient whose condition is dormant has a probability of 0.8 of remaining in that state for the next cycle and a probability of 0.2 of becoming acute. Similarly, there is a probability of 0.7 of remaining in the acute state after one cycle, and a complementary probability of 0.3 for moving into the dormant state.

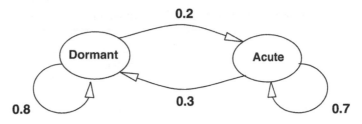

Figure 10.11 State-transition diagram for skin disease.

Let us now perform a cohort simulation of 10 000 patients. Let us assume that they all start in the dormant state. As can easily be seen in Table 10.7, after 13 cycles the number of patients in each state remains the same from cycle to cycle. From this point on, there will always be 6000 patients with a dormant condition and 4000 in an acute condition. All transitions *out* of one state are balanced by transitions *into* it. The process has reached *equilibrium*. The long-run distribution among the various states reaches a *steady state*. Let us now see what happens if all patients begin the process in the acute state. Table 10.8 presents the cohort simulation. Again, after relatively few cycles, the process reaches a steady state. Notice that we have reached the same steady state even if we started from totally extreme initial conditions. Thus, in processes that reach steady state, the initial distribution of patients is not relevant if we observe the process long enough. In some sense, absorbing models also reach an equilibrium where all patients end up in the absorbing state and stay there. Note that not all nonabsorbing models reach equilibrium. Certain conditions must be satisfied by the probability transition matrix in order to reach equilibrium. If these conditions are satisfied, we have a so-called *ergodic chain*, and the equilibrium probabilities of being in each state can be obtained by solving a series of equations that can be generated through matrix algebra. Again, this is beyond the scope of this book.

Finding the steady-state probabilities is useful in many ways. For example, if we know the percentage of time a patient will spend in each state over the lifetime, we can calculate the average quality of life or utility for that patient. The information can be very useful for planning. If different medical resources are needed for patients in different states, the steady-state probabilities can tell us how to allocate proportionately various resources for the different patient groups. We can plan ahead to the steady state and make sure that supply of resources meets demand. Almost all of the applications of Markov models in health care have been in

Table 10.7. Skin disease cohort simulation: I

	State	
Cycle	Dormant	Acute
0	10 000	0
1	8000	2000
2	7000	3000
3	6500	3500
4	6250	3750
5	6125	3875
6	6063	3938
7	6031	3969
8	6016	3984
9	6008	3992
10	6004	3996
11	6002	3998
12	6001	3999
13	6000	4000
14	6000	4000

situations with absorbing states and this will continue to be the focus of this chapter.

10.5 From decision trees to Markov nodes: the Markov cycle tree

We started this chapter by looking at why Markov models are needed. These are situations where the time horizon in a decision problem may not be fixed and events can occur repeatedly over time. Markov models were then presented along with methods to solve them and calculate various measures that could be used in a decision analysis. It is now time to see how the basic decision tree can be combined with Markov models to help us solve the problem without having to deal with messy and unmanageable trees, like the recursive tree in Figure 10.2, especially if we want to extend it beyond three cycles.

In the presentation of calculating Markov models we treated the transition probabilities as known entities that enabled transitions from state to state. We will elaborate on obtaining some of these probabilities later in this chapter. However, for an actual clinical setting, the transition from state to state may involve different paths. In our atrial fibrillation example, a transition from well to dead may occur in several ways: the patient may

Table 10.8. Skin disease cohort simulation: II

Cycle	State	
	Dormant	Acute
0	0	10 000
1	3000	7000
2	4500	5500
3	6500	3500
4	5250	4750
5	5813	4188
6	5906	4094
7	5953	4047
8	5977	4023
9	5988	4012
10	5994	4006
11	5997	4003
12	5999	4001
13	5999	4001
14	6000	4000

die from a fatal bleed, a fatal embolus, or she may die from unrelated causes such as an accident or another disease such as cancer (known as age–sex–race (ASR)-related mortality). Similarly, the transition from well to poststroke can be via a nonfatal bleed or nonfatal embolus. Figure 10.12 presents a probability tree depicting the possible paths from well in one cycle. All causes of death except from a bleed or embolus have been combined into one branch: 'die of other causes.' There will be a similar tree representing the possible transitions from the poststroke state. There is basically no tree for the dead state as no transitions are possible to other states. Hence, there is a possible subtree for modeling the one-cycle transitions from each state. These subtrees can be grafted on to one special node, referred to as a *Markov node*. There is one branch emanating from this node for every possible Markov state. This node, along with the (different) probability trees emanating from it, is called a *Markov cycle tree*. An example of a Markov cycle tree for the atrial fibrillation example is presented in Figure 10.13. Cycle trees enable the decomposition of a complex uncertain situation into smaller, more manageable problems. It lends itself to available data for the various events, whereas data needed for the composite transition probabilities may be very difficult to obtain.

Cycle trees may be evaluated by methods similar to a Markov cohort

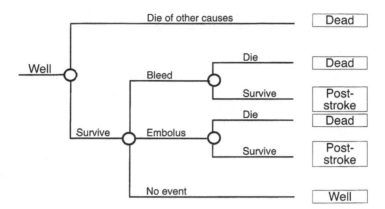

Figure 10.12   Probability tree for well state.

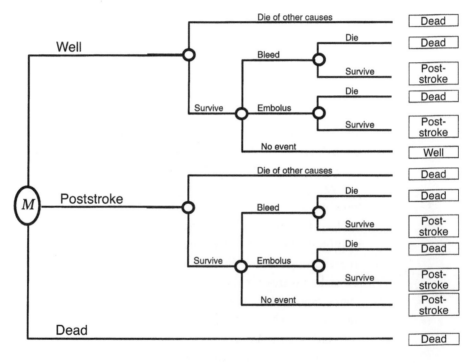

Figure 10.13   Markov cycle tree. *M*, Markov node.

simulation. One only needs the distribution of the initial cohort among the
various states. (In our cohort simulation we assumed all patients started
out in the well state.) The cohort is then partitioned among the states
according to the probabilities of each subtree and traced through the
subtree, yielding a new distribution of the cohort among the states. This

will be the starting distribution for the next cycle. For each cycle we can calculate the cycle sum of utilities, costs, etc. These will be accumulated over all cycles until termination of the process (when nearly the entire cohort is in the dead state). The main difference between this process and the previously described cohort simulation is that it is done on a cohort of a single patient. The breakdown into the states is not by the *number* of patients but rather by the *fraction* of patients. (The cohort simulation could also be done fractionally, but the way it was presented in this chapter is more intuitive and reflects a cohort.)

Once the cycle trees have been determined, there may be a different cycle tree for each branch of the initial decision node. The decision problem can then be represented as the tree in Figure 10.14. The various Markov cycle trees can differ in structure, depth, and in the various probabilities. They can even have different states. However, if this is the case, then the utility structure for the whole problem has to encompass all states across all models. Otherwise, the comparison of expected utilities is meaningless. Most decision analysis software packages include provisions for Markov models in general and Markov cycle trees in particular.

10.6 Estimating transition probabilities*

In the above examples we have used probabilities to describe transitions from state to state. The required probabilities are sometimes directly available from the literature, possibly by means of a probability tree like the one in Figure 10.12. This is true both for constant and time-dependent transition probabilities. If probabilities do depend on time, such as when annual ASR-specific mortality increases with the age of the cohort, and if we know these probabilities, then we can easily incorporate them in the cohort analysis.

Very frequently we have only limited probability data and we have to manipulate them to be able to generate estimates of the various transition probabilities. This requires the introduction of *rates*. We have seen that a probability describes the likelihood that an event will occur in a given time period and its value ranges from 0 to 1. A *rate* describes the number of occurrences of an event per given number of patients per unit of time. For example, data have shown that over 3 years, 60 out of 200 patients have died. The death rate is then 60 per 200 per 3 years, or 20 deaths per 200

---

* This is advanced material and can be skipped without loss of continuity.

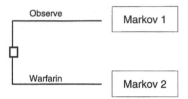

Observe — Markov 1

Warfarin — Markov 2

Figure 10.14   Markov decision tree for atrial fibrillation.

patients per year, or 0.1 deaths per patient per year. Rates range from zero to infinity. A convenient mathematical property of rates, which is not true of probabilities, is that we can add and subtract rates (for the same time interval) and we can divide and multiply a given rate by a factor reflecting risk factors. We can also divide rates by time or by the number of patients, as in the example above. We cannot do these things to probabilities unless they are very small, in which case they behave much like rates. For example, suppose we wanted to reflect the fact that a particular risk group had 10 times the risk of developing a disease as the general population. If the baseline probability in the general population reached more than 10% at some age, we would end up with a probability greater than 100%!

Occasionally, data in the literature will be available as rates and we will need to convert rates into probabilities. If an event occurs at a constant rate r per time unit t, then the probability that an event will occur during time t is given by the equation:

$$P = 1 - e^{-rt} \tag{10.1}$$

This relates nicely to the survival curve, like the one shown in Figure 10.6 (if we label the vertical axis as probability rather than proportion). At any given time point (cycle), the height of the curve is e^{-rt}, which represents the probability of survival to time t. The complement, $1 - e^{-rt}$, is the probability of dying before time t, as described above. On the other hand, if we have a probability and want to convert it to a rate, we use the equation:

$$r = -\frac{1}{t}\ln(1 - P) \tag{10.2}$$

The reason we may wish to convert probabilities to rates is to exploit the additive properties of rates. For example, let the cycle be 1 year ($t = 1$). Suppose we have a constant annual disease-specific mortality probability, $P_D = 0.2$, and that we have mortality rates for the population by age (the 'A' of ASR). We then calculate the disease-specific mortality rate, r_D, using

Equation 10.2. In this case $r_D = -\ln(1 - 0.2) = 0.223$. Let the age-specific annual mortality rate be 0.1, as before. Now we have two mortality forces: age-specific and disease-specific. We can add the two rates to obtain the total mortality rate of $r_D + r_A = 0.323$ and then convert this rate to a total mortality probability using Equation 10.1. This yields $P = 0.276$. This probability can now be used in the appropriate place in a Markov model or decision tree.

A word of caution: when changing the cycle length in an analysis, transition probabilities must be adjusted. If we consider moving from a cycle of 1 year to a monthly cycle, the probabilities *should not* be divided by 12! We have to convert the annual probability to an annual rate using Equation 10.2, divide the annual rate by 12 to obtain the monthly rate, and then convert the monthly rate to a monthly probability by using Equation 10.1. From a practical programming perspective it is useful to be able to vary cycle length without having to adjust all sorts of variables in the model. This can be facilitated by expressing all rates per person year and expressing cycle length in units of years.

10.7 Cohort vs. Monte Carlo simulation: which should I use?

One advantage of the Monte Carlo method, compared to cohort simulation, is that it also yields estimates for the entire frequency distribution of survival values for each state. These enable the estimation of variation around the expected values. However, this is not the most important advantage, nor the one that usually leads analysts to use a Monte Carlo simulation.

The most important reason to use a Monte Carlo simulation arises out of the need to retain variables that determine transition probabilities. Among such variables are aspects of patient history. In such situations, we would like to sidestep the Markov assumption that transition probabilities depend only on the current state. Such variables may include fixed characteristics, such as age, sex, and genetic risk factors. These fixed predictor variables could be accommodated by running the analysis with separate sets of transition probabilities for each relevant subpopulation, and then reaggregating, but it might be more efficient to do a single simulation in which the population characteristics are drawn from a distribution.

More problematic are situations where the variables that influence transition probabilities are characteristics of the prior history, such as previous occurrence of disease, response to treatment, and others. In other words, we may want the transition probabilities in a given cycle to depend on the states experienced in previous cycles. We have seen that devices such as tunnel states can be used to accommodate some such features of case histories in cohort analyses, but each such device adds to the number of states. Imagine a situation in which future transition probabilities depend on the *order* in which clinical events have been experienced, or on other complex functions of past history such as the time between events. The number of states we would have to add to shoehorn such a model into the Markovian template could fill the memories of many desktop computers *c.* 2001. So we use Monte Carlo simulation, which enables us to define transition probabilities as functions of as many variables as we have data on. Such variables, when used in the simulation of an individual patient in a Monte Carlo simulation, are called *tracker variables*. The advantage of Monte Carlo simulation is that we need only retain tracker variables in memory during the simulation of one individual at a time. For each new patient, the tracker variables are 'reset,' and we begin a new simulation.

Using Monte Carlo simulation to model variability in each individual patient's disease history and to model uncertainty in the results is discussed further in Chapter 11.

10.8 Sensitivity analysis

It is inconceivable to address any modeling topic without emphasizing the importance of sensitivity analysis. This definitely holds true for Markov models. After we have obtained various measures, with or without using the models in a decision analysis, we must perform sensitivity analyses on the various parameters used. These include the determination of cycle length, the estimation of transition probabilities among states, estimation of probabilities for cycle trees, and the various costs and utilities for the different states. Even the consideration of adding temporary states or tunnel states can be included in sensitivity analysis. The nature of such analyses is not different from that which has been extensively discussed earlier in the book and will be discussed further in Chapter 11.

10.9 Summary

Markov models provide a framework to model recurring events and to extend models to encompass the lifetime of a patient. These models are useful when a decision problem involves risk over time, when the timing of events is important, and when events may happen more than once. In a Markov model uncertain events are modeled as transitions during defined time intervals (cycles) between defined health states (Markov states). Essential to a Markov model is the Markovian property of 'lack of memory' conditional on the health state: the events subsequent to any cycle depend only on the Markov state of that cycle and not on the history prior to that cycle. In a Markov chain the transition probabilities are constant over time. In a Markov process the transition probabilities may change over time.

Markov process models can be evaluated with a cohort simulation or a Monte Carlo simulation. A Markov cohort simulation considers a hypothetical cohort of patients who are distributed among the possible states and followed over time as they transition among the states from one cycle to the next. The model keeps track of what proportion of the cohort was in which state over time. In a Monte Carlo simulation individual patients are simulated going through various transitions from one cycle to the next and the model keeps track of the number of cycles spent in each state per patient.

Markov models can be used to estimate (partitioned) survival curves, (quality-adjusted) life expectancy (lifetime) costs, and any other cumulative outcome. Heterogeneity of the population can be modeled by increasing the number of states, using temporary states or tunnel states, or by Monte Carlo simulation, in which history is modeled with tracker variables.

Exercises

Exercise 10.1

For a decision analysis you need the 1-year probability of getting diabetes mellitus. In one article you found that the 5-year probability for noninsulin-dependent diabetes mellitus was 0.030. In another article you found that the 4-year probability for insulin-dependent diabetes mellitus was 0.008. Calculate the 1-year probability of getting diabetes.

Exercise 10.2

Breast cancer prevention

There are two new (hypothetical) drugs for women who are at high risk of breast cancer (i.e., women who have a 10-year cumulative incidence of 15%). One of the drugs (PrevCa) has been shown to reduce the risk of breast cancer. However, because of the side-effects associated with PrevCa, 5% of women stop taking this medication each year (and remain off the medication). If women taking PrevCa get breast cancer, they have the same prognosis as those women not taking the drug (i.e., they have a 5-year survival probability of 70%, or 70% are free from any cause of death at 5 years). The other new drug, NewProg, does not reduce the risk of breast cancer, but improves the prognosis of breast cancer if it occurs. Specifically, NewProg reduces the breast cancer-specific mortality rate by 50%. Both drugs must be started before the diagnosis of breast cancer.

A placebo-controlled randomized trial of PrevCa was done in a cohort of women at very high risk of breast cancer. PrevCa was found to increase 10-year disease-free survival (i.e., free of breast cancer and death) from 55% to 65%.

Of the high-risk women who are eligible for treatment with either PrevCa or NewProg, 5% of them will not start any medication because of an aversion to taking pills. For women who elect to take medication, PrevCa is associated with a utility of 0.95 and NewProg is associated with a utility of 0.99. Breast cancer has a utility of 0.8.

(a) For simplicity, assume that the annual probability of death from other causes is constant (i.e., the exponential survival assumption). Assuming that the remaining life expectancy for a similar cohort in the general population is 35 years, what is the annual probability of background mortality?

(b) Assume that the rate of breast cancer is constant over time. For each arm of the clinical trial (PrevCa and placebo), calculate the annual transition probability from no cancer to breast cancer. What is the percent reduction in the rate of breast cancer associated with PrevCa?

(c) Specify the health states and transition probabilities for Markov models that can be used to estimate the health effects associated with PrevCa and NewProg. Assume all probabilities are constant. You may present your answer using a transition probability matrix form or a tree format.

(d) Perform a cohort simulation with your models to estimate the life expectancy and quality-adjusted life expectancy for women who are at high risk for breast cancer and are: (1) treated with PrevCa, and (2) treated with NewProg. Ignore discounting.

(e) What is the expected amount of time spent with breast cancer for each treatment scenario?

Exercise 10.3

Markov madness

Markov madness is a rare disease that afflicts all students of decision analysis who have spent more than 10 h analyzing fictitious health-care scenarios using iterative mathematical models. Fortunately, the majority of afflicted individuals are initially asymptomatic, although 20% immediately exhibit mild confusion and circular reasoning (CR). For persons who are asymptomatic, the annual probability of developing CR is 0.40. During any given year (i.e., within a cycle), if an asymptomatic individual develops CR, there is a 45% chance of becoming asymptomatic again after a very brief and inconsequential episode, a 35% chance of continued CR, a 15% chance of developing complete Markovian psychosis (MP), and a 5% chance of dying of causes other than Markov madness. Asymptomatic persons who do not develop CR remain asymptomatic. For a person who currently exhibits CR, the annual probability of becoming asymptomatic is 0.20, of continued CR is 0.45, of progressing to MP is 0.25, of dying of other causes is 0.05, and of dying of the disease is 0.05. Persons who develop MP can never again become asymptomatic or exhibit CR; their annual probability of dying of other causes is 0.05, and their annual probability of dying of their disease is 0.10.

Assume that transition probabilities are constant from year to year (including mortality probabilities).

(a) Write down the transition matrix for this Markov model, and show your tree.

(b) How many years must pass before fewer than 50% of individuals are asymptomatic?

(c) What is the life expectancy of afflicted individuals?

(d) How many years, on average, do afflicted individuals spend with CR?

(e) Using a discount rate of 3% per year, what is the discounted life expectancy?

(f) What is the probability of dying of Markov madness, as opposed to other causes, over the entire lifetime of an afflicted individual?

(g) Suppose that the probability that an asymptomatic person will remain asymptomatic during a year increases the longer the person has been continuously asymptomatic, up to a maximum of 3 years. Suppose that this probability is 0.6 in the first year, 0.75 in the second year, and 0.9 thereafter. Assume that all other probabilities are unchanged. Develop a revised Markov model to account for this new information, and write down the transition matrix.

(h) Calculate the discounted (using an annual discount rate of 3%) quality-adjusted life expectancy for the model, as modified by the additional assumptions in part (g). Assign quality weights of 0.95 for asymptomatic individuals, 0.8 for CR, and 0.4 for MP.

REFERENCES

Beck, J.R. & Pauker, S.G. (1983). The Markov process in medical prognosis. *Med. Decis. Making*, **3**, 419–58.

Kemeny, J.B. & Snell, J.L. (1976). *Finite Markov Chains*. New York: Springer Verlag.

Sonnenberg, F.A. & Beck, J.R. (1993). Markov models in medical decision making: a practical guide. *Med. Decis. Making*, **13**, 322–38.

11

Variability and uncertainty

Medicine is a science of uncertainty and an art of probability.

Sir William Osler

11.1 Introduction

Decision trees and Markov cohort models, as described and illustrated in the previous chapters, are essentially macrosimulation models. Such models simulate cohorts or groups of subjects. A number of limitations exist to the use of these models. Markov cohort models, for example, have 'no memory,' implying that subjects in a particular state are a homogeneous group without variability. Techniques to overcome these limitations, such as expanding the number of states and using tunnel states, were discussed in Chapter 10. These techniques can get very complex when dealing with extensive variability within a population. Microsimulation using Monte Carlo analysis provides another powerful technique to account for variability across subjects. Microsimulation with Monte Carlo analysis was introduced in Chapter 10 as an alternative method for evaluating a Markov model. In this chapter it will be discussed at greater length in the context of simulating variability.

In the previous chapters we represented uncertainty with probabilities. Implicitly the assumption was that, even though we were unsure of whether an event would take place, we could nevertheless predict or estimate the probability (or relative frequency) it would occur. In essence we were using deterministic models. In reality, however, we are also uncertain of the degree of uncertainty. In other words, rather than dealing with a fixed probability we are actually dealing with a distribution of probabilities. Not only are we uncertain about the probabilities we use in our models, we are also uncertain about the effectiveness outcomes and cost estimates included in the analysis. Thus, every variable value we enter into our models is better represented as a probabilistic (stochastic) variable rather than a deterministic variable. If there is a single uncertain variable, e.g., the relative risk reduction of an intervention, then the 95% confidence interval (CI) of this variable is commonly used to indicate the uncertainty of the effect. Uncertainty in two or more components requires more complex methods, such as Monte Carlo probabilistic sensitivity analysis, which we will discuss in this chapter.

Exploration of the influence of variability and uncertainties in the model is performed with sensitivity analysis. Two fundamentally different reasons exist for doing sensitivity analysis. Variability across subgroups requires that the analyst performs a calculation for each identifiable subgroup to evaluate whether the decision might change depending on the characteristics of the subject/subgroup. Unidentifiable variability and uncertainty require some estimate of the uncertainty of the overall outcome measure of the model.

The immediate goal of analyzing variability and uncertainty is to obtain an interval (or region) of the outcome measure of the model that, with some probability, contains the true value. The ultimate goal is to decide whether the results are adequate for decision making or whether obtaining more information through further research is necessary (Claxton, 1999). This is analogous to questioning whether another diagnostic test is necessary in the clinical setting of diagnosing a disease. Two approaches are possible: that of the frequentist versus that of the Bayesian. The frequentist approach focuses on the probability of the observed data given the hypothesis (P(data | hypothesis)). This approach provides a CI as a function of the data. The Bayesian approach focuses on the probability of the hypothesis given the observed data (P(hypothesis | data)). This approach provides a credible interval as a function of the data combined with everything known prior to the data collection (Manning et al., 1996). In the analogy with diagnostic testing, the frequentist approach focuses on sensitivity and specificity, whereas the Bayesian approach focuses on predictive probabilities.

Many confusing terms and concepts have been used in the analysis of variability and uncertainty. The purpose of this chapter is to clarify the various types of variability and uncertainty and to explain the techniques to analyze them. The focus will be on Monte Carlo methods and our approach is in essence Bayesian. Hopefully this chapter will provide a framework for thinking and communicating about variability and uncertainty. Keep in mind that, even though we attempt to categorize variability and uncertainty, ours is only one perspective and there are many other perspectives. This chapter covers advanced material and as such we would not recommend it as obligatory for a first introduction to decision modeling.

11.2 Types of variability and uncertainty

11.2.1 Variability across subgroups

Variability across subjects, or subgroups of subjects, is known to exist, e.g., varying age, sex, risk factors, and prior events. Although heterogeneity exists, the characteristics are identifiable. Subgroups can be identified based on the subjects' characteristics and these subgroups are relatively homogeneous. In such cases, the analyst needs to explore the implications of this variability (Table 11.1). Variability across subgroups is the type of variability that is typically of concern to clinicians and to the developers of clinical guidelines. For example, when analyzing the optimal imaging workup for suspected coronary artery disease one will want to tailor the decision depending on age, sex, and type and severity of chest pain (Kuntz et al., 1999).

11.2.2 Variability in a population

The public health policy maker will typically want to take decisions for a subpopulation or the population as a whole. In these situations, heterogeneity across subjects may exist, such as varying risk factors and prior events. The ensuing disease history and prognosis may vary as a result of these varying characteristics. If we want to make policy decisions for the whole group, we would need to model the variability in the population at large (Table 11.1). Note that the policy decision does not need to be a uniform management decision for every subject (e.g., prescribe antilipids) but can be tailored (e.g., prescribe antilipids for subjects with an elevated cholesterol who also have at least one other cardiovascular risk factor).

Examples of models that take variability in a population into account and model policy decisions include the Coronary Heart Disease Policy model, the Microsimulation of Screening for Cancer (MISCAN) model, and the PORT Stroke model (Habbema et al., 1984, 1987; van Oortmarssen et al., 1995; Hunink et al., 1997; Samsa et al., 1999).

11.2.3 Stochastic uncertainty

Stochastic uncertainty, or first-order uncertainty, is the uncertainty related to the possible events that may occur over the course of time and is the uncertainty about the actual realized outcome of a strategy for a sample of patients (Table 11.1). In the setting of a trial, stochastic uncertainty is the

Table 11.1. Types of variability and uncertainty in decision models and the corresponding simulation techniques to analyze them

Type	Explanation	Simulation technique	Output
Variability across subgroups	Known heterogeneity across subgroups, e.g., varying age, sex, risk factors, prior events; each subgroup is homogeneous	Sensitivity analyses to predict results for subgroups with identifiable characteristics	Sensitivity graphs for subgroups with identifiable characteristics
Variability in a population	Heterogeneity across subjects in a population, e.g., varying age, sex, risk factors, prior events; decision needs to be made for the population as a whole	Markov cohort analysis with varying initial states or Monte Carlo microsimulation or microsimulation of discrete events, of the study population of size P with heterogeneous subjects	Mean outcome for the study population aggregated across P individuals
Stochastic uncertainty	Uncertainty related to the actual events and outcome for one study population (or one individual if $P = 1$)	Monte Carlo microsimulation of multiple ($n = 1 \ldots N$) cloned (or bootstrapped) copies of the study population of size P	Mean of mean outcomes and standard deviation across N study populations of size P
Parameter uncertainty: fixed effects/random effects	Measurement error of the variable values due to (1) limited sample size of studies but fixed underlying true value (fixed-effects model) or (2) due to limited sample size of studies and heterogeneity of the underlying true value across study populations	Probabilistic sensitivity analysis: Monte Carlo simulation with $s = 1$ $\ldots S$ iterations with each iteration s using one random value from each of the distributions of the variables. Alternative: delta method Estimation of distribution of variable values uses fixed effects or random-effects meta-analysis, as considered appropriate	Mean and standard deviation of S means, each mean derived from N study populations of size P
Model structure uncertainty	Uncertainty with respect to the modeling assumptions	Sensitivity analysis by using different modeling assumptions Weighted combination of alternatives	Yields alternative results or a pooled weighted result

uncertainty associated with the limited sample size. In the setting of prescriptive decision making using models, stochastic uncertainty represents the uncertainty related to the expected outcome in the future. The smaller the sample of subjects for which the decision needs to be made, the larger the uncertainty about the actual realized outcomes. From the public policy maker's perspective, stochastic uncertainty is irrelevant in making decisions for a large population, as would be the case for decisions impacting an entire country. From a hospital administrator's perspective, however, stochastic uncertainty may be very relevant if he/she is concerned about the possibility of a very bad outcome among the small patient group for which the decision is being made.

11.2.4 Parameter (variable value) uncertainty

Rather than dealing with a fixed probability, we usually need to deal with a distribution of probabilities. Similarly, the utility and cost inputs are generally better represented as a probabilistic (stochastic) variable rather than a deterministic variable. This uncertainty is sometimes referred to as second-order uncertainty (Doubilet et al., 1985; Table 11.1).

Sometimes the uncertainty in the variable value (parameter) is thought to arise solely from measurement due to limited sample size of the studies while some fixed underlying true value is assumed to exist. These situations are also referred to as Type B uncertainty in the risk analysis literature (Hoffman and Hammonds, 1994) or fixed effects in the meta-analytical literature. When the measurement error of the variable value (parameter) is due to both limited sample size of studies and due to heterogeneity across study populations, the risk analysis literature speaks of Type A uncertainty (Hoffman and Hammonds, 1994) and the meta-analytical literature of random-effects models (DerSimonian and Laird, 1986).

11.2.5 Model structure uncertainty

Modeling structure uncertainty stems from uncertainty in the model structure and the modeling process. For example, one may question whether a multiplicative versus additive mortality function is the most appropriate (Kuntz and Weinstein, 1995). Not knowing the exact form of the underlying mathematical model may lead to uncertainty. This is uncertainty associated with the assumptions that are made regarding how the model should work (Table 11.1).

Some authors distinguish yet another type of uncertainty, that is, modeling process uncertainty (Brown and Fintor, 1993). This is the overall uncertainty due to the modeling decisions made by the analysts but is actually the aggregation of all the above-mentioned types of uncertainty.

11.3 Analyzing variability and uncertainty

11.3.1 Sensitivity analysis: one-way, two-way, n-way

Sensitivity analysis is used to predict results for subgroups with identifiable characteristics. Sensitivity analysis is generally performed on plausible ranges of the variable values (parameters) using, for example, the 95% CI or some other justifiable range. Univariable (one-way) sensitivity analysis is the best way to check the model and start exploring the robustness of the results of the analysis. Multivariable (two-way, n-way) sensitivity analyses are essential to explore further the robustness of the results. Because many variables generally contain uncertainty, the n-way sensitivity analysis can get out-of-hand and unmanageable. Best-case and worst-case scenarios, in which extreme variable values are chosen first biasing towards and subsequently biasing against the program under consideration, are useful methods to explore the extremes of n-way sensitivity analysis but may lead to conflicting decisions. Conventional univariable and multivariable sensitivity analysis is limited by the subjectivity of the choice of variables to analyze, the chosen range of values considered plausible and meaningful, and the decision as to what constitutes a significant difference in results.

11.3.2 Markov cohort analysis with varying initial states

Modeling variability across individuals in a population may be performed by constructing a (virtual) cohort of subjects representative of the population under consideration. Thus, instead of starting out with, for example, 10 000 cloned copies of one subject or patient, we now divide the 10 000 subjects into subgroups depending on their characteristics such as risk factors and past events. Each subgroup is modeled by letting them start out in the appropriate corresponding health state in the Markov model. As the model progresses over time, the subgroups will go through the corresponding ensuing disease history. Markov cohort analyses with varying initial states can take into account that management decisions may differ depending on risk factors and past history by explicitly modeling the decision conditional on the health state.

An example of a model that uses this approach is the Coronary Heart Disease Policy model which has 540 initial states defined by age, sex, blood pressure, smoking status, lipid levels, and body weight (Hunink et al., 1997). The incidence of coronary heart disease in the model depends on the risk factors and may be different for each subgroup.

A Markov cohort analysis with varying initial states within the population provides a good method to study population variability. These techniques can, however, get very complex when dealing with extensive variability within a population. Microsimulation, using either Monte Carlo analysis or directly with equations, provides an alternative powerful technique to account for variability across subjects.

11.3.3 Monte Carlo microsimulation of variability in a population

A very flexible approach to modeling variability within a population is Monte Carlo microsimulation of a Markov model. The basic underlying principle of Monte Carlo microsimulation is to simulate 'mother nature.' A Monte Carlo microsimulation model flags subjects in order to track their characteristics and individual disease histories. In a practical sense this can be done with tracker variables. Tracker variables can be used to model the initial distribution of age, sex, risk factors, and prior events and are subsequently adjusted as the subjects' age, their risk factor status changes, and events occur during the ensuing disease history. The model tracks individual subjects until some stopping criterion – in most models the patient's death. The tracker variables are used to determine each subject's next set of probabilities of events, the utility for the health state he or she is in, and the corresponding costs associated with that health state.

For example, Figure 11.1 shows a straightforward three-state Markov cohort model with the health states well, sick, and dead. The sick state has been modeled explicitly because it is associated with a lower utility than the well state. Furthermore, once a patient has had an event the model assumes he or she either stays in the sick state or dies. This same simple Markov model can be modeled using only two health states, namely alive and dead, and using a tracker variable for the sick state (Figure 11.2). To accomplish this we can, for example, add a tracker variable to the branch 'event' that counts the number of events that take place over the course of time. If a patient has a first event, the tracker variable changes from a value of zero to a value of one. During the next cycle the subject is known to be sick – he/she is still in the alive state but is now flagged as being sick using the

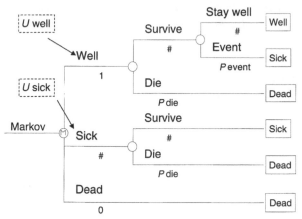

Figure 11.1   Markov model with three states: well, sick, and dead. *U*, utility; *P*, probability.

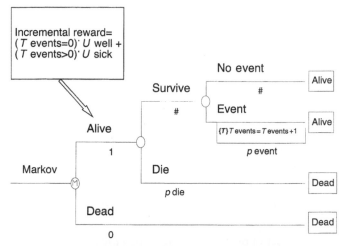

Figure 11.2   The same Markov model as in Figure 11.1, but now using microsimulation with the tracker variable *T* events to model the sick state.

tracker variable, *T* events, which is now larger than zero. The tracker variable is used in all ensuing cycles to adjust the incremental reward by incorporating the appropriate utility, namely that for being sick rather than the utility for well. If during an ensuing cycle another event occurs, the tracker variable increases by 1, but, in this particular example, the incremental reward stays the same, namely that associated with being sick.

In a Monte Carlo microsimulation subjects representative of the population for which the decision needs to be made are followed individually through the model (Figure 11.3). Once you have decided to use tracker variables to flag patients, the calculations need to be done by simulating each individual subject because a conventional cohort analysis cannot, by

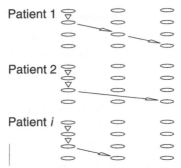

Figure 11.3   The concept of first-order Monte Carlo microsimulation: individual disease histories are simulated one by one.

definition, keep track of the individual disease histories. Depending on what outputs are required, the model may need to keep a record of how many patients were in particular health states over time, the number of specified events per patient, and the accumulated units of effectiveness and costs per patient.

Although this particular example may seem trivial, when modeling multiple risk factors and events the use of tracker variables can be very powerful. In theory one could model everything with tracker variables and only have, for example, the states alive and dead. In practice, a compromise between health states and tracker variables is advisable. Some logical distinction can sometimes be helpful. For example, one could model the underlying disease progression using tracker variables and the events as states. Or one could choose to model the risk factors and naturally occurring events as tracker variables and therapeutic procedures as states.

Monte Carlo microsimulation techniques can be used to model any type of variability or disease history, either initial or over the course of time. This includes modeling, for example, the initial distribution of risk factors for cardiovascular disease (age, sex, blood pressure, smoking status, and lipid levels), past events such as myocardial infarctions and stroke, tumor growth such as the growth of liver metastases, the progression of atherosclerotic disease such as in carotid artery stenosis, and the epidemiology and progression of infectious diseases such as human immunodeficiency virus (HIV: Goldie et al., 2000).

11.3.4 Microsimulation using discrete-event simulation

Microsimulation can also be performed using discrete-event simulation. Discrete-event simulation is a technique developed in industrial engineering to model chains of discrete stochastic events and to model competition for the available resources (Law and Kelton, 2000). Sets of equations can be used to model directly the demographic characteristics and risk factors of the subjects. The life history of each subject is simulated and the development of disease, symptoms, and disease progression can be modeled with equations that track the time to the next event. Instead of dividing time into intervals during which events may or may not occur, as happens in a Markov model, in discrete-event simulation the time to the next event is estimated based on the probability distribution of that event. The variables are then updated to the point in time at which that next event occurs. Such simulations are performed for a large number of subjects creating a file of simulated life histories which can be considered analogous to a population registry. In discrete-event simulation entities (e.g., patients) may interact and compete for resources. Queues and delay times in a queue can also be modeled.

The equations are programmed in a computer simulation which directly simulates the individual life histories by aging the individual, modeling disease progression, and updating the disease status with the incidence and events that have occurred. Similar to Monte Carlo Markov simulation, events are simulated by random draws from distributions describing the probability of an event. As subjects move through the model their expected survival time may change, for example, as a result of detection in a hypothetical screening program that is being analyzed. Events and the use of resources are tracked using equations that include time as a variable. The outputs of the model can be anything that is of interest to predict: survival curves, life expectancy, resource utilization, costs, waiting times, queue length, etc.

Ideally, one would want to verify and validate the model with some real data before modeling interventions. Once the model simulates the current situation realistically, various scenarios and interventions can be evaluated.

Microsimulation using discrete-event simulation has been used extensively to model health programs for screening of cancer (Habbema et al., 1984, 1987; van Oortmarssen et al., 1995). It is also very useful for modeling the potential effects of policy changes or management decisions, such as the effect of buying an additional computed tomography scanner or opening another catheterization laboratory. Discrete-event simulation can even be used to model a pathophysiological system.

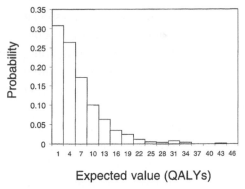

Expected value (QALYs)

Figure 11.4   Probability distribution of the expected value in quality-adjusted life years (QALYs) for 1000 patients.

11.3.5 Monte Carlo simulation of stochastic uncertainty

Performing a Monte Carlo microsimulation of each individual subject in a population has an additional advantage in that it provides us with an estimate of the variance across subjects that is due to pure chance, or stochastic uncertainty (first-order uncertainty). Monte Carlo analysis was discussed previously as a method of analyzing Markov models in Chapter 10. Because we simulate individual subjects, we get a distribution of the possible outcomes across subjects and with that some measure of the degree of uncertainty of the outcome. For example, the simple model presented in Figure 11.2 was run for 1000 patients with an annual rate of dying of 0.1, an annual rate of an event of 0.2, an utility of well of 1.0, and an utility of sick of 0.5. The patients were identical at the outset but they all developed their own disease history as they went through the model. This yielded the distribution of expected value results presented graphically in Figure 11.4. Analysis of these results yielded a mean expected value for this simulation of 6.67 quality-adjusted life years (QALYs), which is also the result of the model from Figure 11.1, with a standard deviation of 5.65 and a 90% CI of 0.6–16.8. Additional outputs can also be calculated with a simulation model such as the mean number of events per subject, which was 1.7 for this run.

A Monte Carlo simulation of stochastic uncertainty should be distinguished from a Monte Carlo microsimulation of variability in a population. The type of decision to be made dictates the type of analysis required. If we are concerned about the decision for one type of individual, we could think of this as a population of size $P = 1$. Performing N simulations of this patient, i.e., analyzing the results for N cloned copies of this patient, will yield measures of stochastic uncertainty associated with the potential outcomes for this subject and other identical subjects. If we are interested in analyzing the stochastic uncertainty of the outcomes for a population taking into account the variability across individuals in the population, we would need to perform N simulations of the population of size P incorporating the variability across the subjects P. This is equivalent to simulating N cloned copies of the study population of size P with its variability and yields N possible aggregate outcomes. The mean and variance across the N aggregate outcomes give us some indication of the uncertainty associated with the outcome and may be of interest to the decision maker. If you want to simulate the results of a clinical trial or clinical cohort and you have data from a representative sample that would be eligible for the trial, then you could use N bootstrap copies of that sample.

Conceptually, Monte Carlo simulation of stochastic uncertainty is analogous to bootstrapping a dataset. The bootstrap technique is a nonparametric method used to draw inferences from a dataset (Efron and Tibshirani, 1993). A bootstrap sample is a random sample, drawn with replacement, from the dataset and equivalent in size. Patients may be represented a number of times in each bootstrap sample. Conceptually a bootstrap sample replicates the drawing of the original sample from the underlying population. The statistic of interest is calculated in every bootstrap sample and the distribution of the statistic across the entire set of bootstrap samples (e.g., $N = 1000$) provides a nonparametric estimate of the stochastic uncertainty of the statistic.

11.3.6 Monte Carlo probabilistic sensitivity analysis

A robust numerical technique to analyze the uncertainty of the variable values in a model is probabilistic sensitivity analysis using Monte Carlo simulation. Monte Carlo simulation to analyze uncertainty may be used for any model, whether it be a decision tree, a Markov model, a regression equation, a model of genetic inheritance, or an astrophysical model of the universe. The basic underlying idea is illustrated in Figure 11.5. Uncertainty of all input variables is modeled with probability distributions of their values. For each run of the model a value of each input variable is picked at random from its distribution. So for the first simulation run of the model we pick at random a value from the distribution of the variable x_1, a value from the distribution of the variable x_2, a value from the distribution of the variable x_3, etc. We run the model with these values and get one set of

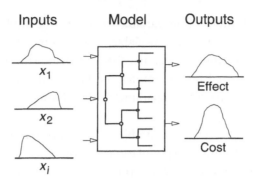

Inputs   Model   Outputs

Effect

Cost

Figure 11.5   The concept of second-order Monte Carlo probabilistic sensitivity analysis.

outputs from the model, for example, one effectiveness outcome value and one cost outcome value. A large number of iterations, $s = 1 \ldots S$ with S, for example, equal to 1000, of this procedure are performed with each iteration using one set of values from the distributions of the variables and each iteration yielding one set of outcome values (Hunink et al., 1998; Halpern et al., 2000). Performing a large number of iterations yields a distribution of effectiveness and cost values. These distributions provide us with a measure of the uncertainty in the results of the model associated with the probabilistic nature of the input variables.

For decision-making purposes within a given setting, the distributions of the input variables should closely reflect the local situation. If data are available from a study representative of the local situation, one can boot-strap the primary data to obtain an estimate of the distribution of the variable values (Briggs et al., 1997; Mennemeyer and Cyr, 1997; Obenchain et al., 1997). For public policy-making purposes the distribution of the input variables is generally best modeled with the combined experience from various representative centers to indicate the uncertainty of the variable values across settings (Doubilet et al., 1985; Critchfield et al., 1986; Parmigiani et al., 1997). Meta-analytical techniques can help derive the appropriate probability distributions (Eddy et al., 1991; Cooper and Hedges, 1994). In general, two approaches can be used. One approach, a fixed-effects model, assumes that the uncertainty of the variable values is due to the limited sample size of the studies but that some fixed underlying true value exists. In contrast, a random-effects model assumes that the uncertainty is due to both the limited sample size of studies and the heterogeneity of the underlying true value across study populations. In general, a random-effects model will yield wider distributions of the input variables and thus larger uncertainty in the overall outcomes.

The distributions of the variable values may be modeled parametrically using some estimate of the available data combined with the judgment of the analyst. Distributions that may be used include the uniform, triangular, normal, lognormal, beta, binomial, and Poisson distributions. Alternatively, one can construct a nonparametric distribution based on the available evidence.

Combining parameter (variable value) uncertainty, stochastic uncertainty, and variability in a population all in one analysis implies performing $S \times N \times P$ simulations, i.e., S iterations to simulate parameter uncertainty of N cloned or bootstrapped copies (to simulate stochastic uncertainty) of a population of size P. Microsimulation of each of the P individuals in a population is used to simulate variability in that population.

11.3.7 Analytical probabilistic sensitivity analysis: the Delta method*

Uncertainty analysis for multiple variables may be performed analytically. This entails deriving equations for the uncertainty in the results using differential calculus. To calculate the uncertainty requires the variance–covariance matrix of the variable estimates. This is only doable if the model is straightforward with a limited number of variables and a reliable data source to estimate the variance–covariance matrix. Analytical methods often become cumbersome and unmanageable with complex models.

Analytical estimates of the overall variance in the results are estimated with the delta method. For example, the variance of the results of a very straightforward model in which the outcome $= P \cdot U$, equals:

$$\text{var}(P \cdot U) = P^2 \, \text{var}(U) + U^2 \, \text{var}(P) + 2 \, P \cdot U \cdot \text{cov}(P, U) \quad (11.1)$$

The equation for the variance of a model with multiple input variables is given in the Appendix to this chapter. If all the variables in the model are independent, the delta method simplifies to a fairly straightforward equation (see Appendix), which would imply that the variance in the results can be estimated by determining the change in the outcome estimate for a small change in each variable value, taking the square of this estimate, multiplying that with the variance of the variable value, and summing the products for all variables.

The delta method and assuming independence of the input variables may provide an initial estimate of the variance in the results. Unfortunate-

---

* This is advanced material and can be skipped without loss of continuity.

ly, the method becomes complex quickly as the number of variables increases and the variance–covariance matrix structure of the variables needs to be estimated.

11.3.8 Analyzing varying model structures

To analyze the uncertainty associated with the use of varying modeling assumptions, the simplest approach is to redo the analysis using alternative assumptions. Performing the analysis first with, for example, a multiplicative mortality function and subsequently with an additive function will shed light on how this assumption affects the results. If the alternative assumption has no major impact on the results, a sentence or two in the report will suffice. If the alternative assumptions affect the decision, there is a choice to be made: either find more evidence to justify the use of one assumption instead of the other or, if this is impossible, present the results of both analyses and let the decision maker decide which of the analyses is the more appropriate based on his/her own judgment. Alternatively we could provide a weighted combination of the results, the weights being proportional to the belief we have in the assumption.

On a more global level one could compare analyses performed by different analysts to determine the influence of varying model structures. An attempt to consolidate the different results depending on the underlying assumptions of the model can provide valuable insights into the decision problem and modeling process (Brown and Fintor, 1993). Such a comparison, especially when performed across different settings and different countries, can demonstrate different perspectives on the decision problem, varying consequences of decisions, differences in costs and effectiveness, and different approaches to coping with uncertainty.

11.4 Uncertainty in cost-effectiveness analysis

Cost-effectiveness analysis, as described in Chapter 9, is increasingly being used to evaluate medical technology and allocate scarce health-care resources. In the previous chapters dealing with cost-effectiveness we considered the input variables to the model deterministic and thus the outputs were also assumed deterministic. Here we will consider how to deal with the uncertainty in both the costs and effectiveness when the input variables are considered probabilistic or the analysis is being performed as a Monte Carlo microsimulation to reflect variability across subjects in the population or stochastic uncertainty. In such models the outputs, in terms of incremental costs and effectiveness gained, are themselves probabilistic rather than deterministic (O'Brien et al., 1994; van Hout et al., 1994; Mullahy and Manning, 1995; Wakker and Klaassen, 1995; Chaudhary and Stearns, 1996; Manning et al., 1996; Briggs et al., 1997; Obenchain et al., 1997; Polsky et al., 1997).

Comparing two health-care strategies is generally done using the incremental cost-effectiveness ratio (CE ratio). The CE ratio is estimated using:

$$CE \text{ ratio} = \frac{\bar{C}_1 - \bar{C}_0}{\bar{E}_1 - \bar{E}_0} = \frac{\Delta\bar{C}}{\Delta\bar{E}} \tag{11.2}$$

where $\bar{C}_1$ and $\bar{C}_0$ are the mean values of the costs using Strategy 1 (the strategy under consideration) and Strategy 0 (the next-best strategy) respectively, $\bar{E}_1$ and $\bar{E}_0$ are the mean values of the effectiveness yielded by Strategies 1 and 0 respectively, and $\Delta\bar{C}$ and $\Delta\bar{E}$ are the mean incremental costs and mean incremental effectiveness gained.

Most analyses evaluating uncertainty in cost-effectiveness studies have focused on presenting the means, CIs, upper and lower bounds, or distribution of the CE ratio. There are, however, several problems with the interpretation of CE ratios and all papers that report distributions or standard deviations or standard errors or CIs of cost-effectiveness ratios should be interpreted with caution (Wakker and Klaassen, 1995; Chaudhary and Stearns, 1996; Polsky et al., 1997; Heitjan et al., 1999).

By presenting CE ratios, information is lost with regard to the distribution across the four quadrants of combinations of $\Delta\bar{E}$ and $\Delta\bar{C}$ and the position within the quadrants (Figure 11.6; van Hout et al., 1994; Stinnett and Paltiel, 1997). (Here we have chosen to plot the effectiveness on the x-axis and the costs on the y-axis, to be consistent with the published literature in this area.) Given a negative CE ratio, for example, it is impossible to distinguish whether this results from a gain in effectiveness at lower costs (superior strategy by dominance, $\Delta\bar{E} > 0$ and $\Delta\bar{C} < 0$, quadrant IV) or a loss in effectiveness at higher costs (inferior strategy by dominance, $\Delta\bar{E} < 0$ and $\Delta\bar{C} > 0$, quadrant II). Reporting the distribution of CE ratios does not allow one to distinguish between these two different situations that have very different implications; i.e., the former strategy should be accepted, the latter rejected. Likewise, given a positive CE ratio, it is impossible to distinguish whether this results from a gain in effectiveness at higher costs ($\Delta\bar{E} > 0$ and $\Delta\bar{C} > 0$, quadrant I) or by a loss in

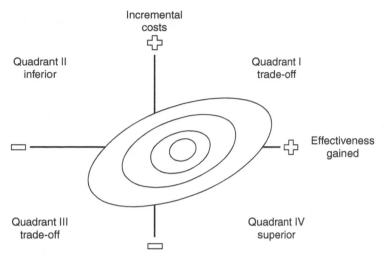

Figure 11.6 The costs-vs.-effectiveness graph with the distribution of results.

effectiveness at lower costs ($\Delta\bar{E} < 0$ and $\Delta\bar{C} < 0$, quadrant III). Depending on the management objectives, one may value these two situations differently. For example, a policy maker faced with a decreasing budget will implement strategies that reduce costs at an acceptable loss in effectiveness, whereas a policy maker faced with an increasing budget will implement strategies that yield a gain in effectiveness at an acceptable cost. Even within the first quadrant (gain in effectiveness at higher costs), there may be different implications for health-care management depending on the purchasable units of health and the associated costs. For example, the fixed cost of a strategy may exceed the available budget, although the ratio of cost and effectiveness may be favorable.

11.4.1 The joint distribution of costs and effectiveness

Uncertainty in costs and effectiveness using the joint distribution of costs and effectiveness displays the variability, or uncertainty, in the relationship between costs and effectiveness and, therefore, in the CE ratio itself. The function clearly distinguishes between the four quadrants of combinations of $\Delta\bar{E}$ and $\Delta\bar{C}$, and it is an informative method to display the relationship between costs and effectiveness. The joint distribution is well defined for every value of costs and effectiveness, which implies that even for a difference in effectiveness of close to zero, or equal to zero, the method may be applied (Fieller, 1932). The joint distribution of costs and effectiveness can be represented graphically in various ways using a scatterplot of $\Delta \bar{C}$ versus $\Delta \bar{E}$, a three-dimensional histogram (the x- and y-axes representing the $\Delta \bar{E}, \Delta \bar{C}$ plane and the z-axis representing the relative frequency with which a particular combination of $\Delta \bar{E}, \Delta \bar{C}$ occurs which yields a sort of mountain landscape), or as iso-probability contour lines in a two-dimensional contour plot (the bird's-eye view), as illustrated in Figure 11.6. In this context each data point of the joint distribution may be considered to be analogous to the expected outcome in a cloned (or bootstrapped) copy of the population under consideration.

11.4.2 Linear combinations of effectiveness and costs

An alternative to working with the joint distribution of $\Delta \bar{E}$ and $\Delta \bar{C}$ is to optimize some weighted linear combination of effectiveness and costs. This approach treats effectiveness and costs as components of a multiattribute outcome function. The relevant weight is generally society's threshold willingness to pay for the gain of one unit of effectiveness (G), or its inverse. One can, for example, maximize net health benefits (Stinnett and Mullahy, 1998) with:

$$\text{Net health benefits} = \text{effectiveness} - \text{cost}/G \tag{11.3}$$

Net health benefits can be interpreted analogously to effectiveness adjusted for the associated costs expressed in units of health by taking into consideration society's threshold willingness to pay. A program's net health benefit compares the health gain expected from the program (effectiveness) with the health gain required to justify the cost incurred (cost/G). If the net health benefit of one intervention exceeds that of another, i.e., if the incremental net health benefit exceeds zero, we can conclude that the intervention is cost-effective compared to its comparator given the threshold willingness to pay.

Similar to the net health benefit, we could alternatively maximize the net monetary benefit with:

$$\text{Net monetary benefit} = \text{effectiveness} \cdot G - \text{cost} \tag{11.4}$$

Net monetary benefits can be interpreted analogously to costs but includes the effectiveness expressed in terms of monetary units by taking into consideration society's threshold willingness to pay. If the net monetary benefit of one intervention exceeds that of another (the incremental net monetary benefit exceeds zero), we can conclude that the intervention is

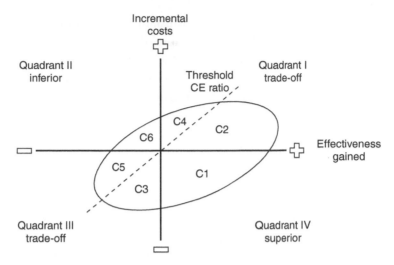

Figure 11.7   The six components of the joint distribution of costs and effectiveness. CE, cost-effectiveness. Reproduced from Hunink, M.G.M., Bult, J.R., de Vries, J. & Weinstein, M.C. (1998). Uncertainty in decision models analyzing cost-effectiveness: the joint distribution of incremental costs and effectiveness evaluated with a nonparametric bootstrap method. *Med. Decis. Making*, **18**, 337–46. Copyright © 1998. Reprinted by permission of Sage Publications, Inc.

cost-effective compared to its comparator given the threshold willingness to pay.

Finally, one can minimize the net cost–benefit (Manning et al., 1996) with:

$$\text{Net cost–benefit} = \text{cost} - \text{effectiveness} \cdot G \qquad (11.5)$$

The net cost–benefit is simply the reverse of the net monetary benefit and can be interpreted analogously to costs but includes effectiveness expressed in monetary units by taking into consideration society's threshold willingness to pay.

Simulating variability and uncertainty will yield a distribution of effectiveness and cost outcomes and thus a distribution of any of the linear combinations. The distributions of the linear combinations of effectiveness and costs are straightforward to calculate and interpret when analyzing the effects of variability and uncertainty in a model. They are very powerful when analyzing variability and uncertainty among multiple strategies, as is often the case with the evaluation of diagnostic tests. The concept can be used very efficiently for the calculation of criteria that a new test or treatment would need to attain to be cost-effective compared to an existing technology (Phelps and Mushlin, 1988; Hunink et al., 1999; Muradin and Hunink, 2001). Furthermore, the concept can be extended to include a weighted combination of the effectiveness and costs when more than one subject is affected by the decision, as would be the case when we consider an intervention for a pregnant woman and her fetus.

11.4.3 The acceptability curve

Each of the linear combinations has the disadvantage that society's threshold willingness to pay is included in the estimate but this disadvantage can be dealt with by performing and presenting the analysis for various values of G as, for example, with an acceptability curve (van Hout et al., 1994). Having estimated the joint distribution of $\Delta\bar{E}$ and $\Delta\bar{C}$ or some linear combination of effectiveness and costs, we can construct an acceptability curve. The acceptability curve plots the relative frequency or probability that the strategy is cost-effective compared to the alternative for varying threshold values of the CE ratio (G). This implies summing the relative frequencies of three components (Figure 11.7) of the joint distribution (van Hout et al., 1994; Hunink et al., 1998):

$\Delta\bar{E} \geq 0$ and $\Delta\bar{C} < 0$ (component 1 in quadrant IV)
$\Delta\bar{E} > 0$ and $\Delta\bar{C} \geq 0$ and the CE ratio $\leq G$ (component 2 in quadrant I)
$\Delta\bar{E} < 0$ and $\Delta\bar{C} \leq 0$ and the CE ratio $\geq G$ (component 3 in quadrant III)

Summing the relative frequencies of these three components of the joint distribution is equivalent to calculating the relative frequency of the distribution of the incremental net health benefits with values larger than zero, the incremental net monetary benefit larger than zero, or the incremental net cost–benefit smaller than zero.

The starting value of the acceptability curve (Figure 11.8) equals the sum of components 1 and 3 for a threshold CE ratio of zero, which is the sum of the joint distribution in quadrants III and IV, i.e., the region in which the program is cost-saving compared to its comparator. As the threshold CE ratio increases (Figures 11.7 and 11.8), component 2 increases and the acceptability curve rises. Simultaneously, however, component 3 of the distribution decreases and causes the acceptability curve to drop. Depending on the position and shape of the joint distribution, these two effects may cancel out or cause the curve to either increase or decrease. For large values of G the curve levels off to the relative frequency of the joint distribution in quadrants I and IV, i.e., the region in which the program increases effectiveness.

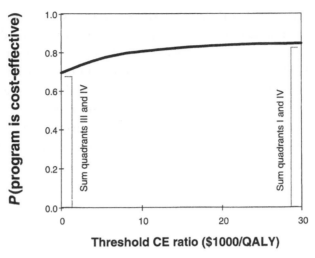

Figure 11.8   The acceptability curve. CE, cost-effectiveness; QALY, quality-adjusted life year.

11.5 Summary

When using mathematical models to estimate the expected value of alternative options we need to explore our assumptions and evaluate and present the effect of variability and uncertainty.

Variability may be known heterogeneity across subgroups and the optimal decision may be determined for each subgroup separately through sensitivity analysis. When analyzing a decision for a population as a whole we may be concerned about the variability across subjects in the population. This type of variability can be analyzed with a Markov cohort analysis with varying initial states, with (first-order) Monte Carlo microsimulation of the individual disease histories, or with discrete-event simulation.

Uncertainty in our models includes stochastic, parameter, and model structure uncertainty. Stochastic uncertainty is the uncertainty related to the actual events and realized outcome for one study population (or one individual) and can be estimated through Monte Carlo microsimulation of multiple cloned (or bootstrapped) copies of that study population. Stochastic uncertainty is irrelevant from the perspective of the public policy maker but may be relevant for, for example, a hospital or health maintenance organization administrator making a decision for a group of individuals. Parameter (variable value) uncertainty is due to the measurement error of the variable values in the model caused by the limited sample size and heterogeneity of the studies from which the values were derived. Parameter uncertainty can be evaluated with probabilistic sensitivity analysis by performing a second-order Monte Carlo simulation, each iteration using one random value from each of the distributions of the variables and the simulation producing distributions of the outcomes. Model structure uncertainty is related to the modeling assumptions with regard to the used mathematical model and can be evaluated by performing sensitivity analysis using different assumptions.

Variability and uncertainty in cost-effectiveness analyses can best be presented with the joint distribution of costs and effectiveness or using a multiattribute outcome such as net health benefits.

Appendix

The delta method

Mathematically, the overall variance of function $f(X)$ with vector $\mathbf{X} = X_1, X_2 \ldots X_i \ldots X_n$ equals:

$$\text{var}(\bar{f}) = \left(\frac{\overline{\partial f}}{\partial \mathbf{X}}\right)^T \text{var } \hat{\mathbf{X}} \left(\frac{\overline{\partial f}}{\partial \mathbf{X}}\right) \tag{11.6}$$

If all the variables $\mathbf{X} = X_1, X_2 \ldots X_i \ldots X_n$ in the model $f(X)$ are independent, the delta method simplifies to a fairly straightforward equation:

$$\text{var}(\bar{f}) = \sum_i \left(\frac{\overline{\partial f}}{\partial \mathbf{X}_i}\right)^2 \text{var } \hat{\mathbf{X}}_i \tag{11.7}$$

Exercises

Exercise 11.1

Using decision analysis software build the two models shown in Figures 11.1 and 11.2. Check that the two models produce the same results. Now superimpose various types of distributions for the variable values and redo the analysis.

Exercise 11.2

Why is stochastic uncertainty a smaller problem for public health policy makers compared to clinical decision makers?

Exercise 11.3

Demonstrate that an incremental CE ratio, that is under the threshold ratio (G) for society's maximum willingness-to-pay ($\Delta cost/\Delta QALY < G$), is in mathematical terms the same, as an incremental net health benefit (NHB) that is larger than 0 ($\Delta NHB > 0$).

What are the advantages of using NHBs instead of incremental CE ratios?

REFERENCES

Briggs, A.H., Wonderling, D.E. & Mooney, C.Z. (1997). Pulling cost-effectiveness analysis up by its bootstraps: a non-parametric approach to confidence interval estimation. *Health Econ.*, **6**, 327–40.

Brown, M.L. & Fintor, L. (1993). Cost-effectiveness of breast cancer screening: preliminary results of a systematic review of the literature. *Breast Cancer Res. Treat.*, **25**, 113–18.

Chaudhary, M.A. & Stearns, S.C. (1996). Estimating confidence intervals for cost-effectiveness ratios: an example from a randomized trial. *Stat. Med.*, **15**, 1447–58.

Claxton, K. (1999). The irrelevance of inference: a decision-making approach to the stochastic evaluation of health care technologies. *J. Health Econ.*, **18**, 341–64.

Cooper, H. & Hedges, L.V. (1994). *The Handbook of Research Synthesis.* New York: Russell Sage Foundation.

Critchfield, G.C., Willard, K.E. & Connelly, D.P. (1986). Probabilistic sensitivity analysis methods for general decision models. *Comput. Biomed. Res.*, **19**, 254–65.

DerSimonian. R. & Laird, N. (1986). Meta-analysis in clinical trials. *Control. Clin. Trials*, **7**, 177–88.

Doubilet, P., Begg, C.B., Weinstein, M.C., Braun, P. & McNeil, B.J. (1985). Probabilistic sensitivity analysis using Monte Carlo simulation. A practical approach. *Med. Decis. Making*, **5**, 157–77.

Eddy, D.M., Hasselblad, V. & Shachter, R. (1991). *Meta-analysis by the Confidence Profile Method: The Statistical Synthesis of Evidence.* New York: Academic Press.

Efron. B. & Tibshirani, R.J. (1993). *An Introduction to the Bootstrap.* New York: Chapman & Hall.

Fieller, E. (1932). The distribution of the index in a normal bivariate population. *Biometrika*, **24**, 428–40.

Goldie, S.J., Kuntz, K.M., Weinstein, M.C., Freedberg, K.A. & Palefsky, J.M. (2000). Cost-effectiveness of screening for anal squamous intraepithelial lesions and anal cancer in human immunodeficiency virus-negative homosexual and bisexual men [see comments]. *Am. J. Med.*, **108**, 634–41.

Habbema, J.D.F., van Oortmarsen, G.J., Lubbe, J.Th.N. & van der Maas, P.J. (1984). The MISCAN simulation program for the evaluation of screening for disease.

Computer methods and programs. *Biomed.*, **20**, 79–93.

Habbema, J.D.F., Lubbe, J.Th.N., van Oortmarsen, G.J. & van der Maas, P.J. (1987). A simulation approach to cost-effectiveness and cost–benefit calculations of screening for the early detection of disease. *Eur. J. Oper. Res.*, **29**, 159–66.

Halpern, E.F., Weinstein, M.C., Hunink, M.G.M. & Gazelle, G.S. (2000). Representing both first- and second-order uncertainty by Monte Carlo simulation for groups of patients. *Med. Decis. Making*, **20**, 314–22.

Heitjan, D.F., Moskowitz, A.J. & Whang, W. (1999). Bayesian estimation of cost-effectiveness ratios from clinical trials. *Health Econ.*, **8**, 191–201.

Hoffman, F.O. & Hammonds, J.S. (1994). Propagation of uncertainty in risk assessments: the need to distinguish between uncertainty due to lack of knowledge and uncertainty due to variability. *Risk Anal.*, **14**, 707–12.

Hunink, M.G.M., Goldman, L., Tosteson, A.N. et al. (1997). The recent decline in mortality from coronary heart disease, 1980–1990. The effect of secular trends in risk factors and treatment. *J.A.M.A.*, **277**, 535–42.

Hunink, M.G.M., Bult, J.R., de Vries, J. & Weinstein, M.C. (1998). Uncertainty in decision models analyzing cost-effectiveness: the joint distribution of incremental costs and effectiveness evaluated with a nonparametric bootstrap method. *Med. Decis. Making*, **18**, 337–46.

Hunink, M.G.M., Kuntz, K.M., Fleischmann, K.E. & Brady, T.J. (1999). Noninvasive imaging for the diagnosis of coronary artery disease: focusing the development of new diagnostic technology. *Ann. Intern. Med.*, **131**, 673–80.

Kuntz, K.M. & Weinstein, M.C. (1995). Life expectancy biases in clinical decision modeling. *Med. Decis. Making*, **15**, 158–69.

Kuntz, K.M., Fleischman, K.E., Hunink, M.G.M. & Douglas, P.S. (1999). Cost-effectiveness of diagnostic strategies for patients with chest pain. *Ann. Intern. Med.*, **130**, 709–18.

Law, A.M. & Kelton, W.D. (2000). *Simulation Modeling and Analysis*, 3rd edn. Boston: McGraw-Hill Higher Education.

Manning, W.G., Fryback, D.G. & Weinstein, M.C. (1996). Reflecting uncertainty in cost-effectiveness analysis. In: *Cost-effectiveness in Health and Medicine*, ed. M.R. Gold, J.E. Siegel, L.B. Russell & M.C. Weinstein, pp. 247–75. New York: Oxford University Press.

Mennemeyer, S.T. & Cyr, L.P. (1997). A bootstrap approach to medical decision analysis. *J. Health Econ.*, **16**, 741–7.

Mullahy, J. & Manning, W. (1995). Statistical issues in cost-effectiveness analyses. In: *Valuing Health Care*, ed. F.A. Sloan, pp. 149–85. Melbourne: Press Syndicate of the University of Cambridge.

Muradin, G.S.R. & Hunink, M.G.M. (2001). Cost and patency rate targets for the development of endovascular devices to treat femoropopliteal arterial disease. *Radiology*, **218**, 464–9.

Obenchain, R.L., Melfi, C.A., Croghan, T.W. & Buesching, D.P. (1997). Bootstrap analyses of cost effectiveness in antidepressant pharmacotherapy. *Phar-*

macoeconomics, **11**, 464–72.

O'Brien, B.J., Drummond, M.F., Labelle, R.J. & Willan, A. (1994). In search of power and significance: issues in the design and analysis of stochastic cost-effectiveness studies in health care. *Med. Care*, **32**, 150–63.

Parmigiani, G., Samsa, G.P., Ancukiewicz, M. et al. (1997). Assessing uncertainty in cost-effectiveness analyses: application to a complex decision model. *Med. Decis. Making*, **17**, 390–401.

Phelps, C.E. & Mushlin, A.I. (1988). Focusing technology assessment using medical decision theory. *Med. Decis. Making*, **8**, 279–89.

Polsky, D., Glick, H.A., Willke, R. & Schulman, K. (1997). Confidence intervals for cost-effectiveness ratios: a comparison of four methods. *Health Econ.*, **6**, 243–52.

Samsa, G.P., Reutter, R.A., Parmigiani, G. et al. (1999). Performing cost-effectiveness analysis by integrating randomized trial data with a comprehensive decision model: application to treatment of acute ischemic stroke. *J. Clin. Epidemiol.*, **52**, 259–71.

Stinnett, A.A. & Mullahy, J. (1998). Net health benefits: a new framework for the analysis of uncertainty in cost-effectiveness analysis. *Med. Decis. Making*, **18**, S68–80.

Stinnett, A.A. & Paltiel, A.D. (1997). Estimating CE ratios under second-order uncertainty: the mean ratio versus the ratio of means. *Med. Decis. Making*, **17**, 483–9.

van Hout, B.A., Al, M.J., Gordon, G.S. & Rutten, F.F. (1994). Costs, effects and C/E-ratios alongside a clinical trial. *Health Econ.*, **3**, 309–19.

van Oortmarssen, G.J., Boer, R. & Habbema, J.D. (1995). Modelling issues in cancer screening. *Stat. Methods Med. Res.*, **4**, 33–54.

Wakker, P. & Klaassen, M.P. (1995). Confidence intervals for cost/effectiveness ratios [see comments]. *Health Econ.*, **4**, 373–81.

Proactive decision making: a way of life

Decisions have to be made and if they are not made actively, they will be made by default.

Milton C. Weinstein

The main purpose of this book is to provide insights and tools which can aid decision making in health care. As Hammond, Keeney, and Raiffa did in their book *Smart Choices* (Hammond et al., 1998), we advocate a *proactive* approach to decision making. The mnemonic PROACTIVE is useful to help remember the steps that should be considered during the decision-making process (Table 12.1), as represented by the terms:

Problem
Reframe
Objective
Alternatives
Consequences and chances
Trade-offs
Integrate
Value
Explore and evaluate

Although we have applied the proactive approach to medical decision making, it can be applied equally well to any decision we make. The same letters can also jog our memory to remember the advantages and limitations of our approach, to consider other approaches, challenges for the future, and to recall other aspects of the decisions we make in life (Table 12.2).

The P stands for path, process, problem, and perception

The *path* we have advocated in this book is a proactive approach to decision making. This path applies just as much to decision making in health care as to life in general. One of the hallmarks of a proactive

Table 12.1. Summary of the PROACTIVE approach to decision making

	Step	Types and perspectives	Tools
Step 1 PRO			
P Problem	Define the problem	What will happen if I do nothing? Is there a problem?	'Go to the balcony' Visualize with a consequence table, sketch, or scheme
R Reframe	Reframe from multiple perspectives	Consider perspective of patient, physician, department, hospital, payer, society	Communicate with those involved in the decision Step to their side Understand their perspective
O Objective	Focus on the objective	Consider diagnostic certainty, medical effectiveness, microeconomics and macroeconomics, psychosocial, political, ethical, and philosophical aspects	Ask those involved 'Why? What's the goal?' Distinguish means objectives and fundamental objectives
Step 2 ACT			
A Alternatives	Consider all relevant alternatives	Wait-and-see, intervention, obtain information Different combinations, sequences, and positivity criterion of diagnostic tests	Logical and lateral thinking Brainstorm before critiquing
C Consequences Chances	Model the consequences and estimate the chances	Model disease and events Estimate the corresponding probabilities	Balance sheet Decision tree Bayesian probability revision Meta-analysis Markov, Monte Carlo, microsimulation models
T Trade-offs	Identify and estimate value trade-offs	Value the outcomes Life expectancy Quality of life Monetary costs	Balance sheet Meta-analysis Utility assessment Cost analysis
Step 3 IVE			
I Integrate	Integrate the evidence and values	Qualitatively Quantitatively	Balance sheet Average out: calculate expected value Fold back: apply decision criterion to choose Multiattribute outcomes
V Value	Optimize expected value	Maximize desirable outcomes Minimize undesirable outcomes	
E Explore Evaluate	Explore assumptions Evaluate uncertainty	Evaluate variability Evaluate stochastic parameter, and model structure uncertainty	One-way, two-way, three-way sensitivity analysis Probabilistic sensitivity analysis Monte Carlo analysis and microsimulation

Table 12.2. PROACTIVE decision making: alternative meanings of the mnemonic

P	Path	Take a proactive path
	Process	Decision making should be an explicit conscious process
	Problem	Define problems explicitly
	Perception	What you observe is your perception
R	Reframe	Consider the problem from multiple perspectives
	Reflect	Reflect on your reality
	Reality	Your perception of the problem is merely a bootstrap of reality
O	Objective	Focus on your objective
	Opposites	Reconcile opposite conflicting objectives
A	Awareness	Be aware, make conscious decisions
	Alternatives	Expand your alternatives
	Active	Be active but know that you do not control the outcome
C	Consequences	Visualize and structure the consequences
	Chances	Estimate the chances
	Connectedness	Be aware of the connectedness of all things
	Chaos	Life is a network on the boundary between order and chaos
T	Trade-offs	Make your trade-offs explicitly and wisely
	Tao	Accept and understand the Tao of modern medicine
I	Integrate	Integrate the evidence and values
	Intuition	Integrate rationality and intuition, your head and your heart
	Interwoven	Recognize the interwovenness of all things
	Interaction	Recognize the dynamic interplay, the interactions
V	Value	Optimize expected value. Know your values
	Vision	Develop a vision, have a dream
E	Explore	Explore your assumptions
	Evaluate	Evaluate variability and uncertainty
	Expectations	Integration of evidence-based medicine and patients' values

approach to decision making is that the decision-making *process* becomes transparent. It becomes an explicit conscious process. In fact, the insight gained during the process is probably more important than the actual numbers that are calculated and sometimes only a few steps of the process are enough to resolve the problem.

Every decision *problem* should first be defined and formulated explicitly. It helps to 'go to the balcony,' as it were (Ury, 1993), that is to distance yourself emotionally (at least for a while), and to visualize the problem with a consequence table, sketch, scheme, or some other tool such as a current reality tree (Goldratt & Cox, 1992; Goldratt, 1994, 1997). Try to get an overview of the situation as if you were an outsider. The simple act of defining the problem explicitly can actually point out serious consequences that you were ignoring, or alternatively the triviality of what we thought was a problem. In fact, formulating problems explicitly makes many problems melt away.

It is important to recognize that your definition of a problem is but one *perception* of the problem. In fact, what we perceive may be very different from what another person perceives. What we observe, see, hear, and feel is our own perception and probably says more about ourselves than about the phenomena we observe. We put on spectacles, as it were, with a color filter and only see one set of colors; or we tune in to a particular wavelength and only hear the chosen frequency. The decision-making tools that we have advocated in this book may actually help us look at problems through multiple filters and thereby overcome preconceived notions of proper action. Systematically going through multiple perspectives is the first step towards broadening your view on the problem. In spite of the fact that decision-making tools help us broaden our view on the problem, we need to keep in mind that decision analysis itself reflects a particular perception of how decisions ought to be made (Berg, 1997).

You see only what you look for, you recognize only what you know. (Sosman)

The R stands for reframe, reflect, and reality

Because of the variation in perceptions, it is important to *reframe* problems, and life for that matter, from multiple perspectives. In medical decision making we need to consider various players: the patient, physician, department, hospital, payer, and society and subsequently choose the relevant one(s). In doing so, we need to communicate with those involved in the decision: we need to step to their side (Ury, 1993) in order to understand their viewpoint.

The very act of formulating the problem and considering it from various perspectives makes us *reflect* about the situation. Reflecting on what we do in medicine is the main theme of fields such as clinical decision analysis, clinical epidemiology, evidence-based medicine, and medical technology assessment. Doing less and reflecting more, both in health care and in life in general, would serve us well.

Reflecting on our problems and on *reality* can be overwhelming because of the complexity of it all. Visualizing and structuring our perceived reality, making a model, helps us make problems explicit and helps organize the bits and pieces of information. In this book we strongly advocate using models to tackle decision problems because of the enormous advantages associated with structuring the problem and organizing the information which in turn helps communicate about the problem. A limitation of any model, however, is that it is merely a model and as such only an abstraction of reality. This not only applies to decision models, statistical and epidemiological models, and balance sheets but also to models in physics, astronomy, economics, and weather forecasting. Every model you make is but a mere reflection of your perception of the truth (Capra, 1975). In fact, you can consider each model a bootstrap of reality. If we bootstrap often enough we'll get a pretty good approximation of the truth but it will never be quite the real thing. The 'map is not the territory' is the well-known saying.

As far as the laws of mathematics refer to reality, they are not certain; and as far as they are certain, they do not refer to reality. (Albert Einstein)

The O stands for objective and opposites

A very important step in every decision-making process is to define your *objective* and then focus on it. The objective can be defined in terms of diagnostic certainty, medical effectiveness, micro- or macroeconomic resource use, psychosocial outcomes, political incentives, ethical concerns, and philosophical issues. Communicating with those involved in the decision is vital. You need to know what their interests are. Ask them: 'Why? Why is this a problem? What do you hope to obtain? What are your interests? What is your goal?' (Goldratt & Cox, 1992; Ury, 1993). We have emphasized the distinction between means objectives and fundamental objectives. Commonly physicians will focus on means objectives: for example, decreasing lipid levels to avoid cardiovascular events is typically a means objective whereas the fundamental objective is increasing life expectancy and quality of life.

Often we find ourselves struggling with conflicting *opposite* objectives. The objective of health care is generally to increase length and quality of life, but these two objectives may be at odds with each other. For example, bypass surgery for claudication is associated with an immediate risk of mortality while the objective is to cure the patient's symptoms. Similarly, the objective of public policy makers in the health-care arena is to increase health-care benefits and limit costs. These two objectives are often conflicting. In day-to-day clinical practice we commonly find ourselves in a conflict between doing more and doing less, e.g., it may be a simple conflict such as: do we continue with the ultrasound examination until we have scanned every abdominal organ in detail or do we focus on just the gallstones that appear to be the cause of the patient's symptoms? It may also be a more complex underlying conflict, such as: do we provide every patient with the most advanced sophisticated technology vs. focusing on social priorities in the face of limited resources? As long as conflicts between opposite objectives exist, tension, arguments, misunderstanding, and lack of cooperation will exist (Goldratt, 1994). In general we need to find some balance between conflicting objectives. For example, in health care we clearly need to find a balance between high-quality care and the associated price tag. A proactive approach to the decisions we make in health care helps us reconcile the underlying conflicting objectives.

The A stands for awareness, alternatives, and active

The greatest advantage of a proactive approach to decision making is the *awareness* it develops of the problem, objective, alternatives, consequences, and trade-offs involved. Putting the information on the table and making the problem explicit facilitates logical thinking and communication about the decision. It's like playing chess on a board instead of in your head: on the board it is so much easier to see what happens!

We have advocated expanding the *alternatives* through logical and lateral thinking. Important generic alternatives to consider in every decision, be it a clinical, public policy or a personal decision, are intervening, doing nothing, and getting more information. Getting more information should be thought of in very broad terms: this may mean performing a test for a clinical decision, distributing a questionnaire in a sample of the population for a public policy decision, or asking someone's opinion for a personal decision. Going logically through all the different combinations, sequences, and positivity criteria of diagnostic tests generally leads to an enormous amount of diagnostic strategies. Add various options for treatment and the number of strategies can become overwhelming. The process of doing this, however, commonly leads to breakthrough strategies that turn out to be the best options. Sometimes this is the only step that is really needed for a good decision: after some brainstorming you may come up with an obvious winner.

We advocate an *active* approach to decision making. Keep in mind, however, that even though you have actively made what seemed the best decision, things can always turn out differently than you would have liked and what you expect. A characteristic of making decisions under uncertainty is that, despite careful analysis, the realized outcome may still be a poor outcome. This does not mean that the decision was a bad one! It means that in spite of an active approach to the decision, in spite of all the careful trade-offs made, things turned out differently than expected or you just had plain simple bad luck. So even though you may be active in making your decisions, remember that you do not have complete control over the outcomes.

The C stands for consequences, chances, connectedness, and chaos

Visualizing and structuring the *consequences* and *chances* associated with your choices is very helpful in getting an idea of what may happen in the future. Over the past years statisticians, epidemiologists, and decision analysts have developed increasingly sophisticated tools to do this. In this book we have described tools such as Bayesian revision, balance sheets, decision trees, Markov models, Monte Carlo models, and microsimulation. In spite of the increasing sophistication, however, every model remains a simplification of reality. It is but one bootstrap of the real thing. Reality is far more complex then the models we make.

In reality all things are inter*connected* (Capra 1996). In the human body there is seldom a clear-cut one-on-one cause–effect relationship. The body is an interconnected set of systems and all these systems are needed for the whole. The cause of disease is multifactorial: genes, nutrition, lifestyle, environment, and psychological factors all play a role. And even these factors are interconnected: for example, a particular genetic constitution may lead to a predisposition to eat more which, given a particular environment, will lead to overweight, which in turn may lead to mild depression and the tendency to develop even worse eating habits. The decisions we make in health care are also connected: advising moderate alcohol consumption to reduce the incidence of cardiovascular disease will at the same time increase the incidence of motor vehicle accidents and the incidence of alcoholic liver cirrhosis.

Often the connectedness is *chaotic*: a small, seemingly inconsequential event may cause a cascade of events that eventually lead to a major event later (Capra, 1996). This can happen on the scale of one individual, within an organization such as a hospital, or in the health-care system as a whole and it can have either a positive or negative effect. For example, a minor injury such as a twisted knee may seem fairly inconsequential but may actually have caused a minor meniscal tear which, if neglected, can lead to a less active lifestyle because of the mild pain on exercise which may lead to overweight which, together with the sedentary lifestyle and the already present hereditary traits, may lead to the build-up of atherosclerotic plaque which eventually can lead to a carotid artery stenosis and a few years later the patient develops a stroke. On the level of the hospital, for example, it may be an intern who suggests implementing a decision tool to help triage emergency room patients between further imaging workup vs. sending them home, which turns out to be a success, which subsequently leads to implementation of a larger information-communication program with decision aids by the radiology department to improve the utility of imaging patients, which may eventually lead to the implementation of a hospital-wide information-communication program, which eventually may lead to enormous improvements in the care delivered. In this way, every decision we make leads to a cascade of sometimes predictable but often unpredictable events. It is precisely this type of snowball effect that can spiral in a positive (or negative) direction and in so doing transform a health-care organization or system. In our view, one of the challenges in the future will be to develop models that capture the seemingly chaotic behavior of health and disease in individuals and populations in order to get more insight into the potential effects of our decisions.

Life is a network on the boundary between order and chaos. (Fritjof Capra)

The T stands for trade-offs and Tao

Medical decisions commonly involve *trade-offs*. The most pertinent ones that we have discussed in this book are the trade-offs between length of life and quality of life, between an upfront risk to reduce the risk of an event later, and between costs and benefits. A main advantage of a proactive approach to decision making is that it makes these trade-offs explicit. It increases awareness of the trade-offs involved in the decision and awareness leads to conscious decision making.

Balance sheets help us organize the information and can be used directly to make the trade-offs (Hammond et al., 1998). Using utility assessment, the trade-offs between length of life and quality of life can be approached explicitly. The unit quality-adjusted life year (QALY) integrates length of life and quality of life in one multiattribute outcome in which the trade-off between length of life and quality of life is made by integrating them into one metric. Although this has clear advantages, there are also limitations to the use of QALYs as utility measures. The underlying assumptions are that health-state utilities reflect preferences under uncertainty and they reflect time trade-offs. If we measure time preference independently of quality of life, we can also include this in our utility estimates. But time preference and quality of life are likely to be interconnected. Consider, for example, a state of extreme disability, such as might follow major cardiac surgery or survival from a major automobile accident. The psychological assessment of this state (utility) likely depends on whether the state is temporary, and we can reasonably expect the patient to recover, or whether the state is permanent disability. Thus, the utility of the state is not independent of the time to be spent in it. How this can be tackled in a practical way that ensures that our utility measures genuinely reflect all the trade-offs involved remains a challenge for the future.

A question often asked of decision analysts is whether their analyses have changed practice. In a sense, clinical decision analysts are often considered to be scientists making sophisticated models in an office set far away from daily practice. Decision models are commonly viewed with some skepticism as to their practicality. The two first authors of this book, however, are in fact active practicing doctors: the one a family practitioner, the other a vascular radiologist. We have found the tools we have described in this book helpful in our practice. But we will immediately add that we do not make a decision tree for every patient who consults us. On the contrary; it is more the insights that we have gained from thinking according to the proactive approach that have been helpful. In developing decision models with our clinical colleagues we have found that the process of working together through the various steps facilitated awareness and open communication about the evidence and values involved. Through the questions we ask, our clinical colleagues may be triggered to take a different view on their daily practice, to reflect on their assumptions, to ask other questions in their next patient encounter, and to search for evidence. The next time we talk with this colleague they will reflect on our questions in a different way and very likely will ask us questions, point to evidence, or express patient's values that in turn will lead us to reevaluate our ideas and our models. And so the process of interaction continues, stimulating a stream of conscious decision making in health care and stimulating a flow of increasing knowledge and awareness of the evidence, values, and trade-offs involved in health-care decisions. This flow of increasing knowledge and awareness of decision making is an irreversible trend in medicine reflected in, for example, the emergence of fields such as clinical epidemiology, clinical decision analysis, meta-analysis, evidence-based medicine, and medical technology assessment and the appearance of the associated journals, collaborations, professional societies, and websites. It is, in fact, a reflection of the age we live in, the knowledge economy, and the knowledge society and as such proactive decision making is the natural way in which health care should develop. One could call it the *Tao* of modern medicine.

Those who follow the natural order flow in the current of the Tao. (Fritjof Capra)

The I stands for integrate, intuition, interwoven, and interaction

Although decision analysis is generally considered a rational analytical approach to decision making, the underlying philosophy is to *integrate* the rational analytical aspects of a decision problem, i.e., the evidence, with the psychological subjective aspects, i.e., our values. Integrating the evidence and values may be done qualitatively based on the balance sheet or quantitatively by calculating the expected value of each option (Hammond et al., 1998).

Even though decision analysis advocates rational decision making, the final decision is generally not based on one hard number from the analysis. The process itself is probably more important than the final result and the insight gained during the process usually has more effect than the numbers that are calculated. Having taken into account all the information you have found during the process and after looking at the problem from various different viewpoints in multiple ways, you finally need to use your judgment and *intuition* to decide whether the analysis sufficiently reflects reality, whether the intangibles have been sufficiently considered, which evidence and values apply to the situation at hand, whether the crucial information is available, and finally whether your decision should be based on the results. In this sense, a proactive approach to decision making attempts consciously to reconcile rationality and intuition, that is, what is going on in our heads with that which is going on in our hearts (Figure 12.1).

Due to the limitations of written text, we have presented our decision-making approach as a sequential process. In practice the steps are often *interwoven*, considered in parallel, and the process itself is cyclic in nature. Frequently we will find that, after having considered various perspectives and objectives relevant to the decision, we have to redefine our problem. Similarly, thinking about the consequences and trade-offs may jog our mind to rethink the objectives and redefine the problem, or it may bring us to think of other alternatives. Structuring the consequences in the form of a decision model generally goes hand-in-hand with finding the evidence. The model needs to be adjusted over and over again to reflect the available

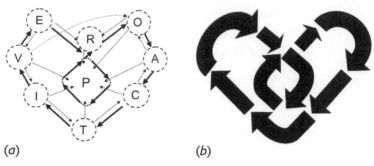

(a)   (b)

Figure 12.1   The PROACTIVE approach to decision making is an interactive dynamic cyclic process. (*a*) The steps are interwoven, considered in parallel, and cyclic in nature. (*b*) The art of decision making is to integrate the evidence and values, and to integrate rationality (represented by the diamond) and intuition (represented by the heart).

data. But the available data also need to be adjusted so that they fit the model structure. During the steps of integrating the information and optimizing the expected value, we may find ourselves reconsidering our objectives and thinking of alternative management options. While exploring our assumptions and evaluating uncertainty, we may conclude that our initial estimates for the evidence and outcome values need to be adjusted. And having come to what seemed the end of the process, namely the decision itself, we frequently find ourselves faced with a related or re-defined decision problem that has now become the more pertinent problem and a new cycle of the process begins.

Not only are the steps of the proactive approach interwoven with each other, the whole process is an *interactive* one with those in clinical practice and public health policy. As we gather information from our colleagues in clinical practice and health policy, our questions may trigger them to think differently about their daily decisions. This will lead to new insights about the decision problem which in turn will trigger us as decision analysts to change our models of the problem and the estimates of the data. In fact, it is a continuing dynamic cyclic process, the process evolving and changing over time as we gather new information, obtain new insights, and interact with all those involved in the decision.

All of nature is interconnected, interwoven, an inseparable network of interactions, a dynamic web of interrelated events. (Fritjof Capra)

The V stands for value and vision

In discussing modeling the consequences of our choices and making trade-offs we emphasized the distinction between *probabilities* and *values*. Probabilities reflect the available evidence of the prevalence of disease and events that may occur. For the most part, this type of evidence is based on observed events and is data collected from cohort studies and randomized controlled trials. This is especially true for policy studies. In clinical decision making, decision makers must occasionally adjust published data to account for characteristics of a particular patient, or, if no published data seem relevant, the decision maker must rely on subjective probabilities that reflect our belief and best judgment about the likelihood of the events of interest.

Values reflect the desirability we attach to a particular outcome. In medical decision making, quality-adjusted life expectancy and costs are widely used to represent the values of outcomes. Although we have emphasized the distinction between probabilities and values, these two are sometimes interconnected. For example, life expectancy is commonly used as an outcome measure in a simple decision tree. If we were to model the same problem with a Markov model, we would use the annual mortality probability in our model as a piece of the evidence rather than as a value. Furthermore, modeling probabilities and values can never be seen as totally separate exercises. In a practical sense, when we estimate an outcome value we have to know what path in the decision model the outcome applies to and this in turn will depend on the probability estimates available. Furthermore, utility and value judgments are very likely influenced by the context of the judgments. Unfortunately, these context effects make prescriptive utility assessment very complex, and to keep things simple and manageable, we make assumptions that, to some degree, violate descriptive realities. This is another reason why caution is justified in applying the results of a decision analysis to the decision at hand, and why judgment and intuition should be brought into consideration.

Essential to the use of decision analysis is to know what values to optimize and to make them consistent with our objective. If potentially conflicting objectives are to be optimized then multiattribute outcomes can be particularly helpful. For example, multiattribute utility models combine various attributes of health-related quality of life into one outcome. Quality-adjusted life expectancy is a multiattribute outcome combining length and quality of life into one unit. Net health benefit is a multiattribute outcome combining cost, effectiveness, and society's willingness-to-pay. A limitation of quality-adjusted life years and net health benefits is that these multiattribute outcomes are linear combinations of the attributes. In reality interactions may exist between the length of life and quality of life and between effectiveness and costs, analogous to the quality-of-life attributes in a multiattribute utility model. The challenge for the future is to explore multiattribute outcomes that are good reflections of our fundamental objectives.

In clinical decision analysis we generally use life expectancy adjusted with the subjective preference of the associated quality of life to reflect the values we attach to the outcomes. In cost-effectiveness analysis we also include costs to reflect society's undesirability of the outcome. Decision analysis is based on the premise that a rational human being should choose the option that maximizes the expected value if value is expressed as a desirable outcome and minimizes expected value if it is expressed as an undesirable outcome. In practice the decisions we make may be very different from what the expected value calculation prescribes as optimal. Sometimes this is because our heuristics and biases influence how we interpret the available information. When heuristics and biases influence our decision making, a decision analysis is particularly helpful. Sometimes the decision model doesn't capture some additional feature of concern. For example, even if an extensive decision and cost-effectiveness analysis shows that a new technology such as lung transplantation is too expensive to justify the gains in terms of QALYs, the minister of health may still decide to allow the technology to be implemented for political or ethical reasons. Finally, the results of the decision analysis may be so extreme that they indicate that we need to rethink our values.

The authors of this book have a varying *vision* of how the described tools can and will be implemented in the future. In the 1970s clinical decision analysis was introduced as a clinical tool that would improve the day-to-day decisions made by physicians for the care of individual patients. A clinical decision analysis consulting service was even started (Plante et al., 1986; Pauker and Kassirer, 1987; Pauker, 1988), but such services did not become widely available. In fact, decision trees are rarely used in clinical practice. To be helpful, decision models need to encompass an extensive review of the available evidence and the models need to be reliable. Both the data review and the model development take time to accomplish: not something that can be done in the context of a 10-min office visit. Furthermore, in clinical practice diagnostic and therapeutic actions are often interwoven, which is difficult to model and for which the necessary data are generally unavailable. Soft data, such as visual impressions, psychosocial information, and logistical consequences, are commonly very important to the pragmatic decision maker and are very difficult, if not impossible, to quantify. All-in-all, clinical practice is a complex and fluid reality which is difficult to grasp in a decision model (Berg, 1997).

Decision models do, however, play an important role in the development of clinical practice guidelines for commonly recurring problems and in the development of (research) protocols. Furthermore, the basic concepts of decision analysis, such as the principle of Bayes theorem, the weighing of risks and benefits, and integrating evidence with patient preferences, are permeating into clinical practice. Currently information is becoming far more accessible through online literature databases, trial registries, review journals, and collaborations specifically focusing on reviewing and summarizing the available evidence. Such developments facilitate evidence-based proactive decision making, whether with or without the use of a decision model. Furthermore, decision support tools are becoming available on the web and in hospital information systems. For such tools to be really useful, however, they will need to be developed with intricate involvement of the users in such a way that both the users and the decision support tool develop and transform together (Berg, 1997).

Decision modeling has been extensively used in technology assessment and its contributions have been the most helpful in setting priorities for health care. Cost-effectiveness of health care interventions is increasingly being used for the allocation of resources. As we develop our modeling techniques and get more reliable evidence, it is likely that decision models will more and more be used to demonstrate the cost-effectiveness of new technologies. Furthermore, decision modeling to demonstrate cost-effectiveness is currently commonly used not as an alternative to performing a clinical trial but rather as an adjunct to such a trial. The clinical trial is then used to demonstrate, for example, the efficacy and costs of a new technology over a short time frame, whereas the decision model is used to extend the results to the lifetime of the patients, to generalize to other settings, and to explore the broader epidemiological and macroeconomical consequences of the intervention. Finally, simulation models are increasingly being used to determine the incremental value of obtaining information from further research, especially if this involves large-scale randomized controlled trials, and to determine whether the delay and the financial cost of further research are justified (Claxton, 1999).

The E stands for explore, evaluate, and expectations

In the last step of the proactive approach we *explore* the robustness of the decision and *evaluate* variability, stochastic uncertainty, and uncertainty of the probability and value estimates through various forms of sensitivity analysis. Performing a sensitivity analysis is an essential step of every decision, whether the decision is based on a discussion, a balance sheet, a decision tree, or some sophisticated Markov Monte Carlo microsimulation model. The basic question 'what if?' needs to be addressed to be confident of the decision. Not only is this an essential step but it is also what makes modeling so useful. A computer can be set to repeat the analysis over and over again to explore what the results would be if an assumption or input variable were to be different than we initially estimated. Exploring the effect of uncertainty is one of the major advantages of decision models and simulation.

Our *expectations* for the future are that proactive decision making will become more and more ingrained in physicians' way of thinking. We do not expect that the future physician will be drawing decision trees. We do, however, expect that the already initiated trend towards evidence-based decision making in medicine will continue, that the cognizance of and respect for patients' values and preferences will impact medical decisions more and more, and that setting priorities in health care will be based on both costs and benefits. With the rapid development of information and communication technology, we expect that obtaining the relevant information and implementing decision aids will become feasible. User-friendly tools and interfaces will be developed which will make it easy to use decision support tools in practice. In the area of technology assessment we expect that decision modeling and computer simulation will be used prior to performing clinical trials in order to refine the research question and fine-tune research protocols. Furthermore, we expect that decision modeling and simulation will be used alongside clinical trials in order to extend beyond the trial results with respect to both the time frame and setting. Finally, we expect that proactive decision making and simulation modeling will be used to determine the value of obtaining information through further research which will help set priorities in research.

In summary

The implementation of proactive decision making in medicine based on integrating evidence and values is an irreversible path consistent with the current transformation towards a knowledge-based society. The tools we have presented in this book are a handful of very useful tools but we are convinced that more and more will develop with time. The path we advocate is awareness and explicitness about the problem, objectives, trade-offs, evidence, and values involved in the decisions we make. In the face of uncertainty, the interconnectedness of events, and the chaotic complexity of our reality, the best we can do is reflect on reality by visualizing, structuring, organizing, and modeling that reality even though we know that it will never capture the real thing. At the same time we need to recognize that every decision is only in part based on evidence. Every decision should also be based on our values. The art of decision making is to integrate the evidence and values. The art of living is to integrate the head and the heart.

REFERENCES

Berg, M. (1997). *Rationalizing Medical Work: Decision Support Techniques and Medical Practices.* Cambridge, MA: MIT Press.

Capra, F. (1975). *The Tao of Physics.* Boston, MA: Shambala.

Capra, F. (1996). *The Web of Life: A New Understanding of Living Systems.* New York: Doubleday.

Claxton, K. (1999). The irrelevance of inference: a decision-making approach to the stochastic evaluation of health care technologies. *J. Health Econ.*, **18**, 341–64.

Goldratt, E.M. (1994). *It's Not Luck.* Great Barrington: North River Press.

Goldratt, E.M. (1997). *Critical Chain.* Great Barrington: North River Press.

Goldratt, E.M. & Cox, J. (1992). *The Goal: A Process of Ongoing Improvement.* Great Barrington: North River Press.

Hammond, J.S., Keeney, R.L. & Raiffa, H. (1998). *Smart Choices: A Practical Guide to Making Better Decisions.* Boston, MA: Harvard Business School Press.

Pauker, S.G. (1988). Clinical decision making rounds at the New England Medical Center. *Med. Decis. Making*, **8**, 55–71.

Pauker, S.G. & Kassirer, J.P. (1987). Medical progress. Decision analysis. *N. Engl. J. Med.*, **316**, 250–8.

Plante, D.A., Kassirer, J.P., Zarin, D.A. & Pauker, S.G. (1986). Clinical decision consultation service. *Am. J. Med.*, **80**, 1169–76.

Ury, W. (1993). *Getting Past No. Negotiating Your Way from Confrontation to Co-operation.* New York: Bantam Book.

Index

Page numbers in bold indicate figures and tables